T
MEDICINE ON THE INTERNET 2000

Edited by
JAMES B. DAVIS

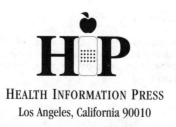

HEALTH INFORMATION PRESS
Los Angeles, California 90010

Health and Medicine on the Internet 2000

ISBN #1-885987-18-8

Disclaimer

The publisher's best efforts have gone into creating this book, and great care has been taken to maintain the accuracy of the information contained in this book. However, the publisher does not guarantee the accuracy, adequacy or completeness of any information and is not responsible for any errors or omissions or any consequences arising from the use of the information contained in this book. Also, the publisher specifically disclaims, without limitation, any implied warranties of merchantability and fitness for a particular purpose with respect to listings on the book. In no event shall the publisher be responsible or liable for any loss of profit or other commercial damages, including but not limited to special, incidental, consequential or any other damages in connection with or arising out of furnishing, performance, or use of this book.

All information contained in this book is subject to change. Mention of a specific product or company does not imply an endorsement. The information you find on the internet should never replace the advice of a trained health professional. If you have any questions about your health, you should always consult a qualified health professional.

All of the images in this book have been obtained from online sources. The caption accompanying each illustration identifies its online source. Text and images available over the internet and other online services may be subject to copyright and other rights owned by third parties. Online availability of text and images does not imply that they may be reused without the permission of rights holders, although the Copyright Act does permit certain unauthorized reuse as fair use under 17 U.S.C. §107. Care should be taken to ensure that all necessary rights are cleared prior to reusing material distributed over the internet and other online services. Information about reuse is available from the institutions that make their materials available online.

Trademarks

The words in this book for which we have reason to believe trademark, service mark, or other proprietary rights may exist have been designated as such by use of initial capitalization. However, no attempt has been made to designate as trademarks or service marks all personal-computer words or terms in which proprietary rights might exist. The inclusion, exclusion, or definition of a word or term is not intended to affect, or to express any judgement on, the validity or legal status of any proprietary right which may be claimed in that word or term.

Health Information Press
4727 Wilshire Blvd., Suite 300
Los Angeles, California 90010 U.S.A.
1-800-MED-SHOP

http://hipbooks.com/

Printed in the United States of America

TABLE OF CONTENTS

INTRODUCTION

If you were like me, when you were a kid one of the first voluntary math problems you did was to calculate the age you would be in the far-distant "Year 2000." And then, when you completed the calculation, you frankly did not believe you would ever really be *that* old! At that time, the "Year 2000" belonged to the realm of science fiction. . . However, now that the Year 2000 is upon us, you are perhaps as shocked as I at how quickly the time has gone by.

On the other hand, although 2000 has arrived here quickly, the interim has been packed with astounding and unprecedented changes and technological advances. Of course, one of the most obvious examples of this is the popularization of home computers and the blast-off of the Internet during the past decade. According to Win Treese, author of "The Internet Index," 760 U.S. households gain access to the Internet *every hour*.[1]

The Internet, too, has grown remarkably in the last five years —and indeed in the last 18 months! This lesson was brought home to us as we set about updating the first edition of *Health and Medicine on the Internet*. Not only was it humbling to add that daunting "2000" to the end of the title, but we also soon realized how much denser and more sophisticated the World Wide Web had become in the relatively short time that had elapsed since publication of the first edition. Web pages themselves are, in general, much more attractive, comprehensive and user-friendly, and the number of them is also rapidly multiplying. The World Wide Web is one global "jungle" that is not experiencing deforestation, but rather it boasts a healthy rate of growth, as well as a great deal of territory and many unusual and exciting inhabitants to be explored and experienced. There are many thousands of health and medical sites on the web, and this number continues to grow.

The question is, how do you sort through all of the countless resources to find the most helpful and accurate health information? In an effort to help people locate the areas of information and communities of support relevant to their health needs, we first created this guide. The updated edition of *Health and Medicine on the Internet* has added many new sites, as well as updated descriptions, and increased categorization. In fact, despite our efforts to prune and tame this wild "jungle" so that it would be a manageable size, we had to expand *Health and Medicine on the*

Internet 2000 from a previously chunky 600-page book to a hefty 900+ page volume.

For our purposes, we presume that the reader already has a working knowledge of how to access and "surf" the Internet. It is also assumed that the reader's primary interest is to tap into a specific pocket of health care information, and that he or she approaches this goal with a short-sighted, task-oriented view. If you or a loved one have just been diagnosed with a disease, most likely your concern is to find out as much as possible about the disease and treatment, as easily and as quickly as possible. You probably don't want to waste time determining which websites are commercial, which are geared to patients, which are geared to medical specialists, and which are out-dated. Instead, you want to go directly to a page that speaks to people like yourself; a page that is full of relevant, reliable, helpful, up-to-date and easy-to-understand information. This book can help you to identify the sites that can best suit your needs.

Say you went to the doctor complaining about the pains in your chest you experienced after carrying home some groceries. The doctor asks you questions, gives you an EKG procedure, and then tells you he believes that you have suffered a myocardial infarction. After the initial fright subsides, suddenly there are dozens of questions brimming inside you: *But I'm only 40 years old,* you think, *and I'm a woman! Isn't it only "Type-A," overweight men over 60 who get heart attacks? How many other women does this happen to? Could it be something else? Should I get a second opinion? What actually is a heart attack, anyway? Why does it happen? How can I make sure it won't happen again? What can I expect in coming months? Can I live a normal life? What kind of treatment is standard? How much will it cost? What will my medical insurance cover? Are there any alternative therapies that may be helpful? What kind of diet is recommended?*

Your physician may not have time to answer all of these questions, and you may not know anybody else to ask who has knowledge about women and heart disease. However, with a little direction, the Internet can serve as a convenient and knowledgeable partner so that you can find the answers to these questions and arm yourself with the valuable information you need to know about this condition in order to minimize your fears and improve your health.

On the World Wide Web, you can browse through FAQs (frequently asked questions) to find the answers to the most general questions about the disease or condition. Or, many times you can e-mail your own question to an online expert to receive an electronic response. You can also post your question on a public bulletin board where it might be read by someone who has experienced the same thing and who is willing to share his or her experience and offer some advice. Or, you can look through clinical data published by the government or academic organizations to begin evaluating the approximate severity or classification of your condition. (One caution, here: you should *never* substitute what you learn from Internet sources for the medical advice of a trained, qualified physician or specialist who you visit in person and who is completely familiar with your medical history.)

Clinical textbooks, patient education sheets, photographic and radiographic images, diagrams, videos, audio files, interactive tours, quizzes and links to related topics. . . the material you can obtain from the Internet takes many forms, is usually free, and arrives instantly on your computer screen as you sit at home or at work.

Health and Medicine on the Internet 2000 is divided into 70 chapters, beginning with *Abuse* and ending with *Women's Health*. Each chapter is broken down into several subtopics that are arranged alphabetically. Every site listed includes the World Wide Web address (also known as the URL or Universal Resource Locator) and a description of what you will find there. There are even illustrations of selected sites. At the beginning of each chapter, we've listed related topics: other chapters where you might find additional information of interest to you. Finally, an index is provided at the end of this book in case you are not sure of where to start looking.

While browsing on the Internet is certainly recommended, *Health and Medicine on the Internet 2000* was designed so that you would not have to "stumble" upon a site that is of relevance to you. Rather, by using this book, you can identify it quickly, type the address into your computer, and visit it in moments. . Then you can link to related sites and save valuable time.

We have checked out every site in this book to verify its address and contents, but there may be cases where the website has moved or been discontinued. Usually, a message will appear on your screen to tell you what has happened and, if the site has moved, to tell you the new URL or provide a link that takes you there. Because URLs can be rather cryptic, make sure you have typed it in accurately. Capitalization and spelling are important. If you still do not get where you are trying to go, type just the beginning part of the address, which will take you to the domain, or computer which acts as host to the website of interest. From that point, you can often work your way down to arrive at the site that caught your eye.

For instance, the correct address to reach the online pamphlet, "Facts about Women and Heart Disease" is *http://www.pharminfo.net/disease/cardio/HD_women.html*. By typing in only *http://www.pharminfo.com/*, you will arrive at the homepage of the drug information resource, PharmInfo Net. From there, you can select "Disease Information: Cardiovascular" which presents you with a list of different resources related to heart disease, one of which is the desired destination. This way, if any of the URLs has changed, you can often still get what you want by starting at the initial domain and working forward, logically.

You needn't have a diagnosed medical condition to find *Health and Medicine on the Internet 2000* a valuable reference. Maybe you want to learn about acupuncture treatment to quit smoking, or maybe you are wondering what kind of vaccinations you need to travel overseas, or maybe your child is working on a project for school and wants to know how the brain works... Maybe you are interested in learning about cloning, or you are thinking of making your own living will and need some instruction —whatever your health or medical science interest may be, you will undoubtedly find it and many other topics addressed in this guide. We hope you have fun with it, and that it makes your encounter with the World Wide Web a pleasure.

Reference

1. Treese, Win: "The Internet Index," No. 24, May 31, 1999. Online. Available: *http://www.openmarket.com/intindex/99-05.htm*. 27 September, 1999.

ABUSE

Child Abuse

See also: Children's Health/Pediatrics.

Administration for Children and Families

http://www.acf.dhhs.gov/

Part of the U.S. Department of Health and Human Services, the ACF is responsible for many federal programs promoting the economic and social well-being of families and children. Site contains descriptions and links to the many programs supported by ACF, including those to prevent abuse of children.

Center for Children in Crisis

http://www.shadow.net/~cpt/

Homepage for this agency whose mission is to protect abused and neglected children, and to provide treatment to incest victims and their families.

Child Sexual Abuse

http://www.cs.utk.edu/~bartley/sacc/childAbuse.html

Definition of sexual abuse, signs and symptoms, and suggestions on how to support and protect the child.

Child Sexual Abuse

http://www.commnet.edu/QVCTC/student/LindaCain/sexabuse.html

Site provides legal information on child sexual abuse, statistics, resources, books, journals and publications, directory of agencies, services, and self-help groups; and personal accounts of child sexual abuse.

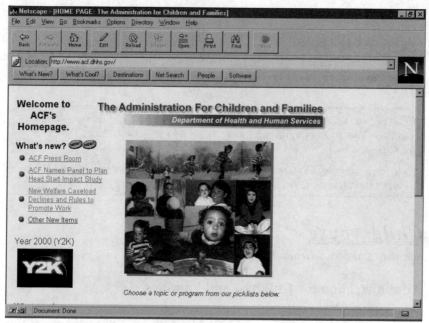

The Administration for Children and Families. *http://www.acf.dhhs.gov/*

Children's Safety Network: National Injury and Violence Prevention Resource Center

http://www.edc.org/HHD/csn/

Provides assistance to organizations seeking to reduce unintentional injuries as well as violence to children and adolescents. Offers online publications and publications available through the mail, as well as resources and links.

Dr. Marc Feldman's Munchausen Syndrome, Factitious Disorder, & Munchausen by Proxy Page

http://ourworld.compuserve.com./homepages/Marc_Feldman_2/

Describes these mental disorders and provides articles about them.

Hopeful Hands

http://www.CoachCenter.com/hopeful.html

Spiritual healing for survivors of child abuse.

Just in Case

http://www.discribe.ca/childfind/educate/jic/victim.hte

Guidelines to help parents identify if their child is the victim of sexual abuse or exploitation.

Mothers Against Munchausen Syndrome by Proxy Allegation

http://www.msbp.com/

This group seeks to protect parents who are falsely accused of MSBP, and to reveal the ulterior motives of the accusers (e.g., protection from allegations of medical malpractice). Site offers links to legal help, media articles, defensive living if your child is in a hospital, discussion group and more.

Mothers Against Sexual Abuse

http://208.236.140.168/index.html

Information on child sexual abuse, including signs, symptoms, resources and a child molestor identification hotline.

Munchausen by Proxy/Factitious Syndrome by Proxy

http://www.mindspring.com/~louisalasher/

Information on this dangerous form of abuse in which caretakers exaggerate and/or fabricate and/or induce symptoms and/or illness in others. The primary purpose of this behavior is to gain attention for themselves. Includes a quiz to check your knowledge of the syndrome and the potential for treatment.

Munchausen by Proxy Syndrome

http://home.coqui.net:80/myrna/munch.htm

Site describes MBPS and how to identify it. From *The Pediatric Bulletin.*

National Clearinghouse of Child Abuse and Neglect Information

http://www.calib.com/nccanch/

Information for professionals on child abuse, neglect, and child welfare. Provides links, access to database and statistics.

Recovered Memory of Sexual Abuse: Scientific Research and Scholarly References

http://www.jimhopper.com/memory

Discussion about amnesia for child abuse, including summaries of professional research and publications on the topic.

Research and Training Center in Rehabilitation and Childhood Trauma

http://www.nemc.org/rehab/homepg.htm

From the New England Medical Center. Mission is to increase knowledge about the causes, treatment, and outcomes of injuries to children. Offers tips on injury prevention and violence intervention.

Sexual Assault Information Page: Incest and Child Sexual Abuse

http://www.cs.utk.edu/~bartley/index/childSexualAbuse/

This site provides many links for survivors of incest and child sexual abuse. It includes statistics, research, recovery resources and support.

A Short Guide for Employees Suspecting Child Abuse

http://www.limestone.edu.on.ca/Pubs/Cah/Cah_Summary.Html

What to do if a child discloses abuse. Posted by a school district in Ontario, Canada.

The Survivors' Voice

http://www.survivorsvoice.com

Newsletter addressing issues of child abuse.

Yes ICAN (International Child Abuse Network)

http://yesican.org

The mission of the Network is to work to break the cycle of child abuse world-wide. Website provides articles, book recommendations, inspiring stories and links, and it hosts several chat room discussions and a bulletin board.

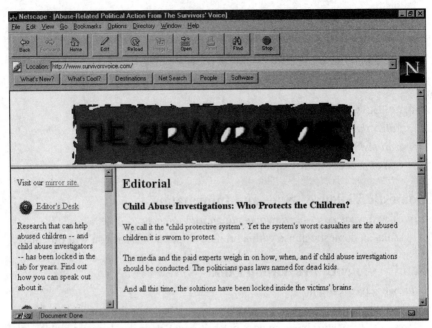

The Survivors Voice. *http://www.survivorsvoice.com/*

Domestic Violence

Blain Nelson's Abuse Pages
http://blainn.cc/abuse/

A former offender shares his story of abuse and recovery, as well as the stories of others in an attempt to educate, prevent and end abusive behavior, and to assist others in recovery. Articles, links, and more.

Cancer in Our Homes: Domestic Violence
http://www.mlode.com/~ra/ra8/index.html

Commentary on domestic violence. Includes words of support, definitions, common myths, interventions and a description of the cycle of abuse.

Domestic Violence
http://www.en.com/users/allison/dvpage.html

Facts about domestic violence, warning signs, advice for those trying to leave an abusive partner and for those who are trying to help someone who is in an abusive relationship, and links.

Domestic Violence Resources
http://www.feminist.org/other/dv/dvinter.html

List of and links to Internet resources pertaining to the topic of domestic violence. Also includes sites on preventing violence against women in general.

Domestic Violence Shelters
http://dir.yahoo.com/Society_and_Culture/Crime/Crimes/Domestic_Violence/Organizations/Shelters/

List of shelters from Yahoo.

Domestic Violence - Sites and Information
http://www.cs.utk.edu/~bartley/index/domesticViolence/

Links on domestic abuse with a brief description of what you will find there.

Family Violence Prevention Fund
http://www.igc.org/fund/

Includes pages on violence against women globally, health care and workplace responses to domestic abuse, news of celebrities and their involvement in domestic violence allegations or the fight against domestic violence, and a quiz to test your knowledge.

Kate's Domestic Violence Pages
http://www.ocs.mq.edu.au/~korman/feminism/Domestic_Violence/

Includes advice and where to get help, as well as links to research, statistics, fact sheets, pamphlets, newspaper and magazine articles available on the web, and ways you can respond to domestic violence.

State DV Coalitions
http://www.cybergrrl.com/dv.html

Phone numbers of domestic violence coalitions, by state.

Elder Abuse
See also: Aging/Gerontology.

Elder Abuse
http://www.calregistry.com/resources/eldabpag.htm

How to identify if you or someone else is the victim of elder abuse; links.

Elder Abuse Prevention and Treatment Resources Page
http://www.aoa.dhhs.gov/abuse/

Includes fact sheets, news, policy and reports on elder abuse from sources such as the White House, Administration on Aging, the Social Security Administration and other groups.

Elder Abuse Prevention: Information and Resource Guide
http://www.oaktrees.org/elder/

Recognizing and intervening in situations where the elderly are suffering from neglect, or from physical, emotional and financial abuse. Spanish version of pages are under development. Includes links, organized by state.

National Center on Elder Abuse
http://www.gwjapan.com/NCEA/

This site contains many resources for professionals and the public regarding abuse of the elderly. Includes basic fact sheets, and elder abuse reporting numbers, as well as publications, data, and information about laws related to elder abuse.

Nursing Home Abuse
http://www.txlegal.com/nursing.htm

Indicators of neglect and physical or emotional abuse taking place in nursing homes.

Nursing Home Resident's Bill of Rights
http://www.careguide.net/careguide.cgi/eldercare/ecthink/billofri.htm!

Nursing homes are required by law to make a bill of rights/policy statement available to any resident who requests it. This site presents 12 issues that should be covered in such a policy statement.

Vulnerable in a Safe Place: Institutional Elder Abuse
http://www.cjona.org/vulnera.html

This online article from the *Canadian Journal of Nursing Administration* reviews the literature on institutional elder abuse and describes strategies to alleviate pressures which may give rise to abuse.

Male Victims of Abuse

Abuse Hurts Men Too
http://www.stirling.u-net.com/abusemen.htm
   Information, articles and links on husband abuse and male rape.

Doubting Thomas Male Sexual Assault
_http://ourworld.compuserve.com/homepages/Doubting_Thomas/msa00.htm_
   Information on the sexual assault and rape of men. Includes links to organizations, articles, bibliography, and hotline numbers.

Male Abuse Survivors Support Forum
http://www.noahgrey.com/massf/
   Site is for male survivors of sexual, physical, and emotional abuse. It offers message boards, discussion groups, chat rooms, personal stories, poetry and prose writings by survivors of abuse, bookstore and links.

Men and Abuse, Rape
http://www.vix.com/pub/men/abuse/abuse.html
   Information, studies, debates, papers and commentaries on male sexual abuse. Includes sexual abuse of a male child, male rape and prison rape.

Men and Domestic Violence Index
http://www.vix.com/pub/men/domestic-index.html
   Includes pages on husband battering and other forms of male abuse.

Recovery from Abuse

Abuse Recovery Resources
_http://www.chebucto.ns.ca/~aa458/abuse_recovery_resources.html_
   Resources for survivors and information on dissociation.

Karra's Korner
http://www.xroads.com/rainbow/karra.html
   Links for survivors of abuse and those who want to assist them to heal.

Sanctuaries

http://www.geocities.com/Wellesley/2976/sanctuaries.html

This site seeks to assist victims of violence and abuse. It contains stories from survivors, information on rape, abuse and domestic violence, and links devoted to abuse recovery and mental health.

The Sanctuary: Safe Network Community, the Underground Abuse Refuge

http://www.rdr.net/~hack/sanct/

Victims of abuse both past and present can come to this site to relax, talk with and listen to others.

Sexual Offense Recovery Online

http://206.155.34.8/sexualoffenserecovery/

How to find a therapist for treatment. Services for victims and offenders.

Sidran Foundation and Press

http://www.sidran.org/

The Sidran Foundation is devoted to education, advocacy and research to help the early recognition and treatment of trauma-related stress in children and the understanding and treatment of adults suffering from trauma-generated disorders. Includes a number of online brochures and a catalog.

Wounded Healer Journal

http://idealist.com/wounded_healer/

Support for psychotherapists and survivors of abuse.

Ritual Abuse

More Than Conquerors

http://www.morethanconquerors.simplenet.com/index/index.htm

Online support forums created by survivors for survivors of ritual abuse, sadistic abuse, mind control victims, and/or those facing a dissociative condition. Provides a caring place to be heard and believed. Anonymity available.

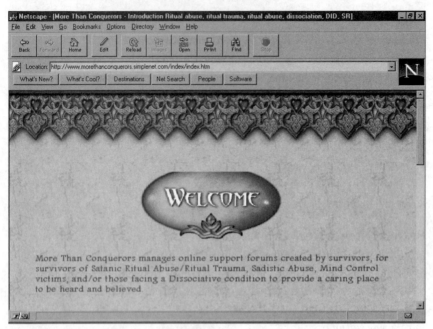

More Than Conquerors. *http://www.morethanconquerors.simplenet.com/index/index.htm*

Sunshine through the Rain
http://enchantedwings.hypermart.net/ritual.html

Symptoms and signs, self-help techniques, triggers, and information on dissociative disorders.

Survivorship Home Page
https://www.ctsserver.com/~svship/

An international forum discussing issues relevant to survivors of ritualistic abuse, torture, and mind control.

Ritual Abuse, Ritual Crime, and Healing
http://www.xroads.com/rahome/rahome.html

Provides support information and encouragement to survivors of ritual abuse. Includes resources, links, frequently asked questions and tips for healing.

Sexual Abuse

Abuse/Sexual Abuse/Incest Resources
http://www.pilot.infi.net/~susanf/ablinks2.htm
   Comprehensive list of resources and links with descriptions.

Anonymous Sexual Abuse Recovery
http://www.worldchat.com/public/asarc/commsymp.htm
   Common symptoms; abuse-related illnesses.

ASARian, Inc.
http://www.asarian.org/
   Links to other various sites on abuse recovery and education. Offers online peer counseling and support, hosts forums for survivors of abuse, and provides electronic services such as web hosting and anonymous web access. Also provides recycled computer equipment for abuse survivors who are unable to afford it.

Essential Information on Abuse, Assault, Rape & Domestic Violence
http://www.mcs.net/~kathyw/abuse.html
   Provides a great deal of abuse, assault and domestic violence resources. Links are rated to show suitability for children.

Living in a Rape Culture
http://pubweb.ucdavis.edu/Documents/RPEP/culture.htm
   Site discusses rape as a byproduct of our culture and social conditioning, and provides information and statistics.

RAINN
http://www.rainn.org/
   RAINN = Rape, Abuse and Incest National Network.

REAL MEN Work to End Violence Against Women
http://www.cs.utk.edu/~bartley/other/realMen.html
   Information about this men's group whose goal is to help society to rethink and work to change traditional stereotypical views of masculinity, and to to eliminate sexism and sexual violence.

Sexual Assault Information Page
http://www.cs.utk.edu/~bartley/saInfoPage.html

Lots of information, from acquaintance rape to pornography, to women's resources links.

Survivors' Page
http://www.sehlat.com/survs.html

Issues relating to sexual abuse.

Treatment for Offenders

Controlling Anger Before It Controls You
http://www.apa.org/pubinfo/anger.html

Online brochure from the American Psychological Association discussing how to understand and manage anger.

Stop It Now!
http://www.stopitnow.com/

The mission of Stop It Now! is to call on all abusers and potential abusers to stop and seek help; to educate adults about the ways to stop sexual abuse; and to increase public awareness of the trauma of child sexual abuse.

Adult Male Sexual Offenders
http://206.155.34.8/sexualoffenserecovery/amale.htm

Through chat sessions and therapy, these pages seek to help offenders to stop.

ADDICTION & RECOVERY

Covered in this chapter: Alcoholism; Cocaine; Drug Information; Drug Policy and Issues; Dual Diagnosis; Emotion Addiction; Family Support; Heroin; Humor & Addiction; Internet Addiction; Marijuana; Methamphetamine; Nicotine; Recovery/Support; Research, Professional and Government Sites; Sexual Addiction.
Related chapter: Mental Health.

Alcoholism

90 Tools for Sobriety
http://www.recovery.org/aa/aa-related/tools.html
Suggestions for staying sober.

AA Grapevine
http://www.aagrapevine.org/
The international journal of Alcoholics Anonymous, which features first-person stories of individuals, information on AA, subscription and submission information, reprint requests and more.

Adult Children of Alcoholics World Service Organization
http://www.adultchildren.org/
Homepage of this 12-step program for women and men who grew up in alcoholic or otherwise dysfunctional homes. Meeting dates, frequently asked questions, events and literature.

Al-Anon/Alateen
http://www.Al-Anon-Alateen.org/
Information, services and principles of this world-wide self-help recovery program for families and friends of alcoholics. Text available in twelve different languages.

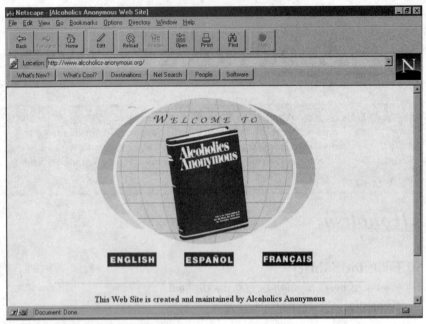

Alcoholics Anonymous World Services. *http://www.alcoholics-anonymous.org/*

Alcoholics Anonymous Information
http://www.aaphoenix.org/aainfo.html
   Homepage of the Phoenix, Arizona AA offers information that is helpful no matter where you live.

Alcoholics Anonymous World Services
http://www.alcoholics-anonymous.org/
   Official site of Alcoholics Anonymous World Services, available in English, French and Spanish. Information on the organization and its philosophy and more.

Alcoholics Victorious
http://www.iugm.org/av/
   Christian support group for recovering alcoholics.

Alcoholism
http://alcoholism.miningco.com/
   Non-AA site that provides a great deal of well-organized information on alcoholism, related issues and recovery resources. Articles on scientific and genetic aspects of alcoholism, nutrition, teen use, drunk driving, workplace issues, and more.

Another Empty Bottle

http://www.alcoholismhelp.com/help/

This site is for friends and family of alcoholics, and it contains discussion areas, chat rooms, a newsletter, help and hotline information, pages for children, and the "Premiere Alcoholism Search Engine."

The Big Book Web Site

http://www.recovery.org/aa/bigbook/ww/index.html

Online version of this Alcoholics Anonymous text and guidebook, with hyperlinks to important sections and highlights.

Daily Reflections

http://www.anaserve.com/~spencers/dailyreflection.html

Thoughtful excerpts from AA publications, for daily contemplation.

A Jewish Response to Alcoholism

http://www.recovery.org/aa/aa-related/jacs.html

Comments encouraging a Jewish component in healing alcoholism.

National Association for Children of Alcoholics

http://www.health.org/nacoa/

This organization seeks to help kids who are hurt by parental alcohol and drug use. Site provides articles, newsletter, information and description of services, and pages written for children.

Online AA Resources

http://www.recovery.org/aa/

Information about Alcoholics Anonymous, including its history, regional resources, online meeting information, and a bibliography. AA resources also available for non-English speakers.

Online Intergroup of Alcoholics Anonymous

http://aa-intergroup.org/

The OIAA was established "to serve cyberspace" and includes a directory of over one hundred online e-mail and real-time AA meetings, including meetings held in different languages, meetings for gay men, lesbians, women, and meetings for many other specific groups and themes.

Online Recovery Resources (Non-AA)

http://www.recovery.org/rec2.html

Links and resources, because AA may not be for everybody.

National Institute on Alcohol Abuse and Alcoholism

http://www.niaaa.nih.gov/

Offers publications and databases, news and events about alcohol abuse and addiction. Site includes the bulletin *Alcohol Alert*, a scientific journal entitled *Alcohol Health and Research World*, pamphlets, reports, research monographs and databases, as well as grant information and links.

Prevention Online (NCADI)

http://www.health.org/

The National Clearinghouse for Alcohol and Drug Information. Access to alcohol and drug facts, research and resources, statistics, online forums and links.

Quizzes to Help Determine Alcohol Dependency

http://www.recovery.org/aa/aa-related/quizzes.html

Includes several self-tests as well as quizzes for family, parents and women.

Relapse

http://www.recovery.org/aa/aa-related/relapse.html

Checklist of symptoms that may lead to relapse.

Self Scoring Alcohol Check-Up

http://www.habitsmart.com/chkup.html

Online quiz provides information on one's drinking habits.

Sober Space

http://www.aa-erie-pa.com/

Includes AA meeting schedules in the U.S., Canada and internationally.

The Twelve Steps
http://www.primenet.com/~katper/12steps.htm

The popular steps are an integral part of Alcoholics Anonymous and other recovery programs.

(Unofficial) Alcoholics Anonymous Page
http://www.halcyon.com/carrick/aa/aa-home.html

Site contains a great deal of information on AA and links to many other recovery sites.

Women for Sobriety Inc.
http://www.womenforsobriety.org/

Self-help program to help women fight alcoholism and other addictions. Features the "New Life Acceptance Program" with 13 principles promoting acceptance and healing through positive thinking, metaphysics, meditation and nutrition.

Cocaine

Cocaine
http://www.mninter.net/~publish/cokepage.htm

Cocaine facts, including history, pharmacology, usage, legal and criminal connection.

Cocaine Anonymous World Services
http://www.ca.org/

Site describes this 12-step fellowship program to help individuals overcome addiction to cocaine. Includes a self-test for cocaine addiction and a link to a CA site in French.

Cocaine/Crack
http://www.drugfreeamerica.org/cocaine.html

Drug information, including appearance, slang names, effects and frequently asked questions.

Drug Information

Addiction, Recovery and Prevention
http://www.idir.net/~irvcohen/

Extensive excerpts from Irving Cohen, M.D.'s book entitled *Addiction: The High-Low Trap.*

Addictions and Life Page
http://www.addictions.org/

Message board discussions, access to recovery resources, and downloadable file of drug related street names/slang terms.

Alcohol and Drugs - General Information
http://www.wellesley.edu/Counseling/selfcare/alcdrug_info.html

Directed toward students, this site describes substances and their effects.

Drogas Informacion en Espanol
http://www.mninter.net/~publish/spanish.htm

El presente panfleto contiene información vital acerca del alcohol y otras drogas, sus efectos psicológicos y la forma en que podemos ayudarnos mutuamente para superar los problemas que causan el alcohol y otras drogas.

Drug Information
http://www.mninter.net/~publish/page3.htm

Database and fact sheets on street drugs, including inhalants, steroids, narcotics, stimulants, depressants, marijuana, hallucinogens and many more.

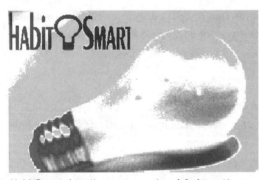

HabitSmart. http://www.cts.com/crash/habtsmrt/

HabitSmart
http://www.cts.com/crash/habtsmrt/

Information and resources addressing addictive behavior, including theories of habits and how to change them. All kinds of addictions are covered, from alcohol to drugs to cigarettes.

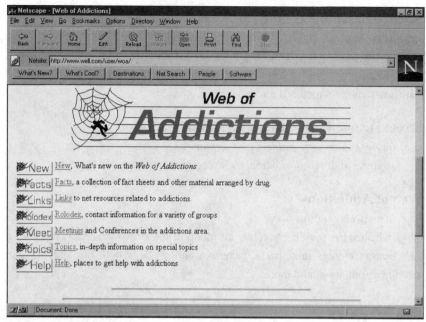

Web of Addictions. *http://www.well.com/user/woa/*

Local NA Helpline Numbers
http://www.na.org/phonelin.htm

Links to local service committee sanctioned Narcotics Anonymous websites all around the globe.

Mike and Terry's House
http://www.syix.com/mleahey/

Narcotics Anonymous news, support, meeting information and more.

Narcotics Anonymous World Services
http://na.org/index.htm

A 12-step program based on the Alcoholics Anonymous format for individuals recovering from any kind of drug addiction.

National Institute on Drug Abuse
http://www.nida.nih.gov/

Part of the National Institutes of Health, the National Institute on Drug Abuse offers links and information about drugs of abuse, publications and research.

Science Based Facts on Drug Abuse and Addiction

http://www.nida.nih.gov/Infofax/Infofaxindex.html

Infofax monographs from the National Institute on Drug Abuse cover the health hazards of specific drugs, understanding addiction, drug abuse survey and statistics, treatment methods and more.

Street Drugs: Photographs and Information

http://www.mninter.net/~publish/photos.htm

Database of drug information, including photographs.

Web of Addictions

http://www.well.com/user/woa/

Dedicated to providing accurate information about alcoholism and other drug addictions. Contains fact sheets, resources and contacts both on- and off-line, meeting information, and more.

Drug Policy and Issues

Drug Enforcement Administration

http://www.usdoj.gov/dea/

The homepage of this agency includes a drug database, description of their programs, online publications, and details on the Freedom of Information Act.

The Drug Library

http://www.druglibrary.org/

Links to sites on specific drug issues, drug laws, drug policy, human rights and the war on drugs.

The Drug Policy Foundation

http://www.dpf.org/

The Foundation is an independent, nonprofit organization that publicizes alternatives to current drug strategies, believing that the war on drugs isn't working.

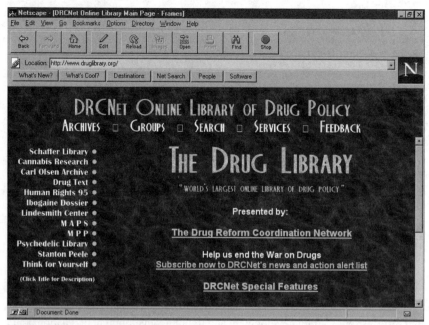

The Drug Library. http://www.druglibrary.org/

International Harm Reduction Association
http://www.ihra.org.uk/default.htm

The IHRA is a professional association of individuals and organizations from around the world who are interested in developing drug policies that will best reduce the harmful consequences of drug use and current drug policies. It offers educational materials and publishes the *The International Journal of Drug Policy.*

The North American Syringe Exchange Network
http://www.nasen.org/NASEN_II/index.html

This organization is dedicated to the creation, expansion and continued existence of syringe exchange programs as a proven method of stopping the transmission of blood borne pathogens in the injecting drug using community.

United Nations International Drug Control Program
http://www.undcp.or.at/

Information on drug abuse around the world, as well as international efforts to reduce both supply and demand.

Dual Diagnosis

See also: Mental Health.

Dual Diagnosis

http://www.monumental.com/arcturus/dd/ddhome.htm

Co-occurring mental illness, drug addiction, and/or alcoholism. Includes newsletter, advocacy, training manuals and links to related sites.

Dual Diagnosis Anonymous

http://www.camft.com/ddameet.htm

Information on DDA meetings and the 12-step process.

Dual Diagnosis Website

http://www.erols.com/ksciacca/

For health care providers, addicts, their families and the general public. Includes articles and chapters to read or download, up-coming events, materials and services for program development and training, development of a national and international treatment program directory, an interactive bulletin board, live chat, subscription to a credentialed listserv, bibliography, search engine, and more.

The Midas Dual Disorders Home Page

http://ourworld.compuserve.com/homepages/Rich_as_Midas/homepage.htm

Although this site serves as a centralized reference for Australian dual diagnosis programs, there are links and information on DD that are useful no matter where you live.

Emotion Addiction

Emotions Anonymous

http://www.mtn.org/EA/

Provides background information on this 12-step program composed of people who are working toward recovery from emotional difficulties. Find a meeting near you.

Family Support

Adult Children of Alcoholics
http://www.recovery.org/acoa/acoa.html

Text files which discuss the common behaviors and problems of adult children of alcoholics; research and resources.

Adult Children Online Resource Page
http://www.intac.com/%7Ewoy/drwoititz/source.htm

Resources for adult children of alcoholics. Includes topics on alcohol, alcoholism, anxiety, parenting, self-help and more.

National Families in Action Online
http://www.emory.edu/NFIA/

National Families in Action is a drug education, prevention, and policy center focusing on preventing drug use, abuse, addiction, and death. Its mission is to help families and communities stop drug use among children by promoting policies "based on science." Information for parents and professionals on drug use and science, the brain, and the law.

Parents+Teachers+DARE Officers
http://www.mninter.net/~publish/parents.htm

Drug education information.

Project Know
http://www.projectknow.com/

A flashy anti-drug site that includes "teen speak," "parent hub," and "school zone."

Red Flags for Drug and Alcohol Abuse
http://www.asam.org/publ/CAGE.htm

Lists observable signs of drug and alcohol abuse, laboratory indicators, and questions to ask to determine if someone has a drug or alcohol problem. From the American Society of Addiction Medicine.

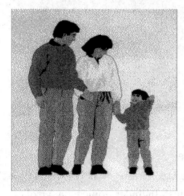

Substance Abuse Information for Parents. http://www.commnet.edu/QVCTC/student/GaryOKeefe/drug facts.html

SAMSHA Looking for Help?

http://www.samhsa.gov/look3.htm

Assistance for your own or for someone else's drug or mental health problems. Site contains help hotlines, directory of treatment facilities, and related information from the Substance Abuse and Mental Health Services Administration.

Substance Abuse Information for Parents

http://www.commnet.edu/QVCTC/student/ GaryOKeefe/drugfacts.html

Information to help parents indentify specific drug use. A risk factor sheet evaluates a child's potential misuse of drugs. Education, prevention, and methods of treatment for substance abuse are also provided.

Heroin

Erowid Heroin Vault

http://www.erowid.org/entheogens/heroin/heroin.shtml

Information on heroin, including research, legislation, treatment, pharmacology, media coverage, resources and links.

Heroin

http://www.health.org/pubs/qdocs/heroin/doaher.htm

Information taken from the Department of Justice's book, *Drugs of Abuse.*

Opiates

http://www.hyperreal.org/drugs/opiates/index.html

Information on heroin, and other opiates.

Humor & Addiction

Do You Have a Thinking Problem?
http://www.users.cts.com/crash/e/elmo/think.htm
   "Has your efficiency decreased due to thinking?"

Humor and Addiction
http://www.users.cts.com/crash/e/elmo/funindex.htm
   How many alcoholics does it take to change a lightbulb?

Guardians of Recovery
http://www.syix.com/mleahey/GOR/sheild.htm
   Satire of those hard-core 12-steppers.

Service-Based Recovery Anonymous
http://www.syix.com/mleahey/SBR/index.htm
   Are you addicted to recovery?

Internet Addiction

Center for On-line Addiction
http://www.netaddiction.com/
   Online-gambling, Internet and cybersex addiction information and tests.

Internet Addiction Disorder
http://www.cmhc.com/guide/iad.htm
   If you're reading this book, you may want to check out this site. . .

Net Overuse Called "True Addiction"
http://www.addictions.org/netaddict.htm
   Article from *U.S.A. Today*.

On-Line Gambling
http://www.people.virginia.edu/~cpb5t/
   Research paper addressing the social, legal and economic impact of online gambling.

Virtual Addiction
http://www.virtual-addiction.com/
>Information and resources on computer and Internet addiction.

You Know You Are Addicted to the Internet When...
http://www.kristasmom.com/p71.htm
>Quiz yourself (humor).

You Might Be Addicted...
http://www.rotfl.com/irc-addict/
>"... to the IRC if you have created a link to this site" (humor).

Marijuana

Cannabis.com
http://www.cannabis.com/
>Information from the pro-use side of the marijuana debate.

Marijuana Facts for Teens
http://www.nida.nih.gov/MarijBroch/Marijteens.html
>Basic questions and answers about marijuana and marijuana use.

Marijuana Information
http://www.drug-abuse.com/information/marijuana/
>Information from the National Institute of Drug Abuse.

Methamphetamine

Crystal Meth Anonymous Online
http://www.crystalmeth.org/
>Basic information, meetings, bulletin boards, e-mail support and other resources.

Factline on Amphetamines

http://www.drugs.indiana.edu/pubs/factline/ampet.html
Information on amphetamine in all its forms.

Methamphetamine Frequently Asked Questions

http://www.kci.org/meth_info/faq_meth.htm
Also includes links to slang names and other meth info sites.

Nicotine

Alt.Support.Stop-Smoking (AS3)

http://www.swen.uwaterloo.ca/~bpekilis/as3
The newsgroup's website and archives.

American Cancer Society Tobacco Information

http://www.cancer.org/services/tobacco/
A search for "tobacco" yields information on its link to lung cancer.

ASH: Action on Smoking and Health

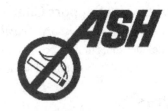

http://www.ash.org/
This organization works to protect the rights of anti- smokers. Site provides cig- arette, tobacco and nicotine information.

Action on Smoking and Health.

CDC's TIPS (Tobacco Information and Prevention Source)

http://www.cdc.gov/tobacco/
Includes research, news, advice for how to quit, educational materials and TIPS for teens.

Environmental Tobacco Smoke

http://www.oncolink.upenn.edu/pdq_html/6/engl/600039.html
Learn about the effects of second-hand smoke.

NicNet

http://tobacco.arizona.edu/

Lots of information on nicotine and tobacco research.

No Smoke Cafe

http://clever.net/chrisco/nosmoke/stop.html?

The chat room and the wall of ex-smokers are only some features of this site for former smokers.

Nicotine Anonymous

http://www.nicotine-anonymous.org/

Online pamphlets and answers to questions such as: *What is nicotine addiction? What are the symptoms? What is Nicotine Anonymous? What are Nicotine Anonymous meetings?* and more information on this 12-step program.

NO SMOKE Software

http://www.smokefreekids.com/nosmoke.htm

Computer software designed to assist individuals to quit smoking.

QuitSmokingSupport.Com

http://www.quitsmokingsupport.com/

Includes tools to help you to quit smoking, encouragement, e-mail discussion groups and lots of tobacco and addiction information.

Quitters

http://www.corral.net/quitters/

Encouragement to quit smoking, information and links.

Smoking and Cancer

http://www.oncolink.upenn.edu/causeprevent/smoking/

Information and links from the University of Pennsylvania Cancer Center's OncoLink. Also features an art gallery of children's anti-smoking drawings.

Tobacco Control Archives

http://galen.library.ucsf.edu/tobacco/

Access document collections which show research on the addictive nature of nicotine, tobacco industry documents, and information on the "Joe Camel" Campaign lawsuit.

Recovery/Support

Note: Search the Internet to find treatment facilities suitable to your own needs. None are included here, since they can't all be mentioned.

Christians in Recovery

http://www.christians-in-recovery.com/

Free access to information and resources, much of it Christian, and a Members Only area which offers private chat rooms, scheduled recovery meetings, e-mail groups, message boards, and 12-step Bible study groups.

Christian Recovery Connection

http://www.tfs.net/~iugm/

A virtual community of believers offering advice and support to those recovering from addictions. Includes scriptures for recovery, advice on finding a church that is "recovery friendly," as well as non-religious recovery information such as recommended diet and more.

Clean and Sober Home for the Homeless Biker

http://pw2.netcom.com/~nitrosmi/skull.html

Clean and sober motorcycle magazine, Sober and Harley Davison chat rooms, biker links, NA and AA information and support.

DOC: Doctors Ought to Care

http://www.bcm.tmc.edu/doc/

The mission of this group is to fight tobacco and alcohol use among youths.

JACS

http://www.jacsweb.org/

For **J**ewish **A**lcoholics, **C**hemically dependant persons and **S**ignificant others.

Join Together: Online

http://www.jointogether.org/jointogether.html

Self-described as a "resource center and meeting place for communities working to reduce harms [from] the use of illicit drugs, . . . alcohol and tobacco."

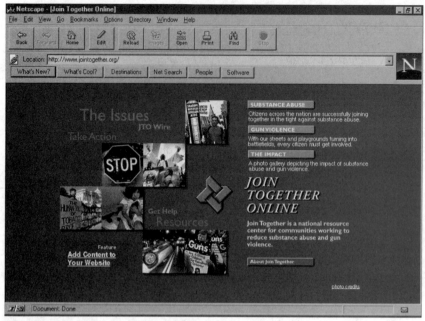

Join Together Online. http://www.jointogether.org/jointogether.html

Prevention Primer

http://www.health.org/pubs/primer/index.htm

Reference tool for "prevention practitioners." Offers summaries of issues and strategies, a brief history of prevention efforts and an overview of key topics, issues, principles, and approaches that have proven successful. The topics are indexed alphabetically. From the National Clearinghouse for Drug & Alcohol Information.

Recovery Is Good for You

http://www.users.cts.com/crash/e/elmo/recovr.htm

Links to recovery sites.

Recovery Medicine Wheel (Native American)

http://www.recovery.org/aa/aa-related/medwheel.txt

Thoughtful interpretation of recovery with a Native American perspective.

Recovery Newsletter

http://www.recoverynewsletter.com/

Subscription information and free issue of this online newsletter written for recovering alcoholics and other addicts. Although it does discuss the 12-steps, it also addresses topics such as health and nutrition, recreation, technology, and more. You'll also find links and information on AA.

Sobriety and Recovery Resources

http://www.winternet.com/~terrym/sobriety.html

Contains a great deal of information, ranging from personal stories and articles to teen substance use, recovery information and newsgroups.

unhooked.com

http://wwww.unhooked.org/

Page presents an alternative viewpoint to the 12-step program; i.e., "sobriety, secularity and self-help." Includes meeting information, discussions, newsletter, art gallery and poetry, treatment information, nutrition and food pages and features.

Research, Professional & Government Sites

Addiction Research Foundation/Center for Addiction

http://www.arf.org/

Combines research, information and community action on alcohol, tobacco and other drugs.

American Society of Addiction Medicine

http://www.asam.org/

A professional organization whose goal is to educate physicians and improve the treatment of individuals suffering from alcoholism or other addictions. It contains practice guidelines, discussion forums, Society publications and more.

Brown University Center for Alcohol and Addiction Studies

http://center.butler.brown.edu/

Research on addiction, links and affiliated projects.

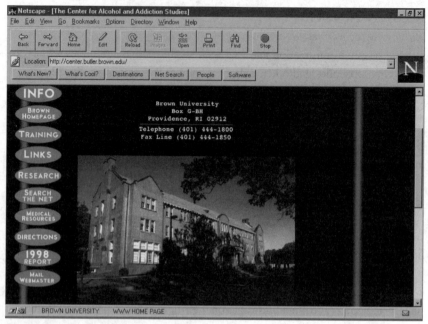

Brown Univ. Center for Alcohol and Addiction Studies. *http://center.butler.brown.edu/*

Bureau of Alcohol, Tobacco and Firearms Home Page
http://www.atf.treas.gov/

The Bureau enforces Federal laws and regulations relating to alcohol, tobacco, firearms, explosives and arson. Site contains news and discusses programs.

Center for Addiction and Alternative Medicine Research
http://www.winternet.com/~caamr/

Contact information available.

Center for Substance Abuse Research
http://www.bsos.umd.edu/cesar/cesar.html

CESAR is a research center affiliated with the University of Maryland that collects, analyzes, and disseminates information on the nature and extent of substance abuse and related problems.

Research Institute on Addictions

http://www.ria.org/

Site describes RIA research and projects. RIA scientists study alcoholism, substance abuse, and related issues such as crime and violence. The Institute offers addiction treatment services through its Clinical Research Center.

Sexual Addiction

Overcome Sexual Addiction

http://www.sexualaddiction.com

Yes, you *can* get too much. . . Sexual addictions can be as damaging as other compulsions. Understand and overcome this self-destructive addiction.

Sexual Compulsives Anonymous

http://www.sca-recovery.org/

Support for sex addicts, based on the 12-step program of AA.

AGING / GERONTOLOGY

Alzheimer's Disease & Dementias

AD Dementia Web Resources
http://www.biostat.wustl.edu/ALZHEIMER/submit.html

Site provides resources for caregivers, offers clinical care guides, research about the aging process, products and services for the aging, links to personal homepages, information on nursing homes and assisted living, and more.

Alzheimer Web
http://dsmallpc2.path.unimelb.edu.au/ad.html

Devoted to research on Alzheimer's disease (AD). Includes links to research centers, summaries of recent research papers, patient information, recommended books, articles and links.

Alzheimer's Association
http://www.alz.org/

Answers to your questions on Alzheimer's, e.g., *What is it? What causes it? What are warning signs? How common is Alzheimer's?* Learn about the diagnosis, current research, medical affects and treatment. Index of local Association chapters and links. Information and resources for caregivers and patients.

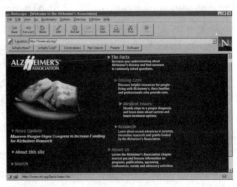

Alzheimer's Association. *http://www.alz.org/*

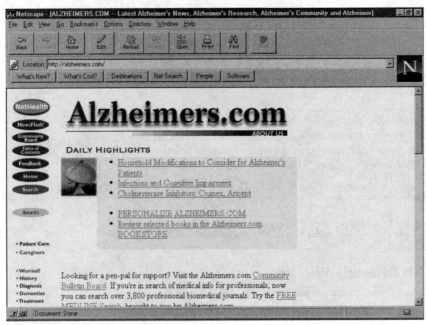

Alzheimers.Com. *http:/alzheimers.com/*

Alzheimer's Bookstore

http://www.alzheimersbooks.com/

Includes detailed descriptions about books on caregiving, family experiences with Alzheimer's, medical books, books about spirituality and other categories.

Alzheimers.com

http://alzheimers.com/

Site provides information about Alzheimer's for the public. Sections covered include how to help someone suffering from the disease, prevention, treatment, diagnosis, risks, history and new research. Additional features include a community bulletin board for caregivers, a description of other types of dementia or illnesses that may be mistaken for Alzheimer's, and a book review section.

Alzheimer's Disease Education & Referral Center

http://www.alzheimers.org/

Provides information on Alzheimer's from the National Institute on Aging. Site allows you to e-mail your own question to be answered by a specialist. Publications and information on new studies and treatments are offered.

Alzheimer's Disease and Other Dementias: Info for Consumers

http://www.health.state.ny.us/nysdoh/consumer/alzheimer/alzeihm.htm

These PDF files contain the contents of the *New York State Task Force on Alzheimer's Disease and Other Dementias, Final Report and Recommendations*, and other Alzheimer's resources.

Alzheimer's Disease Pearls

http://www.mayo.edu/geriatrics-rst/AlzPearls.html

Tips on managing various aspects of care for Alzheimer's patients. Includes a philosophy of care, behavior problems, agitation, delusions and hallucinations, and more.

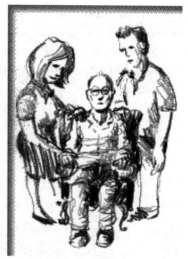

Alzheimer's Disease and Other Dementias. *http://www.health.state.ny.us/nysdoh/consumer/alzeihm.htm*

Alzheimers Network

http://www.jakinbox.com/

Attractive but simple site provides a manageable amount of information on Alzheimer's disease. Links included.

Alzheimer's Support Network

http://gator.naples.net/presents/Alzheimer/

Pages on Alzheimer's disease and wandering; library, monthly newsletter, bibliography and links.

Coping

http://www.isl.net/~hoffcomp/

The objective of this site is to share coping experiences and tips that may be useful to others caring for a loved one diagnosed with Alzheimer's Disease or other forms of dementia.

Dementia Web

http://dementia.ion.ucl.ac.uk/

Includes the Virtual Carer chat room for those caring for individuals with dementia, support and advice for caregivers, and links to research organizations that study dementia.

Early Alzheimer's Disease

http://www.ahcpr.gov/clinic/alzcons.htm

A patient and family guide from the AHCPR describing the early signs and symptoms of Alzheimer's disease. Sources for medical, social, and financial support are listed.

Family Caregiver Alliance Clearinghouse

http://www.caregiver.org/factsheet.html

Information on Alzheimer's, dementia, and other disorders. Also provides family caregiving tips. Fact sheets available in English and Spanish.

Forgetfulness: It's Not Always What You Think

http://www.alzheimers.org/agepage.html

Information sheet explains dementias, and mentions how other treatable problems that older people may have can be mistaken for dementia.

The Nun Study

http://www.coa.uky.edu/nunnet/

This site describes the background and latest results of a longitudinal study of aging and Alzheimer's. The participants were 678 nuns ranging from 75-103 years of age. Updated regularly.

University Alzheimer Center

http://www.ohioalzcenter.org/

Center is connected with Case Western Reserve University. The site provides basic information on Alzheimer's, new treatments (including medications and research regarding the benefits of exercise), links to other Internet resources, description of the ten warning signs of AD, and information about how to participate in the Center's brain autopsy program.

Caregivers

The Caregiver's Handbook
http://www.biostat.wustl.edu/ALZHEIMER/care.html

The entire text of this handbook for caregivers and elderly care-receivers is available online. The table of contents with hyperlinks assists in reaching the section you need most.

Caregiving Online Newsletter
http://www.caregiving.com/

Monthly online newsletter for those providing eldercare. Regular columns include the male caregiver, the working family caregiver, ask the experts, and more.

Dementia: Management of Behavior Problems
http://www.mayo.edu/geriatrics-rst/Behav.html

Information from the Mayo Clinic for caregivers.

Elder Care Navigator
http://www.mindspring.com/~eldrcare/elderweb.htm

Subtitle to this site is "Helping People Navigate the Elder Care Maze."

Eldercare Locator:
How to Find Community Assistance for Seniors
http://www.ageinfo.org/elderloc/

A nationwide directory assistance service designed to help older persons and caregivers locate local support resources for aging Americans.

Eldercare Site
http://www.alzwell.com/

Support and understanding for people who provide care for the elderly. Includes lots of tips, links, and a daily IRC chat channel.

elderlifeplanning.com
http://www.elderlifeplanning.com/

News and information on eldercare services, home care, elder housing alternatives, long term care insurance, caregiver support and more. ElderPlanningCafé Discussion Forum also available.

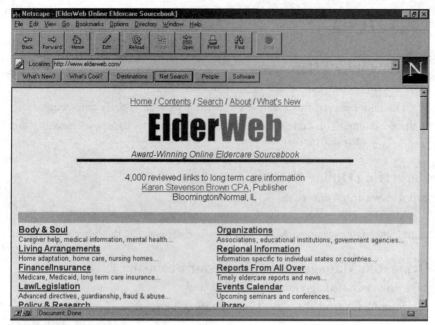

ElderWeb. http://www.elderweb.com/

ElderWeb

http://www.elderweb.com/

A great deal of information, and "4,000 reviewed links to long term care."

Extended Care Information Network

http://www.extendedcare.com/Eldercare/public/main.html

Health care professionals offer information, news and advice on extended care facilities (i.e., nursing homes, assisted living facilities and adult day care) and home care asistance.

Surviving Caregiving

http://www.isl.net/~hoffcomp/Welcome.html#Surviving Caregiving

Practical and supportive information and articles for caregivers, including hospice considerations, home modifications, "respite destinations on the internet," caregivers' survey, and more.

Today's Caregiver Magazine

http://www.caregiver.com/

Bimonthly magazine for the caregiver.

Depression

Aging, Exercise and Depression
http://www.coolware.com/health/medical_reporter/exercise.html
Exercise may lessen the odds of depression for senior citizens.

Depression in the Elderly
http://depression.com/special/special_02_elderly.htm
Depression of the elderly often goes undiagnosed and untreated.

Depression in the Elderly
http://www.psycom.net/depression.central.elderly.html
If you're over 65 and feeling depressed, this site answers many of your questions. Includes a self-administered depression scale and recent research.

General Health & Longevity

Health/Prolongevity/Anti-Aging Resources
http://www.aeiveos.com/resource/index.html
Many topics are covered, including health & longevity, euthanasia, nutrition, traditional and alternative medicine, government sites, and more.

Longevity Game
http://www.northwesternmutual.com/games/longevity/longevity-main.html
Input personal information to receive an estimate on how long you will live, based on research done by the life insurance industry.

Rejuvenation and Longevity
http://www.anti-aging.org/index.htm
Each day, 10,000 baby boomers in the U.S. turn 50 years old. Site advocates use of hormones and other therapies to reduce effects of age-related degenerative diseases. In laymen's terms, it describes the causes and effects of aging and recent research in resisting aging.

Seniors' Health

http://www.healthtouch.com/level1/leaflets/118566/118566.htm

Fact sheets cover health issues of particular concern to the elderly, including heart health, arthritis, nutrition, cancer and more.

Seniors-Site

http://seniors-site.com/

For seniors and their caregivers. There are many topics to choose from, including the usual caregiving and health sites, as well as information on alternative medicine, computers and the Internet, frauds and scams to be aware of, gifts, grandparenting, pets, nutrition, sex, fitness, travel and much more.

Government Sites & Agencies

Administration on Aging

http://www.aoa.dhhs.gov/

Information for older persons, their families, and people interested in aging. Includes health, financial and social issues, and government contacts. It provides statistics, electronic booklets on health and living topics, women and aging, retirement, Alzheimer's disease and much more.

American Association of Retired Persons

http://www.aarp.org/

The AARP is a national association of people over 50 years old that promotes education on aging, as well as advocacy and community action. Find articles on health and aging, managed care, work security, independent living and technology. Also access the searchable AgeLine database which provides summaries of articles appearing in various journals, as well as videos and reports about older people and aging.

Area Agencies on Aging

http://www.aoa.dhhs.gov/aoa/webres/area-agn.htm

Forty-two states and Puerto Rico have Area Agencies on Aging, while the others have State Agencies on Agency. This site links you to the office of the state of your choosing.

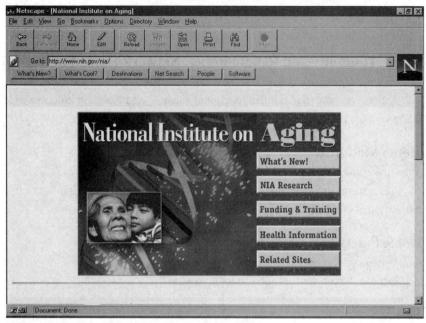

National Institute on Aging. *http://www.nih.gov/nia/*

CDC Senior Health Page

http://www.cdc.gov/health/seniors.htm

Reports from the Centers for Disease Control and Prevention on issues pertaining to the elderly.

National Institute on Aging

http://www.nih.gov/nia/

This is a biomedical research agency of the NIH that promotes healthy aging by supporting biomedical, social and behavioral research and public education. The site describes NIA's research, and offers publications on health and aging topics.

Senior Citizen Network

http://www.info.gov/Info/html/senior_citizens.htm

Links to government agencies and medical assistance programs for the elderly.

Housing & Home Modification

Aging, Disability and Rehabilitation Network Home Page
http://www.asaging.org/networks/adrn/adrnhome.html
Articles on how to maximize functional capacity and maintain independence while you age by making changes in your home and life style.

Home Modification and Repair
http://www.aoa.dhhs.gov/aoa/eldractn/homemodf.html
Adaptations to homes that can make it easier and safer for the elderly to carry out activities such as bathing, cooking, and climbing stairs.

Home Safety and Modification
http://monticello.avenue.gen.va.us/jaba/Library/safety.html
Includes web resources and library holdings.

SeniorSites
http://www.seniorsites.com/
Senior Sites includes links to websites with senior housing resources, information to guide you in selecting a nonprofit housing facility, and a directory of national and state senior housing associations. For seniors who are interested in investigating nonprofit housing and services.

Incontinence

Incontinence
http://www.hc-sc.gc.ca/seniors-aines/seniors/pubs/vigincon.htm
What is incontinence? What causes it? How many seniors experience it? And other questions answered at the Canadian government's Division of Aging and Seniors site.

InContiNet Home Page
http://IncontiNet.com/home.htm
Links and discussion about incontinence and pelvic muscle disorders.

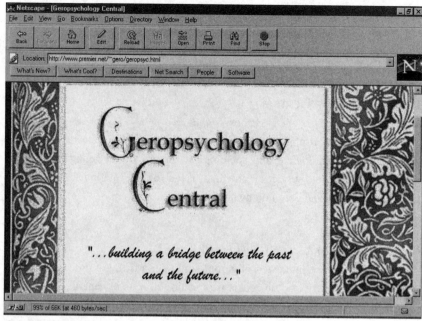

Geropsychology Central. *http://www.premier.net/~gero/geropsyc.html*

Urinary Incontinence
http://wellweb.com/INCONT/URINCON.HTM
  Describes this disorder and how to manage it.

Links

American Physical Therapy Association: Geriatrics Section
http://geriatricspt.org/
  Intended for physical therapists, geriatric clients and their families, students and anyone interested in health care issues relating to older people.

Andrus Gerontology Library
ttp://www.usc.edu/isd/locations/science/gerontology/
  The Andrus Library contains 11,000 book titles, 110 journals, 300 newsletters, videos and other media.

Directory of Web and Gopher Sites on Aging

http://www.AoA.DHHS.GOV/aoa/webres/craig.htm

Sites are arranged by subject, by state, and by organization; or you may perform a keyword search.

Geropsychology Central

http://www.premier.net/~gero/geropsyc.html

Site describes itself as an "online resource devoted to the study of the neurological, psychological and sociological aspects of the aging process." It includes resources and services for seniors, as well as information about and links to geropsychology and gerontology sites.

GeroWeb

http://www.iog.wayne.edu/IOGlinks.html

Site serves those interested in gerontology, geriatrics, the process of aging, services for the elderly, or the concerns of senior citizens in general. Allows you to browse by category and includes the GeroWeb Virtual Library on Aging.

Hardin Meta Directory: Geriatrics

http://www.arcade.uiowa.edu/hardin-www/md-ger.html

Hardin Meta Directory "lists the best sites that list the sites." Lists are broken down into large, medium and small, and are verified regularly.

MedWebPlus: Geriatrics

http://www.medwebplus.com/subject/Geriatrics.html

Rates a large number of geratric websites and takes you to them. Although not visually appealing, a well-organized cross-listing helps you to find the information you want.

Nutrition & Aging

Food and Nutrition Service Online

http://www.fns.usda.gov/fns/

Information about government-supported nutrition assistance programs, such as food stamps.

Jean Mayer United States Department of Agriculture Human Nutrition Research Center on Aging

http://www.hnrc.tufts.edu/

Nutrition and aging resources, scientific and research programs, from Tufts University.

National Policy and Resource Center on Nutrition and Aging

http://www.fiu.edu/~nutreldr/

Bibliography and links to articles relating to nutrition and aging, documents from the Administration on Aging, description of Meals on Wheels programs and more.

Vitamin Dispenser

http://www.healthyideas.com/healing/vitamin/

Select from a number of health problems and receive information on vitamins recommended to help treat each condition. Some problems addressed include age spots, Alzheimer's and wrinkles. Links to other websites are provided.

Online Seniors

Access America for Seniors

http://www.seniors.gov/

Easy-to use government site provides services for seniors online. Includes health and nutrition, employment and volunteer opportunities, taxes, education, leisure and more.

Dr. Frank & Kelly On-Line!

http://www.drfrank.com/

Racey advice for seniors from Dr. Frank, a syndicated newspaper columnist and radio talkshow host, and his partner, Kelly.

Elderhostel

http://www.elderhostel.org/

Offers educational programs for elderly who are interested in learning, travel and adventures.

ElderPage
http://www.aoa.dhhs.gov/elderpage.html
  Information and links for older persons and their families.

SeniorCom
http://www.senior.com/
  Serves the online community for those 50 and over. Includes articles, chats and other services on topics including travel, entertainment, money, health, news, employment, housing, home, and marketplace issues.

SeniorNet
http://www.seniornet.com/
  This sophisticated website provides opportunities for collaborative lifelong education among older adults. It is devoted to teaching older adults how to use the Internet and personal computer. Offers learning centers, support groups, articles, educational programs (including online computer classes), links and more.

Research & Statistics

Center for Aging
http://garnet.berkeley.edu/~aging/
  All about the Center and its programs, publications and resources.

National Aging Information Center
http://www.aoa.dhhs.gov/naic/
  This site collects policy-related materials, demographic and other statistical data on the health, economic and social status of older Americans. Links to many resources and a bibliography of reading materials.

National Archive of Computerized Data on Aging
http://www.icpsr.umich.edu/NACDA/index.html
  Access to research studies and databases covering different aspects of aging.

Sixty-Five Plus in the United States
http://www.census.gov/ftp/pub/socdemo/www/agebrief.html
  Statistics on aging from the U.S. Census Department.

Stroke and Aging Research Project
http://www.columbia.edu/~dwd2/
 Project studies the association between cerebrovascular disease and dementia. Bibliography and links to related sites.

Veterans' Services

Facilities and Leadership
http://www.va.gov/stations97/guide/home.asp?DIVISION=ALL
 Link to VA facilities by state; and where to go for help.

Veterans Health Administration
http://www.va.gov/health/index.htm
 Information on various VA services, including the Diabetes Program, nursing services, and more. Links to VA Internet servers.

Women and Aging

National Center on Women & Aging
http://www.brandeis.edu/heller/national/index.html
 Partnership of over 30 agencies which study various women and aging issues, e.g. financial resources and health practices. Includes a newsletter and other publications, and description of projects NDWA supports.

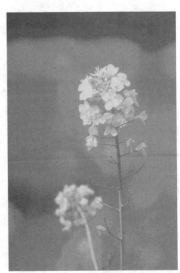

Seniors in Action Women's Issues
http://www.seniors.org/womensissues.asp
 Retirement and health care issues of particular interest to older women.

National Center on Women & Aging. *http://www.brandeis.edu/heller/national/index.html*

ALLERGIES / IMMUNOLOGY

Allergies

Allergies and Asthma

http://www.best.com/~gazissax/chealth3.html

Site provides general information and links to newsgroups and other resources relating to allergies and asthma. It is part of the Children's Health Page website.

Allergy, Asthma and Immunology Online

http://allergy.mcg.edu/

This website is maintained by allergists and contains information and news for patients, their parents, physicians, and "individuals purchasing group health care programs." Information for patients includes an *Asthma Life Quality Test*, when to see and how to find an allergist, information on insect allergies, exercise and additional advice. Information for physicians includes practice parameters and clinical immunology. In addition, an Allergy-Immunology Glossary is provided, as well as helpful links to medical and general resources.

AIR: Allergy Internet Resources

http://www.Immune.Com/allergy/allabc.html

A "starter" collection of links on allergy topics, to help Allergy mailing list members who want to know more about allergies. Includes food allergies, kids allergies, latex allergies, skin allergies, hay fever, stings and more. Also contains access to free allergy discussion list.

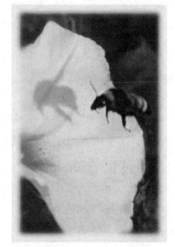

Allergy, Asthma and Immunology Online. *http://allergy.mcg.edu/*

Allergy Online

http://allergy.hno.akh-wien.ac.at/allergy/

The allergology server at Vienna Medical School offers patient and scientific information on allergies, pollen and related topics in English and German. Interesting historical trivia about allergies also provided.

American Academy of Allergy Asthma and Immunology/ National Allergy Bureau Report

http://www.aaaai.org/

Information and resources for professionals, patients and children on allergies, asthma and immunology. Includes a physician referral directory, public information materials, and directory of patient support groups, as well as access to the National Allergy Bureau which provides the media and the public information on pollen and mold aeroallergen levels around the country. Reports are updated three times a week, and particle counts and predominant allergen are provided.

On-Line Allergy Center

http://www.sig.net/~allergy/welcome.html

Helpful information on the relief of a variety of symptoms, including nasal congestion, eye redness/soreness, sneezing, wheezing, coughing, joint pain, intestinal pain, skin rashes/irritation, itching, yeast infections, mood swings, hyperactivity, attention deficit disorder and fatigue. Allergy facts, tips and feature articles as well as news updates are provided for allergy sufferers world-wide.

Links

Immunology (Biosciences)

http://golgi.harvard.edu/biopages/immuno.html

Links to journals, organizations, gophers and more.

Kellogg Immunology Sites

http://www.library.dal.ca/kellogg/internet/immunol.htm

Includes journal links, practice guidelines and links to information for patients.

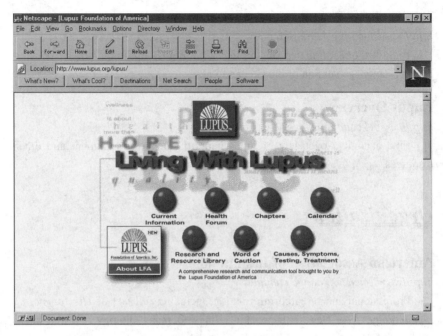

Lupus Foundation of America. *http://www.lupus.org/lupus/*

Microbiology, Immunology and Virology Websites

http://www.microbiology.adelaide.edu.au/general/microwww.htm

Comprehensive list of microbiology, immunology and virology links to university, research and professional organizations all over the world.

Lupus

The Lupus Foundation of America: Living with Lupus

http://www.lupus.org/lupus/

Provides information on lupus, a chronic autoimmune disease which causes inflammation of various parts of the body, especially the skin, joints, blood and kidneys. Site addresses the different types of lupus, causes, complication, diagnosis, treatment, nutrition and diet; and it provides contact information for local chapters. Several forums address different aspects of the disease.

Lupus Home Page

http://www.hamline.edu/lupus/

Includes questionnaire on coping with lupus, mailing lists, articles, a Spanish-language version of the site, and links.

Lupus Overview

http://cerebel.com/lupus/overview.htm

Find a clinical overview of lupus nephritis, nephritis treatment and other resources.

Organizations

American Association of Immunologists

http://www.scienceXchange.com/aai/

Professional and research information, including full text of *The Journal of Immunology*, AAI Newsletter Archive, links to many biology research sites, methods of educating the public, and more.

National Institute of Allergies and Infectious Diseases

http://www.niaid.nih.gov/

News, facts, publications and research updates; clinical research trial information, grant information and more.

National Jewish Center for Immunology and Respiratory Medicine

http://www.njc.org/

The National Jewish Center treats asthma, tuberculosis, emphysema and other respiratory and immune system diseases. This site offers information for health care consumers and professionals on topics such as asthma, chronic bronchitis, and sleep-related breathing disorders.

Poison Ivy

Poison Ivy: An Exaggerated Response to Nothing Much
http://www.bio.umass.edu/immunology/poisoniv.htm
> The cure may be worse than the itch.

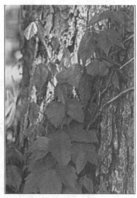

Poison Ivy, Western Poison Oak, Poison Sumac
http://res.agr.ca/brd/poisivy/title.html
> Text and pictures of poison ivy, poison oak and poison sumac. Learn to identify these poisonous plants.

Poison Ivy.
http://res.agr.ca/brd/poisivy/pois.html

Primary Immune Deficiency

Jeffrey Modell Foundation
http://www.jmfworld.com/
> Information on primary (or inherited) immune deficiency. Includes 10 warning signs of PID and links to related sites.

Sjogren's Syndrome

Sjogren's Syndrome Foundation
http://www.sjogrens.com/
> This site acts as information clearinghouse for Sjogren's Syndrome, an incurable autoimmune disorder where the body attacks its own moisture-producing glands causing dry eye, dry mouth, and potentially worse effects.

ALTERNATIVE MEDICINE

Acupuncture & Acupressure

Acupuncture Resource Guide

http://scils.rutgers.edu/~mavcol/acu-yes.html

Provides basic information and lots of links for professionals, researchers, students, and health care consumers.

Acupuncture.com

http://www.acupuncture.com/

Information about acupuncture and other traditional Chinese medicine theories such as herbology, qigong, Chinese nutrition and massage. Also find marketplace, frequently asked questions, and articles; and resources and links for consumers, students and practitioners.

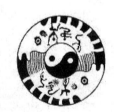

Acupuncture.Com.
http://www.acupuncture. com/

American Academy of Medical Acupuncture

http://www.medicalacupuncture.org/

What is medical acupuncture? Continuing education for professionals, and referral to an acupuncturist in your area.

History of Acupuncture
http://www.healthy.net/clinic/therapy/acupuncture/specifics/history.htm
Describes acupuncture in China and in the Western world.

James Roy Holliday III Guide to Acupressure
http://falcon.cc.ukans.edu/~moriarty/acupressure/acuguide.html
Great site with lots of information and guide to problems and proper points to be stimulated.

Medical Acupuncture Web Page
http://www.med.auth.gr/~karanik/
Includes acupuncture news, basic information on acupuncture, an online acupuncture journal, veterinary acupuncture, acupuncture books and publications, database, research results and papers, professional links and much more. Site available in English or Greek.

The National Acupuncture and Oriental Medicine Alliance
http://www.healthy.net/pan/pa/acupuncture/naoma/index.html
Professional organization with searchable database.

Therapies: Acupuncture
http://www.1healthyuniverse.com/resources/resource.cfm?level=2&previd=6
About a dozen links with brief descriptions of what you will find there.

Traditional Acupuncture
http://welcome.to/april.acupuncture
Acupuncture is used by one-third of the world as a primary means of health treatment. This site describes the philosophy of traditional acupuncture, symptoms and illnesses it can help, methods and tools, and offers case studies and links.

Apitherapy

Bee Online
http://www.apitherapy.org/
Discusses the use of bee venom and other bee products such as royal jelly and bee pollen for healing purposes.

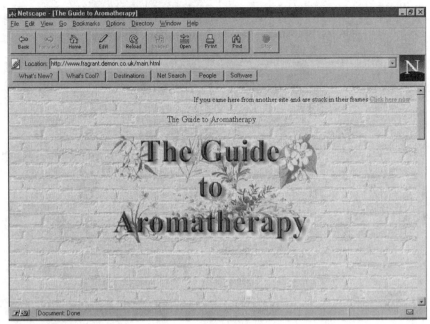

The Guide to Aromatherapy. *http://www.fragrant.demon.co.uk/main.htm*

Aromatherapy

Ancient Healing Art

http://www.halcyon.com/kway/home.htm

Ways to use essential oils, products, blending tips and aromatherapy articles.

The Aromatherapy Network

http://www.aromatherapy.net/

Basic essential oil information, monthly articles focusing on a specific oil and its uses, information about how to learn more, how to expand your knowledge and your understanding of aromatherapy.

The Guide to Aromatherapy

http://www.fragrant.demon.co.uk/main.html

Includes a description of many oils from Ajowan to Zanthoxylum, their sources, how to blend and how to use them, a symptoms guide to therapeutic uses of essential oils, a glossary, courses and events, and more.

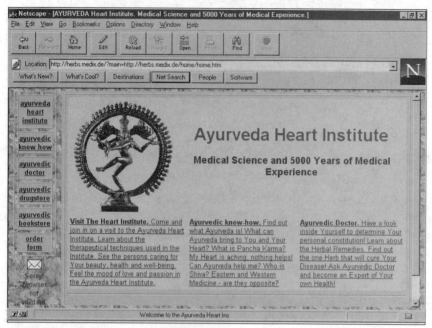

Ayurveda Heart Institute. *http://herbs.medix.de/home/home.htm*

Ayurveda

Ayurvedic Foundations
http://www.ayur.com/

Describes Ayurveda and reasons for using it, as well as provides information on the Ayurvedic Foundations workshops, tapes and counseling. Bulletin board and links to newsgroups and other websites.

Ayurveda Heart Institute
http://herbs.medix.de/home/home.htm

Information about the Institute, Hinduism and Ayurveda; Ayurvedic doctors and an Ayurvedic drugstore where you can get herbal mixes to treat specific problems. Herbal index and a special section on coronary heart disease.

Ayurvedic Health Center Online

http://www.ayurvedic.com/

Introduction to Ayurvedic health including the three doshas and other principles of Ayurvedic healing. Also includes ancient Ayurvedic texts, recommended readings and a bookstore.

Good Care Inc.

http://www.technimed.com/GoodEarth/

Herbs, massage oils, teas, and other products for the Ayurvedic market.

Bach Flowers

Dr. Edward Bach Centre

http://www.bachcentre.com/

Flower remedies: Dr. Edward Bach discovered 38 flowers had healing properties. E.g., holly helps heal hatred and jealousy, while wild rose helps with apathy. Site provides history, description of these flowers, indications, and information on Dr. Bach.

New Bach Flower Therapies

http://Ourworld.compuserve.com/homepages/Neue_Therapien_Dietmar_RKra emer/Newbach.htm

Information and literature on Bach flower therapy, in German and English.

Color Therapy

Aura-Soma

http://berlin.snafu.de/~frank.guschmann/e_index.htm

Aura-soma is described as a "holistic soul therapy in which the vibrational powers of colour, crystals and natural aromas combine with light in order to harmonise body, mind and spirit of mankind." This site provides information, products, a bibliography and links to related sites.

Complementary Medicine

Aesclepian Chronicles
http://www.forthrt.com/~chronicl/homepage.html
Synergistic Health Center's online articles and discussion.

Complementary Medicine Site
http://www.complementary-medicine.com/
Products for practitioners.

General Complementary Medicine References
http://www.forthrt.com/~chronicl/archiv.htm
Links to many complementary medicine resources. Includes general and specific physical/body and mind/spirit medicine resources, e-zines, journals, newsletters, newsgroups, discussion groups, mailing lists and organizations.

Internet Resources: Alternative and Complementary Medicine
http://library.mcphu.edu/resource/alt_med.htm
Includes overview sites, organizations and professional societies, journals, lists and directories.

National Center for Complementary and Alternative Medicine
http://nccam.nih.gov/
Part of the National Institutes of Health, the NCCAM facilitates and conducts research in complementary and alternative medicines. The NCCAM Clearinghouse dessiminates such information to the public. Site includes answers to frequently asked questions and remarks for those considering alternative medical therapies.

Eastern Medicine

American Board of Eastern Medicine Web Site
http://www.easternmedicine.com/american.htm
Professional organization for eastern medicine practitioners. Site offers information on the ABEM, comments on the martial arts, hygiene, phlebotomy and a code of ethics. Provides list of insurance companies that cover eastern medical techniques, colleges where it is studied, and organizations helpful to practitioners.

Chinese Medical News

http://www.dmu.ac.uk/ln/cmn/

Free, bi-monthly publication.

Chinese Medicine

http://www.hanwei.com/culture/medic.htm

Well-written essay addressing cultural aspects of Chinese medicine.

East Meets West International, Inc.

http://www.eastmeetswest.com/

Offers Eastern products to the Western market.

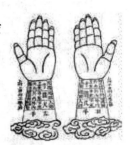

Chinese Medicine.
http://www.hanwei.com/ culture/medic.htm

Eastern Medicine Online

http://www.easternmedicine.com/services.htm

Eastern, Western, homeopathic and naturopathic medicine supplies.

Meditopia!

http://www.meditopia.com/

"Medical Utopia" brings solutions from the East for such ills as breast cancer, depression, Crohn's disease, enlarged prostate, schizophrenia, and more.

National College of Oriental Medicine

http://www.acupunctureschool.com/

Information about this school in Florida.

Feldenkrais Method

Feldenkrais Method Web Pages

http://www.feldenkrais.com/

Describes this method of healing through movement.

Gerson Therapy

Gerson Therapy
http://www.gerson.org/

This site provides information about Gerson therapy, which is a nutrition-based and detoxifying medical treatment for the cure of cancer, heart disease, diabetes and other degenerative diseases.

Herbal Medicine

Algy's Herb Page
http://www.algy.com/herb/index.html

Includes medicinal uses of herbs, how to grow them, a seed exchange, recipes and links.

Botanical.Com
http://www.botanical.com

Lots of information on plants and their medicinal and culinary uses. Includes "A Modern Herbal," indexing more than 800 plants, an index of recipes and an index of poisonous plants. Features articles, an ask-an-expert section, and links.

Henriette's Herbal Homepage
http://metalab.unc.edu/herbmed/

Includes medicinal and culinary herb facts, pictures and a database of plant names, as well as news list archives and shareware programs for those interested in herbs.

Herb Guide
http://www.gardenguides.com/herbs/herb.htm

Features articles on the growth and use of herbs, a scroll-down index of herbs, vegetables and more.

Herbal Alternatives
http://www.herbalalternatives.com/

Information on herbs, vitamins and alternative medicine. Online purchasing.

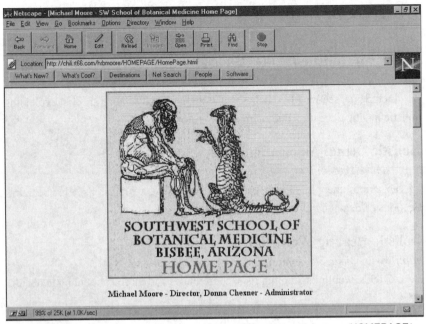

Southwest School of Botanical Medicine. *http://chili.rt66.com/hrbmoore/HOMEPAGE/
HomePage.html*

HerbNET

http://www.HerbNET.com/

Information about herbs, herbal products, remedies, schools, publications and more. Calls itself the most comprehensive herb site on the web.

Pryme Thyme Newsletter

http://members.tripod.com/~starspirit/prymethyme.html

Contains articles related to herbs and herb use.

Reference Guide for Herbs

http://www.realtime.net/anr/herbs.html

Site provides basic information on a couple of dozen common herbs, from alfalfa to yellow dock.

Southwest School of Botanical Medicine

http://chili.rt66.com/hrbmoore/HOMEPAGE/HomePage.html

Medicinal plant images, folios, manuals, journals, and pharmacology resources on the medicinal uses of plants, as well as catalog for this school located in Bisbee, Arizona.

Holistic Medicine

American Holistic Health Association
http://ahha.org/

Includes a searchable database of holistic practitioners, articles explaining holistic health, education and membership information.

Holistic Dental Association
http://simwell.com/hda/

Describes the philosophy of holistic dentistry, which considers the ramifications of dental care on the entire individual.

Holistic Healing Web Page
http://www.holisticmed.com/

Articles, weblinks, mailing lists, conferences and more about holistic health.

Holistic Health Journal
http://holistichealthjournal.com/

Web companion to the printed journal.

Holistic Health Resources
http://tln.lib.mi.us/~cwiggins/home.HTML

Recommended sites and readings that approach health from the holistic perspective. Broken down into physical, emotional, social, environmental and spiritual health (with overlap, by definition).

Holistic Internet Resources
http://www.hir.com/

Guide to practitioners and schools with descriptions and links where relevant, articles and book reviews on holistic health, events and Internet connections.

Holistic M.D.
http://www.consciouschoice.com/holisticmd/index.html

Dr. Ronald Hoffman hosts a syndicated radio program on health, and authors a column on various health issues. Site includes a number of his articles, links and more.

WorldWide Wellness: Internet Resources for Wholeliving

http://www.wholeliving.com/

Uses "intermedia synergy" to unite the world. Provides a directory of goods and services for "whole living," articles, interviews and book/music reviews.

Homeopathy

Homeopaths Without Frontiers

http://www2.antenna.nl/homeoweb/noborder.html

Organization of volunteers that provide international homeopathic medical services.

Homeopathy

http://www.healthy.net/clinic/therapy/homeopat/index.html

Introduction to homeopathy, homeopathic remedies and treatment, and homeopathic research and resources.

Homeopathy Discussions Online

http://www.homeopathyhome.com/cgi-local/bb/Ultimate.cgi

Homeopathic discussion topics include: general discussion, children and parenting, pets and animals, research, Italian-language discussion, professionals and practitioners, and skin diseases.

Homeopathy Home

http://www.homeopathyhome.com/

Resources and frequently asked questions (FAQs), references, mailing lists, and newsgroups regarding complementary medicine and homeopathy.

Homeopathy Introduction

http://lifematters.com/homeointro.html

A series of articles on homeopathy, including: cuts, bruises and burns; colds and flu; homeopathy and pregnancy.

Homeopathy Online

http://www.lyghtforce.com/homeopathyonline/

A journal of homeopathic medicine.

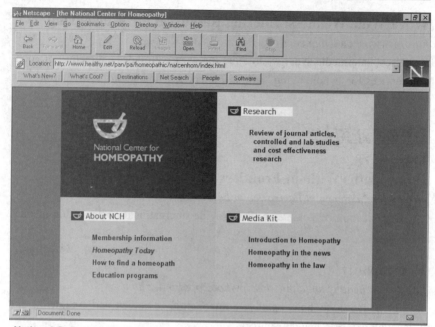

National Center for Homeopathy. http://www.healthy.net/pan/pa/homeopathic/
natcenhom/index.html

Homeoweb Home Page

http://www2.antenna.nl/homeoweb/index.html

Includes homeopathic Internet resources and information on homeopathic medical journals.

National Center for Homeopathy

http://www.healthy.net/pan/pa/homeopathic/natcenhom/index.html

Attractive site discusses membership and educational courses in homeopathy, how to find a homeopath, journal review and basic information on homeopathy.

Hypnosis

Hypnodirect.com

http://www.hypnodirect.com/

Although the primary goal of this site is to help people locate a hypnotist in their area, this site also provides extensive information and resources on hypnosis for the public as well as for professional hypnotists.

Hypnosis.com

http://www.hypnosis.com/

Information and links to hypnosis and hypnosis therapy.

Inner Trance Formations

http://www.cet.com/~alanb/welcome.htm

Addresses how to use hypnosis for self-healing and self-discovery.

Labyrinth Walking

The Labyrinth

http://www.mindspring.com/~daniel12/labyrinth.htm

Describes the use of labyrinths for gaining insight. "At its most basic level the labyrinth is a metaphor for the journey to the center of your deepest self and back out into the world with a broadened understanding of who you are." How to create your own labyrinth, links and resources.

The Sacred Labyrinth Walk: Illuminating the Inner Path

http://www.sacredwalk.com/

Historical information, guidelines, photos and frequently asked questions regarding this ancient meditative path to achieving self-alignment and insight.

Through Mazes to Mathematicians

http://www.math.sunysb.edu/%7Etony/ mazes/index.html

Information on mazes and labyrinths, discussed from the mathematical point of view.

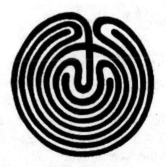

Through Mazes to Mathematicians.
http://www.math.sunysb.edu/%7Etony/ma zes/satmaze.html

A Web of Labyrinths

http://www.mcli.dist.maricopa.edu/smc/ labyrinth/index.html

Historical and spiritual information on labyrinths, activities and a gallery of labyrinths from around the world.

Leeches

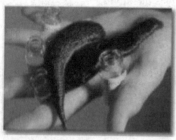

Biopharm Leeches.
http://www.biopharm-leeches.com/

Biopharm Leeches
http://www.biopharm-leeches.com/
Clinical use of leeches.

Bloodletting
*http://www.library.ucla.edu/libraries/biomed
/his/blood/blood1.htm*
Images of bloodletting from UCLA's
biomedical library.

Leech Makes Comeback in Medicine
http://www.ohiohealth.com/leechnews.htm
Article originally published in the November 3, 1997 *Columbus Dispatch.*

Leeches USA
http://www.accurate-assi-leeches.com/leeches/index.html
This company provides leeches for medical use. Find information about the
practice, including how to apply and store leeches and how to dispose of them after
they are used.

Links

Alternative Medicine Homepage
http://www.pitt.edu/~cbw/altm.html
A jumpstation for sources of information on unconventional, unorthodox,
unproven, or alternative, complementary, innovative, integrative therapies such as
folk medicine, herbal medicine, diet fads, homeopathy, faith healing, new age
healing, chiropractic, acupuncture, naturopathy, massage, and music
therapy. Special section on HIV/AIDS.

Ask NOAH About: Alternative (Complementary) Medicine
http://www.noah.cuny.edu/alternative/alternative.html

A great set of links to alternative medicine Internet sites. The different healing approaches are explained and resources are provided. Index by disorder, as well.

Holistic Healing
http://www.inforamp.net/~marcotte/healing.htm

Contains an enormous list of links with brief descriptions. General topics include different healing methods (acupressure to yoga), alternative treatments, directories of pracitioners, organizations, schools, publications, holistic healing for animals, and fraud.

Yahoo's Alternative Medicine
http://www.yahoo.com/Health/Alternative_Medicine/

Covers everything from apitherapy (bee therapy), to music therapy, to yoga.

Massage Therapy

Alive! Therapeutic Massage & Bodywork Reiki Healing Center
http://www.massagetherapy.com/

Includes a brief history of massage, reiki and shamanism. Describes facilities.

The Complete Guide to the Alexander Technique
http://www.alexandertechnique.com/

Learning movement to ease tension and stress. Links.

Healing Touch
http://www0.delphi.com/healingtouch/

Online resources for students of massage therapy. Addresses the history and benefits of massage and provides links to massage schools and an online chat.

Illustrated Guide to Muscles and Medical Massage Therapy
http://danke.com/Orthodoc/

For pain relief and posture alignment in adults, teens and children, this site provides general information and links.

Massage and Healthy Tidbits

http://www.angelfire.com/pa/healthytidbits/

Discusses the benefits and basics of massage, from a massage therapist.

Massage Magazine

http://www.massagemag.com/

Highlights of the current issue and subscription information.

The Massage Therapy Homepage

http://www.lightlink.com/massage/

Articles, links to education resources, products, and massage therapists.

Massage Therapy Web Central

http://www.qwl.com/mtwc/

"Hub" for professional massage therapists.

Massage-One.com

http://massage-one.com/

How to find a massage therapist where you live, as well as schools, history, links, and what to expect.

The Shiatsu School of Canada

http://www.shiatsucanada.com/shiatsu/index.html

Offers degrees and courses in shiatsu, a Japanese form of massage.

Shiatsu: Therapeutic Art of Japan

http://www.doubleclickd.com/shiatsu.html

Addresses this Japanese form of healing through touch.

Somatics on the Web

http://www.somatics.com/links.htm

Some topics include ergonomics, aging, ending chronic pain, back injuries, and more.

Therapeutic Message for Health and Fitness

http://www.doubleclickd.com/theramassage.html

Why does massage work, and what does it do?

Touch Research Institute
http://www.miami.edu/touch-research/
Institute studies the effect of touch and movement therapy on people in all stages of life. Site describes research and events, has a frequently asked questions section, and publishes a quarterly newsletter called *Touchpoints*.

Medical Astrology

Medical Astrology Catalog of Books
http://www.astroamerica.com/medical.html
Explains how astrology as a component of medical care can be helpful. Site provides bibliography.

Meditation

American Meditation Institute
http://www.americanmeditation.org/
Offers workshops in meditation, instructions on how to meditate, frequently asked questions and a newsletter.

Buddhist Meditation and Depth Psychology
http://www.buddhanet.net/depth.htm
Downloadable file of an essay discussing meditation.

Complete Guide to the Transcendental Meditation Programme
http://www.tm.org/
Program claims to help you gain deep relaxation, relieve stress, promote health and creativity, and obtain inner happiness. Site introduces you to the program, provides research results of studies of those who practice TM, answers frequently asked questions and more.

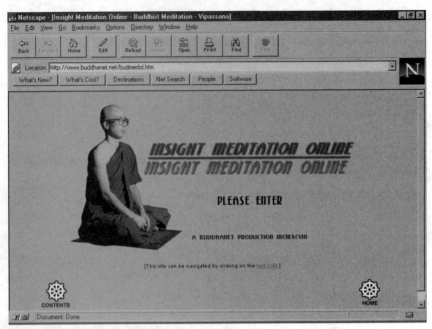

Insight Meditation Online. http://www.buddhanet.net/budmedol.htm

Insight Meditation Online

http://www.buddhanet.net/budmedol.htm

Loving-kindness and insight meditation instruction with downloadable meditation files. Special sections on meditating with children, and meditating in Burma.

Maharishi University of Management

http://www.miu.edu/

This school studies transcendental medicine, yogic flying, and other holistic practices.

Meditation Mount

http://www.meditation.com/

Group meditation as a service to humanity.

Practicing the Presence: A Course in Meditation

http://www.webpak.net/~meditate/

Learn how to get beyond thought and concept with this free online course. For beginning or advanced meditators.

The Real Values of True Buddhist Meditation

http://www.webcom.com/~imcuk/uba khin/VALUES1.html

Buddhist meditation involves training in morality, concentration and wisdom. First part of a six-part essay, with information and links.

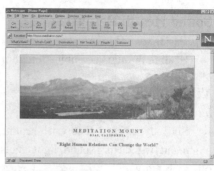

Meditation Mount.
http://www.meditation.com/

Shambhala: Worldwide Network of Meditation Centers

http://www.shambhala.org/

Meditation in the Shambhala tradition uncovers a natural sense of goodness, fearlessness, and humor, a way of personal warriorship, and a vision of enlightened society.

World Wide Web Online Meditation Center

http://www.meditationcenter.com/

Offers a number of meditations with instructions, and frequently asked questions.

Zen Centers

http://www.iijnet.or.jp/iriz/irizhtml/centers/usa.htm

List of Zen Buddhist centers in the United States.

Music and Vibration Therapy

Hemi-Sync

http://www.monroe-inst.com/programs/hemi-sync.html

According to this site, "Hemi-Sync effectively concentrates the inherent resources of your mind, brain and body" for an enormous number of uses, such as greater emotional well-being, better sleeping, deeper transcendent experiences, better mental performance, and easier pregnancy. It claims to work by adjusting vibration frequencies that affect human brain wave patterns.

Sound Health Resources
http://www.soundhealthresources.com/
> Healing through a combination of music and low frequency sounds.

Vibrational Healing
http://www.aloha.net/~vibes/
> Site advocates a theory of healing by bringing body/mind energies into alignment by focusing sound, light, gemstones, aromatic oils, flower essences and other vibratory tools.

Naturopathy

American Association of Naturopathic Physicians
http://www.naturopathic.org/
> Site offers textbook online, *Journal of Naturopathic Medicine*, library, bookstore, links, and a database of naturopathic physicians.

Dr. Quinn's Naturopathic Medicine Page
http://www.drquinn-nd.com/naturopathic.html
> Describes what naturopathic medicine is and its philosophy, the types of treatment that it involves, what to expect when visiting a naturopathic doctor, how naturopathic doctors are trained, and more.

National College of Naturopathic Medicine
http://www.ncnm.edu/
> Information about the college programs and admission. Naturopathic medicine's techniques include modern, traditional, scientific and empirical methods. Six principles of healing form the foundation for naturopathic medical practice, which are: to use the healing power of nature, treat the whole person, do no harm, identify the cause, practice prevention, and act as patient's teacher.

NaturMedia
http://www.geocities.com/WallStreet/1133/
> News and information on naturopathic medicine.

Naturopathic Medicine
http://www.naturopathy.com/

Provides an introduction to naturopathic medicine, therapeutic modalities, symptoms and diseases, and links.

Naturopathic Medicine in the UK
http://www.naturopathy.org.uk/

Definition of and introduction to naturopathic medicine, philosophy, techniques and training, registry and more.

Naturopathic Medicine Network
http://www.pandamedicine.com/

Site offers public and professional resources. Includes chat rooms, natural pharmacy, education links, yellow pages, newsletter, classified ads, and a physician round table.

Oxygen Therapy

Hyperbaric Oxygen Therapy Information Center
http://www.marketnet.com/mktnet/wound/hbo2.html

Site explains hyperbaric oxygen therapy (HBOT), a supplemental therapy and method of providing additional oxygen to the tissues of your body. This increased oxygen delivery is said to further the body's ability to kill germs and to increase healing.

Oxygen and Ozone Therapies
http://www.oxytherapy.com/

Testimonials, frequently asked questions, mailing list, veterinary oxytherapy and much more about this practice.

Publications

Conscious Choice
http://www.consciouschoice.com/

Bi-monthly magazine that reports on environmental issues and natural alternatives in health care, food, and nutrition.

Trance Net
http://www.trancenet.org/front.shtml

Publications and webzines that critically discusses transcendental meditation, cult and new age figures.

Qigong

A Chi Gong (Qigong) Primer
http://www.Acupuncture.com/QiKung/ChiPri.htm

All qigong contains common principles: mind, eyes, movement and breath. Article introduces this system of exercise.

Dave Lo's Yan Xin Qigong Page
http://www.robelle.com/~dlo/qigong/

This site describes qigong, an ancient Chinese art of meditation and physical exercise to promote health, mental well being, martial arts skills and spiritual development. Offers articles and links to qigong resources.

Qi: The Journal of Traditional Eastern Health and Fitness
http://www.qi-journal.com/

Learn about Chinese culture and traditional Chinese medicine in this online journal. Includes links, *t'ai chi* animations, products, quizzes, calendar of events, and a listing of professional teachers and clinics.

Qigong
http://Acupuncture.com/QiKung/QikunInd.htm

Information for consumers, including a brief history of qigong (or chi gong).

Qigong Taiji Healing Art

http://www.erols.com/dantao/index.html

Describes this synergistic Eastern practice that combines elements of qigong, *t'ai chi*, and other traditions to achieve vitality and longevity.

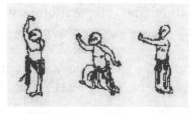

Qigong Taiji Healing Art.
http://www.erols.com/dantao/index.html

QigongCenter.com

http://www.QigongCenter.com/

Site describes workshops and provides articles and links. Join or peruse the qigong mail list.

Reiki

Distant Healing Network

http://homepages.centrenet.co.uk/~rgirling/index.htm

Submit a request, and volunteer Reiki practitioners from all around the world will pray about it, using their healing energy to help you or your loved one.

The International Center for Reiki Training

http://www.reiki.org/

Includes over 70 articles on Reiki, as well as Reiki information for doctors and nurses, legislation pertaining to the practice of Reiki, information on classes, training and workshops, Reiki frequently asked questions and database, Reiki tools, chat, links and more.

Reiki Healing Energy

http://www.whidbey.com/turtle/reiki/

An invitation to explore Reiki. Provides personal experiences and frequently asked questions, as well as links.

Reiki International

http://www.cyb1.com/reiki/default.htm

Explains Reiki principles simply, and discusses how to learn this healing practice.

ReikiOne Information Center
http://www.tamoore.com/reiki/

This website is for the discussion of Reiki energy. Offers books on Reiki, a practitioner/teacher directory, question and answer forum, classified ads, events postings, a distance healing network, and many other items of interest.

Reiki Pages by Light and Adonea
http://www.angelfire.com/az/SpiritMatters/

An interactive book about Reiki. Includes Reiki history, organizations, classes and manuals, explanations of how to do various basic to advanced techniques, articles, links, art, resources (including books, audio/video tapes, research papers, newsletters, newsgroups, mailing lists, message boards, chat rooms) and more.

Traditional Japanese Reiki
http://www.reikilinks.com/

Discusses the original teachings of Reiki master Mikao Usui, 1865-1926. The Usui healing system sought to heal the whole person (body, mind and spirit) by embodying affirmations to be used every morning and evening and providing the student of the system with a means of treating themselves and others using a form of qigong energy that is automatically refreshed from the surroundings. Site includes some Reiki stories, ethics, history and more.

Schools

Holistic Healing Schools
http://www.inforamp.net/~marcotte/healing.htm#Schools

Links to holistic educational sites on the Internet.

Homeopathy Schools
http://www.homeopathyhome.com/directory/usa/training_colleges.html

Listing includes addresses, telephone numbers and websites, where applicable.

NaturalHealers.com
http://www.naturalhealers.com/find.shtml

Find a school by specialty and location.

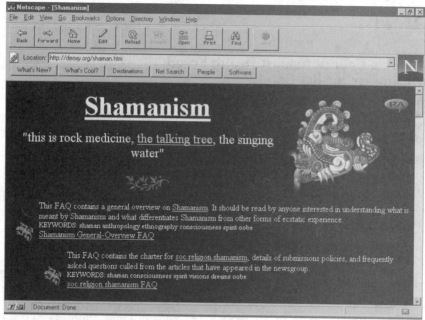

Shamanism. http://deoxy.org/shaman.htm

Shamanism

The Foundation for Shamanic Studies

http://www.shamanism.org/

The Foundation's goals are to advance the teachings, study and preservation of shamanism. It offers workshops and provides information. Site answers questions about shamanism and provides links and an interactive message forum.

Shamanism

http://deoxy.org/shaman.htm

General overview of shamanism, as well as a mixture of information on different South American philosophies and practices, shamanism resources, history, art and music.

Shamanism Frequently Asked Questions

http://www.webcom.com/gspirit/Shaman/so.toc.html

Shamanism, shamanic ectstasy, how to become a shaman, and other issues are addressed.

Skeptics

Georgia Council Against Health Fraud: Healthcare Reality Check
http://www.hcrc.org/

In their own words, the Council: "seeks to combat health quackery through public education. A particular focus of GCAHF is the linking of scientific and medical professionals via the Internet for greater distribution of anti-quackery information." Site offers news, encyclopedia, dictionary, literature, mailing lists and links to this effect.

Quackwatch
http://www.quackwatch.com

A nonprofit corporation whose purpose is to combat health-related frauds, myths, fads, and fallacies. It investigates questionable claims, answers inquiries, distributes and sells publications, reports illegal marketing, generates consumer-protection lawsuits and seeks to improve the quality of health information on the Internet and to attack misleading advertising. Look through long list of articles/discussion to see if specific therapy is discussed (e.g., "magnet therapy").

Veterinary Medicine

Alternative, Complementary and Holistic Veterinary Medicine
http://www.altvetmed.com/

Includes directories and frequently asked questions, information on specific problems (epilepsy, arthritis, fleas, etc.) and treatments, periodicals and other items of interest.

Holistic Veterinary Medicine/Petsynergy
http://www.petsynergy.com/

Information on holistic rabbit, horse, cat and dog pet care, including homeopathy, flea and skin treatments, nutrition, and how to locate a holistic vet.

Veterinary Acupuncture Homepage
http://homepage.tinet.ie/~progers/roghome.htm

Includes research, links and events.

BIOMEDICAL ETHICS

Covered in this chapter: Advance Directives/Do Not Resuscitate; Bioethics; Cloning; Euthanasia & Physician Assisted Suicide; Genetics & Gene Therapy; Human & Animal Research Subjects; Publications.

Related chapters: Death & Dying; HIV/AIDS; Hospice; Insurance & Managed Care; Pain & Pain Management; Sexual & Reproductive Health; Transplantation.

Advance Directives/Do Not Resuscitate

See also: Death & Dying; Pain & Pain Management.

10 Legal Myths about Advance Medical Directives
http://www.abanet.org/elderly/myths.html

Important information that corrects common misconceptions. From the American Bar Association.

Advance Directives
http://eduserv.hscer.washington.edu/bioethics/topics/advdir.html

Questions and answers on advance directives, as well as case studies, additional readings, and related links.

Advance Directives (AARP)
http://www.aarp.org/programs/advdir/home.html

From the American Association of Retired Persons, this site describes advance directives, including their advantages, options and how to get started.

Choice in Dying
http://www.choices.org/

Nonprofit organization helps people to make end-of-life decisions. Contains advance directives, provides counseling and education, advocates for legislation and trains professionals. Site also offers newsletter, press releases and Internet resource links.

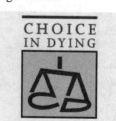

Choice in Dying.
http://choices.org

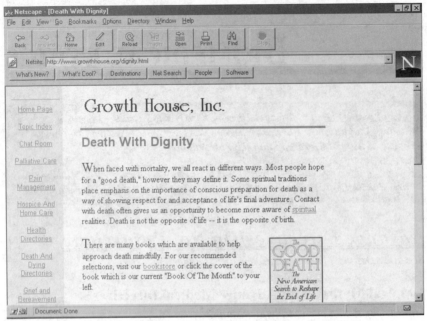

Growth House Death with Dignity. *http://www.growthhouse.org/dignity.html*

Deciding about CPR: Do Not Resuscitate Orders
http://wings.buffalo.edu/faculty/research/bioethics/dnr-p.html

Questions and answers about Do Not Resuscitate (DNR) orders, for patients and their families, from the New York State Department of Health.

Do Not Resuscitate Orders
http://eduserv.hscer.washington.edu/bioethics/topics/dnr.html

Questions and answers on when to administer CPR, and issues that physicians advising a Do Not Resuscitate order should consider.

Dying Well: Defining Wellness through "End of Life"
http://www.dyingwell.org/

This site of hospice and palliative care doctor Ira Byock, M.D., contains his writings (including editorials, articles and book excerpts), bibliography, links, and information about the Missoula Demonstration Project which seeked to study dying and quality at the end of life.

Growth House Death with Dignity

http://www.growthhouse.org/dignity.html

Provides an overview of key issues in the death with dignity and right to die movements, including doctor assisted suicide, voluntary euthanasia, self deliverance, advance directives, durable power of attorney, living wills, Do Not Resuscitate orders, and related matters.

Health Care Advance Directives

http://www.ama-assn.org/public/booklets/livgwill.htm

Online booklet that describes your right to make your own health care decisions. Form and instructions are included.

Hospice Net Advance Directives

http://www.hospicenet.org/html/directives.html

Describes what advance directives and living wills are.

Living Wills Registry (Canada)

http://www.sentex.net/~lwr/

This site advises people on how to create a living will.

Living Wills A to Z

http://www.rights.org/deathnet/LifesEnd/LE_living_wills.html/

Listing of books that examine an individual's right to make informed choices about health care.

Medicare and Advance Directives

gopher://gopher.gsa.gov/00/staff/pa/cic/fed_prog/other/med&adv.txt

Text file from the U.S. Department of Health and Human Services/HCFA that describes and answers questions about patients' rights to make health care decisions. Includes a discussion of living wills and durable power of attorney for health care.

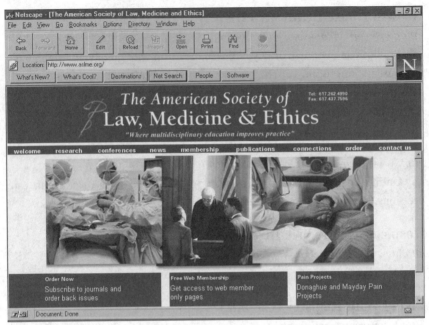

American Society of Law, Medicine & Ethics. http://www.aslme.org/

Bioethics

American Society of Law, Medicine & Ethics
http://www.aslme.org/

Site provides information on membership, access to journals, research information, news and more.

Basic Resources in Bioethics
http://www.georgetown.edu/research/nrcbl/scopenotes/sn15.htm

Listing of organizations, encyclopedias, online databases, bibliographies, series, journals and newsletters related to bioethics; with bibliographical or contact information and links, where appropriate.

Bioethics and Health Care Ethics on the WWW
http://www.ethics.ubc.ca/resources/biomed/

Links to ethics institutions and organizations, online discussion groups, courses and publications.

Bioethics Discussion Pages

http://www-hsc.usc.edu/~mbernste/index.html

Ethicists and the general public are invited to participate in discussions. Recent topics included cloning humans, "social worth" in the allocation of scarce resources, euthanasia, and the right of insurance companies to genetically test their customers.

Bioethics Resources

http://eduserv.hscer.washington.edu/bioethics/resource/index.html

This site provides discussion, advice and resources for professionals on various bioethical issues, including advance directives, confidentiality, breaking bad news, cross-cultural beliefs, end-of-life decisions, informed consent, managed care, maternal/fetal conflict, medical mistakes, and more.

Bioethics.net

http://www.med.upenn.edu/bioethic/cgi/none.cgi

From the Center for Bioethics at the University of Pennsylvania. This site provides an enormous amount of resources including Bioethics for Beginners, a virtual library, surveys, publishing in bioethics, the *American Journal of Ethics and Medicine*, and roundtable discussions of specific topics.

Center for Medical Ethics and Mediation

http://www.wh.com/cmem/

The Center is an educational association that provides training, research, consultations and mediations for health care professionals and organizations in an effort to enhance skill development in conflict resolution and ethical decision-making. Site provides codes of ethics and tools for devising a code of ethics; and allows you to e-mail information on an issue for mediation.

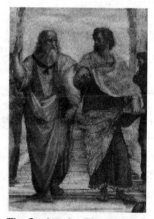

The Center for the Study of Bioethics

http://www.mcw.edu/bioethics/

From the University of Wisconsin, this site describes course work (including web-based courses), offers a Bioethics Online abstract service,

The Society for Bioethics and Classical Philosophy, at the Center for the Study of Bioethics. http://www.mcw.edu/bioethics/sbcp.html

selected bioethical web resources and connects to the Society for Bioethics and Classical Philosophy.

Codes of Ethics Online: Health Care
http://csep.iit.edu/codes/health.html

Includes debate over physical and mental disabilities, a long list of organizations, and descriptions of different codes of ethics.

The Doctor's Dilemma
http://www.expomed.com/ethics.htm

An interactive role-playing software program for doctors to explore their approach to medical ethics. Situations involve issues such as AIDS, end-of-life support, informed consent, artificial insemination, and others.

Ethics in Biomedicine
http://www.mic.ki.se/Diseases/k1.316.html

Lots of good information and links to be found at this site by the Karolinska Institute.

Ethics in Science
http://www.chem.vt.edu/ethics/ethics.html

Science ethics resources, including articles, essays and a bibliography.

European Database on Medical Ethics
http://www.gwdg.de/~uelsner/euroeth.htm

Includes the Euroethics searchable database, a listing of bioethical conferences and events, related documents, e-mail and links.

Library of Bioethics and Medical Humanities Texts and Documents
http://wings.buffalo.edu/faculty/research/bioethics/texts.html

Articles and other resources compiled by the University of Buffalo Center for Clinical Ethics and Humanities in Health Care.

Medical Humanities
http://endeavor.med.nyu.edu/lit-med/medhum.html

From the NYU School of Medicine, this site includes a literature, arts and medicine database, archives and directories.

Medical Oaths and Declarations

http://ch.nus.sg/CH/students/oaths.html

Provides a collection of medical declarations in current use, including the Hippocratic Oath, the International Code of Medical Ethics, and many others.

MedWebPlus: Bioethics

http://www.medwebplus.com/subject/Bioethics.html

Links to a number of bioethics sites on the Internet, by topic.

National Reference Center for BioEthics Literature

http://www.georgetown.edu/research/nrcbl/

Claims it is the world's largest collection related to ethical issues in medicine and biomedical research. Site provides books, journals, newspaper articles, legal materials, regulations, codes, government publications, and other relevant documents concerned with issues in biomedical and professional ethics.

On-line Science Ethics Resources

http://www.chem.vt.edu/ethics/vinny/ethxonline.html

Links to online resources and ethical codes of conduct.

Sheffield Institute of Biotechnological Law and Ethics

http://www.shef.ac.uk/uni/projects/sible/sible.html

This site was created in response to the legal and ethical problems generated by developments in biotechnology.

Cloning

Cloning: A Special Report

http://www.newscientist.com/nsplus/insight/clone/clone.html

"Dollymania" has advanced a great deal in two years. This sight provides the latest highlights in cloning, written for the public.

Cloning Ethics

http://vetc.vsc.edu/vuhs/apbio/clone/

Discusses both sides of the cloning issue, provides information on cloning technology, history and related sites.

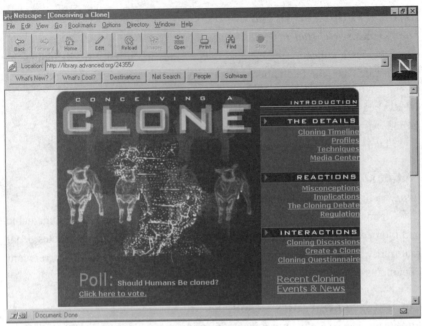

Conceiving a Clone. http://library.advanced.org/24355/

Conceiving a Clone
http://library.advanced.org/24355/
    Details and discussion on cloning of humans and other creatures.

Human Cloning and Re-engineering
http://cac.psu.edu/~gsg109/qs/
    "The goal of this web site is the dissemination of information on human embryo cloning research and related topics, with special attention directed to the moral implications."

Human Cloning Foundation
http://www.humancloning.org/
    This organization believes human cloning has many health and social benefits and should not be banned.

NPR Talk of the Nation: Cloning
http://www.realaudio.com/contentp/npr/ne7f24.html
    Audio file of National Public Radio news program and interview on cloning.

Yahoo! Cloning Links

http://dir.yahoo.com/Science/Biology/Genetics/Cloning/

Cloning of humans, cloning ethics, and related issues.

Euthanasia & Physician Assisted Suicide

Before I Die

http://www.wnet.org/archive/bid/index.html

Site accompanies a PBS program of the same name, and contains personal accounts of death and terminal illness, as well as sidebars, essays and viewpoints which discuss issues such as physician-assisted suicide.

Doctor Assisted Suicide

http://web.lwc.edu/administrative/library/suic.htm

Resources and links to journal and newspaper articles, books, Internet sites, media broadcasts and more. Also discusses relevant legislation.

ERGO!'s Euthanasia World Directory

http://www.finalexit.org/index.shtml

The Euthanasia Research and Guidance Organization site offers information on voluntary assisted suicide for the terminally and irreversibly ill who are suffering unbearably. Find news stories, right-to-die societies, essays, frequently asked questions and related sites.

Euthanasia in Holland

http://www.euthanasia.org/dutch.html

The Netherlands is the only nation where euthanasia is practiced openly. This site describes how it works in this country, where it is defined as the termination of life by a doctor at the express wish of a patient who is suffering unbearably.

Practical Issues in Physician Assisted Suicide

http://www.acponline.org/journals/annals/15jan97/pipas.htm

Reprint of article originally appearing in the *Annals of Internal Medicine.*

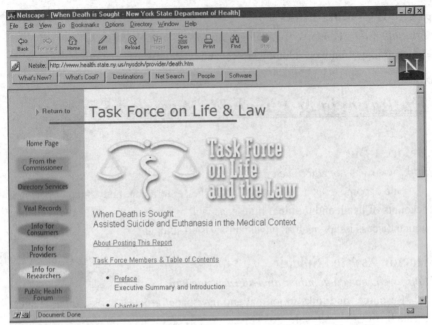

When Death Is Sought. http://www.health.state.ny.us/nysdoh/provider/death.htm

When Death Is Sought

http://www.health.state.ny.us/nysdoh/provider/death.htm

Contains the New York State Task Force on Life and the Law report entitled, *When Death Is Sought: Assisted Suicide and Euthanasia in the Medical Context.* Additional information for the public and researchers available.

Genetics & Gene Therapy

The Council for Responsible Genetics

http://www.gene-watch.org/

The CRG's mission is to educate the public about social and environmental implications of new genetic technology, and to advocate for the socially responsible use of these technologies. Program areas include genetic discrimination, patenting of life forms and the genetic engineering of food.

Gene Therapy for Human Patients: Information for the Public
http://www.nih.gov/od/orda/cover.htm

Basic information for nonscientists about experiments intended to cure disease through transplantation of genes into nonreproductive (somatic) human cells.

Genethics
http://www.changesurfer.com/Hlth/Genes.html

Links. Includes syllabi and educational programs; the Human Genome Project; gene therapy; gene testing, confidentiality and discrimination; biological patents and eugenics.

Genethics Literature Online
http://www.ethics.ubc.ca/brynw/genlit.html

Excerpts, articles and links to information on the following: gene therapy and genetic engineering, cloning, testing confidentiality, genetic counseling, DNA banking and bioprospecting, commercialization, law, eugenics, transgenics, human research and research tools.

Genetics and Ethics Home Page
http://www.ethics.ubc.ca/brynw/

Link to the Human Genome Project, journals, genethics literature, discussion groups, research, public action groups, genetics and the law, conferences and more.

Institute for Human Gene Therapy
http://www.med.upenn.edu/ihgt/

General information on gene therapy, seminars and training, basic science and clinical trials. Lots of information, presented modestly.

Human & Animal Research Subjects

Alternatives to Animal Testing
http://www.sph.jhu.edu/~altweb/

For academic, government and industry scientists, as well as the regulated community. Provides scientific information about new methods, research and resources. General information includes frequently asked questions, discussion groups, and a glossary. Professional information includes research and grants, a calendar of upcoming meetings, regulations and more.

Animal Rights Resource Site

http://arrs.envirolink.org/

Learn about animal rights. Provides frequently asked questions, organizations, issues, and much more.

The Dilemmas of Experimenting on People

http://www.techreview.com/articles/july97/morenolinks.html

Articles and information on protecting humans from research, including some papers issued at the time of the 50th anniversary of the Nuremberg trials.

Human Subjects/Participants and Research Ethics

http://www.psych.bangor.ac.uk/deptpsych/Ethics/HumanResearch.html

Points to consider in a discussion of the ethical use of human subjects in research experiments. Includes policy documents and position papers, ethics committees and institutional review boards, and related servers and directories.

Resources on Nonconsensual Human Experimentation

http://www.dc.peachnet.edu/~shale/humanities/composition/assignments/experiment.html

Includes documents of human experimentation, information on the Tuskeegee experiment, experiments by Nazis, drug and mind control experiments, and more.

Publications

Ethics Connection: Issues in Ethics

http://www.scu.edu/Ethics/publications/iie/

Quarterly journal from the Markkula Center for Applied Ethics. Site provides information on the Center and on practicing ethics, links, as well as online issues, cyberforum and subscription information.

Eubios Journal of Asian and International Ethics

http://www.biol.tsukuba.ac.jp/~macer/EJAIB.html

Online journal of the Asian Bioethics Association. Its goal is to review and update news and trends in bioethics (including medical ethics, bioethics, and issues arising from advancements in biotechnology) around the world, and it does so by reviewing approximately 1000 articles per issue. Special focus is given to issues raised by genetic and reproductive technologies.

Journal of Medical Ethics

http://www.bmjpg.com/data/jme.htm

Current contents, archives, and subscription information for this journal which features original articles addressing the ethical aspects of health care, as well as conferences, book reviews, editorials, correspondence, news and notes.

BIOMEDICINE

Anatomy

Anatomy of the Human Body
http://rpisun1.mda.uth.tmc.edu/mmlearn/anatomy.html

Click on the brain, elbow, arm, hand, knee and ankle of "dummy" to call up various radiological images of that location.

The Articulation Page
http://www-adm.pdx.edu/user/bio/articula/home.html

Articulation is the putting together a skeleton, piece by piece. This site serves as a how-to guide for putting together a posed skeleton.

The Atlas of the Human Body
http://www.ama-assn.org/insight/gen_hlth/atlas/atlas.htm

This site was created by the American Medical Association to provide patient information. Selecting a system or body part from the original menu brings you to a page that provides basic information on its anatomy and function.

ATLAS-Plus
http://www.med.umich.edu/lrc/Atlas/atlas.html

Uses digitized images, computer graphics, sound, animations and text to teach basic concepts and principles of human anatomy. The three courses are: Gross Anatomy, Histology and Embryology.

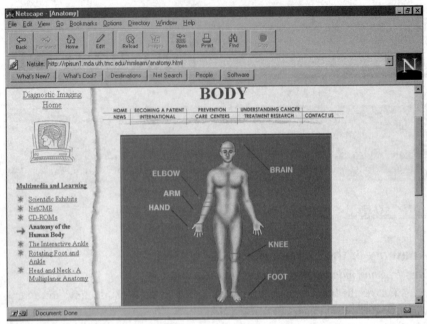

Anatomy of the Human Body. *http://rpisun1.mda.uth.tmc.edu/mmlearn/anatomy.html*

The Digital Anatomist Program

http://sig.biostr.washington.edu/projects/da/

A learning tool for students and clinicians, this site contains online interactive atlases of the brain, knee and thoracic organs.

HistoWeb

http://www.kumc.edu/instruction/medicine/anatomy/histoweb/

Images of tissues and cells.

Neuroanatomy Study Slides

http://www.mcl.tulane.edu/student/1997/Kenb/neuroanatomy/
readme_neuro.html

This study tool provides three views (unlabelled, labelled and marked) of 25 slides showing spinal cord, medulla, midpons, high pons, midbrain, diencephalon and other views of the brain.

The Virtual Body

http://www.medtropolis.com/vbody/

An elaborate interactive presentation of human anatomy. You must download Macromedia's Shockwave Player Plugin (instructions provided at the site) to view.

The Visible Human

http://www.nlm.nih.gov/research/visible/visible_human.html

The goal of the National Library of Medicine's Visible Human project is to create complete, anatomically detailed, 3-dimensional representations of the male and female human body. Currently the project is collecting transverse CT, MR and cryosection images of representative male and female cadavers at one millimeter intervals. Facts, articles and numerous projects based on viewing these images can be found at this site.

Biochemistry

Biochemistry and Molecular Biology

http://golgi.harvard.edu/biopages/biochem.html

Loads of links, alphabetized by subject and provider.

Biochemistry Tutorials and Guides

http://www.graylab.ac.uk/cancerweb/educate/biochem.html

Links to various biochemistry sites on the web.

BioChemNet

http://schmidel.com/bionet.cfm

General biology, chemistry, biochemistry, molecular chemistry information and news. Great assortment of links.

General, Organic and Biochemistry

http://ull.chemistry.uakron.edu/genobc/

Provides the highlights of a textbook with practice exams, many animations, and course syllabi.

Graphics Gallery

http://www.accessexcellence.org/AB/GG/

Contains a series of labelled images with accompanying text. Topics include gene function, genetics, building blocks (molecules, cells and tissues), chromosomes and cell division, biotechnology, viruses and cell processes.

HyperCLDB

http://www.biotech.ist.unige.it/cldb/indexes.html

Hypertext access to Interlab Project's Cell Line Data Base which shows the cell culture availability of over 3,300 human and animal cell lines.

Journal of Molecular Biology

http://www.academicpress.com/jmb

A weekly journal that publishes original scientific research concerning studies of organisms or their components at the molecular level. Table of contents, abstracts and supplementary information are available free at this site, and subscription information is also available.

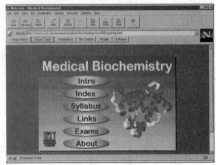

Medical Biochemistry. http://www.kumc. edu/research/medicine/biochemistry/bioc800/ opening.html

Medical Biochemistry

http://www.kumc.edu/research/ medicine/biochemistry/bioc800/ opening.html

Site provides slides, animations and interactive molecular modeling modules that accompany a course at the University of Kansas Medical Center. Links to related sites, medical journals, medical dictionaries and lay-oriented general medicine sites are offered.

Medical Biochemistry Exams

http://bob.usuf2.usuhs.mil/biochem/exams/exams.html

Online exams test your knowledge of protein and carbohydrate biochemistry, nutrition and more.

Molecular Graphics Art Shows

http://www.scripps.edu/pub/goodsell/mgs_art/index.html

Artistic interpretations of biochemical structures. Site shows images of original artwork appearing in two juried shows, with brief text identifying the artist and explaining what is illustrated.

National Institute of General Medical Sciences

http://www.nih.gov/nigms/

This NIH Institute supports biomedical research that is not targeted to specific diseases, but focused on understanding life processes and advancing disease diagnosis, treatment and prevention efforts.

NetBiochem

http://www.auhs.edu/netbiochem/NetWelco.htm

A complete medical biochemistry site for the computer. Covers many biochemical topics, from Fatty Acid Metabolism to Purines and Pyramidines, with accompanying multimedia enhancements, quizzes and review tables.

Physiology and Biophysics - World Wide Web Virtual Library

http://physiology.med.cornell.edu/WWWVL/PhysioWeb.html

Includes biomedical and physical science links.

Periodic Table of the Elements

http://ull.chemistry.uakron.edu/genobc/periodic/

Click on any element to obtain elemental information (e.g., atomic number, atomic weight, oxidation status, melting and boiling point, and more).

Biotechnology

BioABACUS

http://www.nmsu.edu/~molbio/bioABACUShome.htm

Searchable database of abbreviations and acronyms used in biotechnology.

BioTech

http://biotech.icmb.utexas.edu/

An interactive educational resource and biotechnology reference tool.

BioTechniques
http://www.biotechniques.com/

Online journal and BioMall for the biological sciences.

Biotechnology
http://www.cato.com/biotech/

This section of the World Wide Web Virtual Library contains over 1000 URLs specific to biotechnology, pharmaceutical development and related fields.

Biotechnology Information Center
http://www.nal.usda.gov/bic/

A service of the National Agricultural Library of the U.S. Department of Agriculture, this site contains news and links to biotechnology topics.

Biotechnology Links
http://schmidel.com/bionet/biotech.htm

Part of BioChemNet's extensive listings.

Center for Biotechnology
http://life.bio.sunysb.edu/biotech/

Part of the State University of New York at Stony Brook, the Center is a link between the biomedical industry and a network of research, business development, and educational resources. Site describes various Center research projects, educational programs and associated organizations.

Genetic Engineering
http://www.geocities.com/Athens/Olympus/4338/index.html

Discusses the advantages and disadvantages of genetic engineering.

Health Services/Technology Assessment Texts
http://text.nlm.nih.gov/

From the U.S. National Library of Medicine. Search AHCPR Guidelines, Technology Assessments, ATIS (HIV/AIDS Treatment Information Service) publications, NIH Clinical Studies, NIH Consensus Development Programs and other databases.

International Centre for Genetic Engineering and Biotechnology Home Page

http://base.icgeb.trieste.it/

The Centre is an international organization dedicated to the safe use of biotechnology, "with special regard to the needs of the developing world." Research, resources, training and services are available at this site.

National Center for Biotechnology Information

http://www.ncbi.nlm.nih.gov/

Lots of information and resources, including access to the GenBank Sequence Database, the Human Genome Project, research and more.

World Wide Biotech Information

http://www.aba.asn.au/links.html

Starting points for searching for biotech information on the web.

Genetics

Cooperative Human Linkage Center

http://www.chlc.org/

Site provides genetic maps and provides information on genetic markers. Also allows access to CHLC publications and project information.

Hereditary Disease Foundation

http://www.hdfoundation.org/

Nonprofit, basic science organization dedicated to the cure of genetic diseases.

Human Genome Project

NIH site: http://www.nhgri.nih.gov/HGP

DOE site: http://www.ornl.gov/hgmis/publicat/

This is an international research project whose general goal is to map the human genome and to locate the estimated 50,000 to 100,000 different genes within it. The U.S.Human Genome Project is sponsored jointly by the National Institutes of Health and the Department of Energy. These sites describe project goals; summarize the progress done thusfar; address ethical, legal and social implications; provide historical and bibliographical information, and provide links to many related resources.

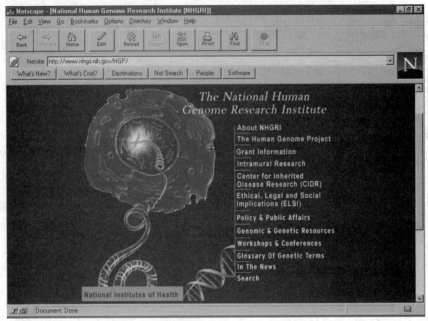

National Human Genome Research Institute. *http://www.nhgri.nih.gov/HGP/*

Genethon: Human Genome Research Centre

http://www.genethon.fr/genethon_en.html

Genethon's projects include a DNA and cell bank, map of the human genome, gene identification, and genotyping services, as well as others. Site describes these projects and presents public data and information.

National Human Genome Research Institute

http://www.nhgri.nih.gov/HGP/

The Institute's mission is to run the Human Genome Project (see above), and this site contains HGP and grant information, discussions of ethical, social and legal implications, a glossary of genetic terms, a list of resources, news and more.

Primer on Molecular Genetics

http://www.ornl.gov/hgmis/publicat/primer/intro.html

Online publication explains genetic fundamentals and human genome information. Lots of information, with hypertext links and illustrations.

Links

Biomedical Information Resources and Services

http://www.mic.ki.se/Other.html

Biomedical information resources and services by subject. Includes sites on specific diseases and disorders, as well as sites related to molecular biology, ethics, history and occupation.

BioSites

http://galen.library.ucsf.edu/biosites/

A current listing of important Internet resources in the biomedical sciences. Sorted by topic (over 75) and alphabetically.

Medical Informatics

American Medical Informatics Association

http://www.amia.org/

Answers questions about AMIA operations, meetings, membership, and publications.

Bioplanet

http://www.bioplanet.com/

The bioinformatics homepage includes articles, frequently asked questions, a bulletin board and other bioinformatic resources, jobs postings and a place to post your resumé.

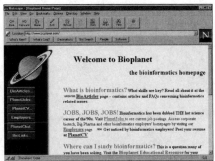

Bioplanet. *http://www.bioplanet.com/*

Health Informatics World Wide

http://www.imbi.uni-freiburg.de/medinf/mi_list.htm

Provides a complete list of web resources relating to medical informatics, sorted by country.

How to Become a Bioinformatics Expert

http://www.TechFak.Uni-Bielefeld.DE/bcd/ForAll/Econom/study.html

Describes what the profession involves and its potential as a career (good). According to the site, "bioinformatics combines the tools and techniques of mathematics, computer science and biology in order to understand the biological significance of a variety of data."

Journal of Informatics in Primary Care

http://www.ncl.ac.uk/~nphcare/PHCSG/Journal/index.htm

Online journal for medical informatics includes back issues with papers, articles, news, conference reports, and subscription information.

Medical Informatics and Medicine

http://www.cs.man.ac.uk/mig/resources/

Medical informatics involves the storage, retrieval and use of biomedical data and computer technology to solve problems and create models of biomedical systems.

BLOOD / HEMATOLOGY

Anatomy & Images

Atlas of Hematology

http://www.med.nagoya-u.ac.jp/pathy/Pictures/atlas.html

View thumbnail images of a variety of blood stains, which may be enlarged to screen size. Images show healthy blood, as well as samples of iron deficiency anemia, leukemia, lymphoma, and about a dozen other blood disorders.

Blood Outline

http://www.mc.vanderbilt.edu/histo/blood/

An introduction to blood and its components.

Cells of the Blood

http://www-micro.msb.le.ac.uk/MBChB/ bloodmap/Blood.html

Identify the basic blood cells such as neutrophils, eosinophils, monocytes, lymphocytes, basophils and erythrocytes, and learn more about their function.

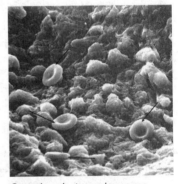

Scanning electron microscope image identifying erythrocytes, as seen at: **Blood Outline.**
http://www.mc.vanderbilt.edu/histo/ blood/RBC-SEM.jpg

Index of Hematology Cases

http://www.uchsc.edu/sm/pmb/medrounds/ hemeindex.html

Medical rounds, online. Consider several cases and participate in discussion.

Red Cells

http://www.pathguy.com/lectures/rbc.htm

Part of Ed's Pathology Notes, provides links to pathology images (including pictures of red blood cells), study notes, and more.

Anemias

See also: Sickle Cell Disease, later in this chapter.

Anemia

http://www.adam.com/ency/article/000560.htm

Information on fourteen different kinds of anemia.

Anemia: An Approach to Diagnosis

http://www.ohsu.edu/cliniweb/handouts/anemia.html

Outline for clinicians.

Anemia: Medical Self-Care

http://www.healthy.net/library/books/healthyself/womens/anemia.htm

Written for the general public. Describes the different kinds of anemias, symptoms, and self-care procedures.

Anemia, Pernicious

http://www.rxmed.com/illnesses/anemia,_pernicious.html

Describes pernicious anemia, its symptoms, causes and treatment.

Aplastic Anemia

http://dpalm2.med.uth.tmc.edu/edprog/00000146.htm

Etiology, incidence, diagnosis, pathophysiology and treatment of aplastic anemias.

Iron Deficiency in Adults:
A Comprehensive Management Guide

http://www.ironpanel.org.au/Acontents.html

Article intended for licensed medical practitioners.

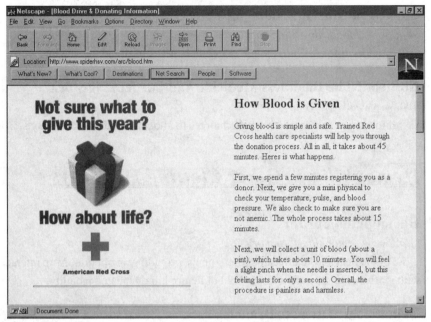

Giving blood is simple and safe. Trained Red Cross health care specialists will help you through the donation process. All in all, it takes about 45 minutes. Heres is what happens.

First, we spend a few minutes registering you as a donor. Next, we give you a mini physical to check your temperature, pulse, and blood pressure. We also check to make sure you are not anemic. The whole process takes about 15 minutes.

Next, we will collect a unit of blood (about a pint), which takes about 10 minutes. You will feel a slight pinch when the needle is inserted, but this feeling lasts for only a second. Overall, the procedure is painless and harmless.

Blood Drive & Donating Information. http://www.spiderhsv.com/arc/blood.htm

Blood Donation & Transfusion

American Association of Blood Banks
http://www.aabb.org/
Facts about blood, blood donation, transfusions, education, training, and Association information.

America's Blood Centers
http://www.americasblood.org/
Click on a state to find your nearest blood center and other blood facts.

Blood Donation Process
http://www.itxm.org/CBB/donorreg.htm
Simple explanation of what happens when you volunteer to give blood.

Blood Drive & Donating Information
http://www.spiderhsv.com/arc/blood.htm
From the American Red Cross.

Blood Transfusion: Knowing Your Options

http://www.bloodtransfusion.com/

Provides information as to the risks and benefits of blood transfusion.

NoBlood! The Bloodless Medicine and Surgery Network

http://www.noblood.com/

Information and research on alternatives to allogeneic blood transfusions.

Hemophilia & Other Clotting Disorders

Haemophilia Forum

http://www.hemophilia-forum.org/

For medical and health care professionals, providing an opportunity to interact with world-wide specialists in the field of hemophilia. Updated monthly.

Hematologic Diseases Branch

http://www.cdc.gov/ncidod/dastlr/hematology.htm

The goal of the Branch is to work to reduce the complications of hemophilia and other bleeding and clotting disorders. It does this through surveillance, educating of public and health care practitioners, and by supporting research.

Hemophilia

http://www.geocities.com/WallStreet/1450/

Links to hemophilia sites on the Internet. Over 25,000 Americans suffer from this disorder, and an estimated 85 percent of hemophiliacs born before 1982 may be HIV positive. Site is dedicated to these individuals.

Hemophilia: A Genetic Disease

http://communityhigh.org/usr/graham/hemophilia/

The origin, etiology and progression of hemophilia, written for laypeople.

Hemophilia Home Page

http://www.web-depot.com/hemophilia/

Good information on hemophilia, its relationship to AIDS, organizations, mailing lists, newsletters, legislative information, gene therapy and other treatments. Includes a section on women with bleeding disorders.

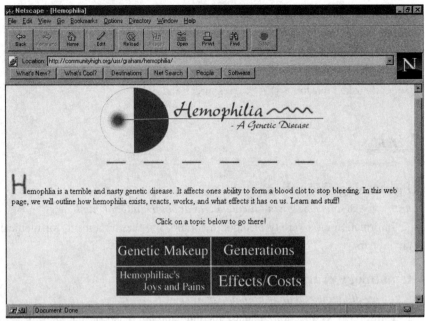

Hemophilia: A Genetic Disease. http://communityhigh.org/usr/graham/hemophilia/

National Hemophilia Foundation

http://www.hemophilia.org/

Information on bleeding disorders, resources, research and programs searching to find a cure for hemophilia.

Understanding von Willbrand Disease

http://www.wfh.org/von_w.html

Explains this genetic disorder, in which the protein required for blood to coagulate properly is absent.

von Willbrand's Disease

http://www.mindspring.com/~mattrk/

Information on this clotting disorder which is 100 times more common than hemophilia.

World Federation of Hemophilia

http://www.wfh.org/

Information and resources on hemophilia. Includes library and links, news updates, articles and press releases, information for patients and family members, frequently asked questions (FAQs), resources and links.

Links

Haematology Handbook

http://www.swsahs.nsw.gov.au/livhaem/Handbook/Handbook.html

Information on a variety of blood disorders and their treatment, for medical practitioners.

Hematology & Blood Diseases

http://www.lib.uiowa.edu/hardin/md/hem.html

Hardin MD's collection of small, medium and large lists of Internet links.

Hematology, MedMark

http://medmark.org/hem/hem2.html

Extensive list of hematology resources. Broken down into associations/societies, centers/institutes/labs, departments/divisions, information for consumers, journals/news/publications, general/unclassified, and guides/guidelines.

Hematology Resources

http://www.cc.emory.edu/PEDS/HEMONC/hem.htm

Links to general hematology sites, galleries of images, journals, sickle cell disease and other blood disorders.

Hemic and Lymphatic Diseases

http://www.mic.ki.se/Diseases/c15.html

Section on hematological diseases includes many links to sites on anemias, neutropenia, Job's syndrome, blood coagulation disorders and purpura. Also includes general hemic disease links.

MedWebplus Hematology

http://www.medwebplus.com/subject/Hematology.html

A large number of links, organized by topic.

Lymphedema

Lymphedema Etiology, Prevention & Treatment

http://lymphedemaservices.com/info.html

Lymphedema is chronic edema of the extremities due to lymph node disorders or lymph vessel blockage. This site describes the disorder in layperson's terms. Includes anatomy and pathology, prevention, incidence, presentation and treatment.

National Lymphedema Network

http://www.lymphnet.org/

The Network is a nonprofit organization to educate and advise lymphedema patients, health care professionals and the general public.

Publications & Professional Societies

American Journal of Hematology

http://www.interscience.wiley.com/jpages/0361-8609/

Basic information on this journal and how to subscribe. Available in print and online versions.

American Society of Hematology

http://www.hematology.org/

Information about this society which seeks to promote diffusion of information on blood, blood-forming tissues, and blood diseases. Also includes access to the journal *Blood*, educational materials on a large variety of topics, ASH news and meeting information.

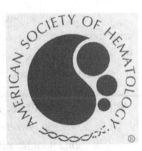

American Society of Hematology.
http://www.hematology.org/

Blood: The Journal of the American Society of Hematology

http://www.edoc.com/blood/

Site contains article abstracts, table of contents, and subscription information. Subscription allows you to view journal online.

Blood Weekly

http://www.newsfile.com/1b.htm

Weekly newsletter with news reports, research, journal articles and summaries available online. Sample issue is available. Subscription information provided.

Blood Cells, Molecules & Disease

http://seconde.scripps.edu/

Current and back issues of this quarterly journal are available at this site.

Sickle Cell Disease

Baby Net: Sickle Cell Disease

http://babynet.ddwi.com/tlc/pregnancy/siklcell.html

Public health information sheet.

Sickle Cell Anemia

http://wellweb.com/INDEX/QSICKLE.HTM

Information for parents on sickle cell disease in newborns and infants.

Sickle Cell Defiers

http://defiers.com/

"Turning fear into action." Devoted to improving the quality of life for those with sickle cell disease, through exchange of information and support. Site created by the sickle cell community for the sickle cell community. Contains stories, chat room and bulletin board, research reports, books and more.

Sickle Cell Disease: A Guide for Parents

http://text.nlm.nih.gov/ahcpr/sickle/www/scdptxt.html

An online booklet with valuable information and a glossary.

Sickle Cell Disease Association of America

http://SickleCellDisease.org/

National organization devoted to solving problems caused by sickle cell disease. Site describes SCDAA mission, member organizations, and provides information on the disease, research updates, educational materials and programs.

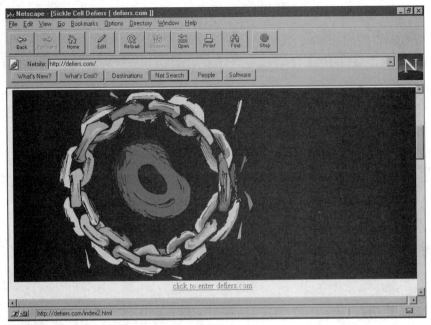

Sickle Cell Defiers. http://www.defiers.com/

Sickle Cell Disease: Beyond the Pain

http://uhs.bsd.uchicago.edu/uhs/topics/sickle.cell.html

A comprehensive approach to care for people with sickle cell disease.

Sickle Cell Foundation of Georgia, Inc.

http://www.mindspring.com/~sicklefg/

Explains the disease and its prevalence in layperson's language. Describes the Foundation's education, screening and counseling programs, and links to sickle cell in the news.

Sickle Cell Information Center

http://www.emory.edu/PEDS/SICKLE/

Patient and professional education, news, research updates and sickle cell resources.

BONES / ORTHOPEDICS

Bone Resources

Belgian Orthoweb International Homepage
http://www.belgianorthoweb.be/index_uk.htm

A comprehensive guide to orthopedics. Includes professional meetings, organizations and news, review articles, patient information, questions and answers, web links and much more.

Bone and Joint Resources
http://www.orthop.washington.edu/bonejoint/zzzzzzzz1_1.html

Hypertext articles on different topics, such as shoulder, low back pain, arthritis, and others.

Bone Home
http://www.bonehome.com/

Site calls itself an "online magazine in orthopaedics." Offers case studies, courses, protocols, images, links, software and other products related to bone care.

Common Orthopedic Disorders
http://www.drmendbone.com/disorders.htm

Contains information on conditions of the knee, shoulder, and hip.

Osteovision
http://www.osteovision.ch/

Interactive information center in the bone field discusses bone and calcium metabolism. Links, announcements, job opportunities and slide collections.

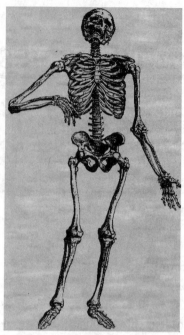

Wheeless' Textbook of Ortho-paedics. *http://www.medmedia.com/*

Wheeless' Textbook of Orthopaedics

http://www.medmedia.com/

Click on a part of an image of a skeleton to get information about that bone, common injuries to it and how to manage them. In addition, site offers research abstracts, radiographics and links.

WorldOrtho

http://www.worldortho.com/

Orthopedics, sports medicine and trauma handbooks, as well as related websites. Contains feature articles, photo gallery, links to electronic textbooks and online quizzes, inventions and more.

Links

LinkOrthopaedics

http://www.dundee.ac.uk/orthopaedics/link/welcome.html

"The scope of Orthopaedics is interpreted in the broadest sense and so links are included to sites covering such diverse topics as biomaterials, biomechanics, biomedical engineering, ergonomics, fracture fixation, functional anatomy, joint replacement, kinesiology, occupational therapy, orthotics, physiotherapy, prosthetics, rehabilitation, sports science and wheelchairs." Sites are listed by country and name, as well as by category.

MedWebplus Orthopedics

http://www.medwebplus.com/subject/Orthopedics.html

Links to organizations, diseases, and orthopedic-related sites.

Orthogate Web Links
http://owl.orthogate.org/
A comprehensive collection of links to orthopedic sites.

Organizations

Academic Orthopaedic Society Home Panel
http://www.a-o-s.org/
Book reviews, case presentations and news for those involved in teaching orthopedics.

American Academy of Orthopaedic Surgeons
http://www.aaos.org/
Contains information for the public on how to find a surgeon as well as a number of patient brochures. Information for members includes discussion groups, library, medical education, research and legislative watch.

American Shoulder and Elbow Surgeons
http://www.aaos.org/wordhtml/ases/homeases.htm
Membership information, local chapters, and interesting sites.

ISAKOS
http://www.isakos.com/
The International Society of Arthroscopy, Knee Surgery, and Orthopedic Sports Medicine homepage offers information on their Annual Congress.

OWL Organizations Page
http://owl.orthogate.org/org.html
Links to organizations related to orthopedics from all around the world.

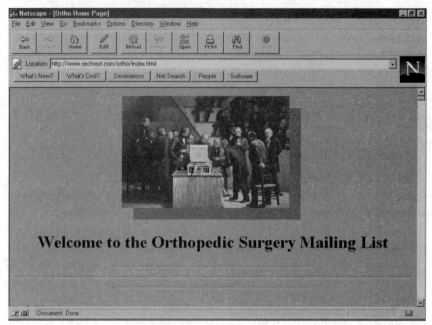

Orthopedic Surgery Mailing List. http://www.sechrest.com/ortho/index.html

Orthopedic Surgery

Anesthesia for Orthopedic Surgery
http://www.anes.ccf.org:8080/pilot/ortho/orthintr.htm

Learning "module" for residents beginning their orthopedic anesthesia rotation. Provides a great deal of information on procedures and techniques.

Orthopaedic Surgery on the Web
http://www.swmed.edu:80/home_pages/OrthoSurg/OrthoSites.html

Colleges, universities, societies, news and discussion groups, educational resources, clinics and institutions related to orthopedics.

Orthopedic Surgery Mailing List
http://www.sechrest.com/ortho/index.html

Site provides information on the orthopedic mailing list, but also membership directory, newsgroups, orthopedic surgery grand rounds, FTP site, and numerous related links. To subscribe, send e-mail to: *orthopedic-request@weston.com* with the following message: "SUBSCRIBE *Yourfirstname Yourlastname.*"

Orthotics

Biomechanics Magazine

http://www.biomech.com/

"The Magazine of Body Movement and Medicine." Includes links and archives, as well as products.

Biomechanics World Wide

http://www.per.ualberta.ca/biomechanics/

This site covers the huge field of biomechanics and offers a large section of orthopedics links from around the world. A discussion forum, posting of career opportunities and research news, institute and laboratory sites, as well as associations are provided for many sub-topics, including orthopaedics.

Orthotic and Prosthetic Information

http://www.opoffice.org/

Access site for three organizations: the American Orthotic and Prosthetic Association, The American Board for Certification in Orthotics and Prosthetics, and the American Academy of Orthotists and Prosthetists.

Orthotics and Prosthetics Online

http://www.oandp.com/

Information for medical professionals and patients. Patient care, product information, consulting, rehabilitation, and links to organizations, research sites and more. Site features profiles, which are actually case studies with discussion, a listserv, classified ads and more.

PandO.Net! Prosthetic and Orthotic Network

http://www.pando.net/

Information and resources for the prosthetics and orthotics communities. Some features include a community directory to patient care, organizations, and suppliers; a book store, newsletter, forum and classified ads.

Osteoporosis

See also: Women's Health - Osteoporosis.

National Osteoporosis Foundation

http://www.nof.org/

The causes of osteoporosis, as well as prevention, detection, and treatment. Information for medical professionals and patients.

National Institutes of Health Osteoporosis and Related Bone Diseases National Resource Center

http://www.osteo.org/

Discusses osteoporosis and related disorders including Paget's disease of bone and *osteogenesis imperfecta*. Includes section on osteoporosis and men, and an area for professionals.

Optimal Calcium Intake

http://text.nlm.nih.gov/nih/cdc/www/97.html

Recommendations by age, sex and condition.

Osteoporosis Information and Resources

http://www.pslgroup.com/OSTEOPOROSIS.HTM

Medical news, osteoporosis links, discussion groups and related sites.

Podiatry

Foot and Ankle Web Index

http://www.footandankle.com/

"Ask the foot doctor" about your medical problems, find a podiatrist in your area, learn about foot care and link to related sites.

A Foot Talk Place on the Net

http://www.foottalk.com/

The primary goal of this site is to provide the general public with information on podiatry and foot disorders. In addition, use it to locate a podiatry clinic near you, view images, and connect to other foot-related sites.

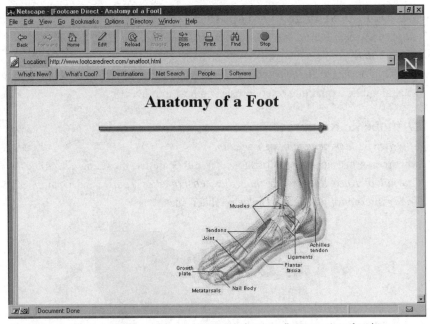

*Anatomy of a Foot at: **Footcare Direct:** http://www.footcaredirect.com/anatfoot.htm.*

Footcare Direct
http://www.footcaredirect.com/

Learn the basics of foot care, from anatomy of a foot to finding the right shoes, as well as information on specific problems such as bunions, shin splints, flat feet and warts.

Orthotic Podiatry
http://www.nwpodiatric.com/indexab.html

Site has information on foot care, including diabetes, a self test, and a doctor search, as well as the latest in research and products.

Publications

Internet Journal of Orthopedic Surgery and Related Topics
http://www.rz.uni-duesseldorf.de/WWW/MedFak/Orthopaedie/journal/

Quarterly journal that publishes recent clinical and research advances in the field of orthopedic surgery.

JAMA Patient Page - Osteoporosis

http://www.ama-assn.org/sci-pubs/journals/archive/jama/vol_279/no_18/ pp0513.htm

The *Journal of the American Medical Association* has gathered articles for the general public explaining osteoporosis and how to prevent it.

Orthopedic Resources

http://www.slackinc.com/bone/bone.htm

Access to four different orthopedics publications, including *The American Journal of Knee Surgery*, *Orthopedics*, *Orthopedics Today*, and *Orthopaedics Today International Edition*. Links to related sites.

Brain & Brain Disorders

Acquired Brain Injuries

Brain Injury Association, Inc.
http://www.biausa.org/

Topics addressed include anatomy of a brain injury, life after a brain injury, the cost of brain injury, brain injury prevention, treatment and rehabilitation, kids' corner, resources and a national directory.

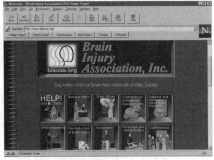

Brain Injury Association, Inc.
http://www.biausa.org/

Brain Injury Center
http://www.braincenter.org/

Acquired brain injury is any injury to the brain including stroke, trauma, anoxia, infection, and tumors. Information and support for patients and their families.

Perspectives Network
http://www.tbi.org/

For survivors of acquired brain injury, their families, caregivers, friends and health professionals. Information, resources, survivor tools, frequently asked questions and support.

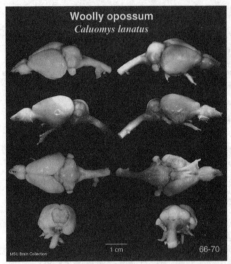

Wooly Opossum Brain from the: **Comparative Mammalian Brain Collection.**
http://www.neurophys.wisc.edu/brain/specimens/marsupalia/woollyopossum/index.html

Yves' Acquired Brain Injury

http://www.geocities.com/HotSprings/2059/

Story of one man's ABI and rehabilitation, and links to sites of interest.

Anatomy

Comparative Mammalian Brain Collection

http://www.neurophys.wisc.edu/brain/

Interesting site displays the brains of over 100 different species of mammals (including humans).

Layman's View on Brain Chemistry

http://www.maui.net/~jms/brainuse.html

This site discusses neurotransmitters, i.e., the chemicals in the brain that process perception and emotions, and effect personality. Information about brain size, brain tumors, and more. Written for laypeople, in large type.

Whole Brain Atlas

http://www.med.harvard.edu:80/AANLIB/home.html

CT, MRI and SPECT/PET images of the normal brain and the brain of patients suffering from various disorders, including cancers, degenerative diseases such as Alzheimer's, and inflammatory diseases such as multiple sclerosis. Access to the Atlas Navigator, an amazing site for those with the ability to read Java.

Aneurysms

3-D Visualization of Brain Aneurysms
http://everest.radiology.uiowa.edu/nlm/app/aneur/brain/aneur.html
Three case studies with different views of brain aneurysm.

Aneurysm and Arteriovenous Malformation Support
http://www.westga.edu/~wmaples/aneurysm.html
Site that is collecting personal stories of patient's and/or families' experiences with aneurysms, in order to offer others support and information. "Narratives may cover anything the author feels is pertinent to his/her aneurysm experience."

Aneurysm Information Project
http://www.columbia.edu/~mdt1/
List of resources available at the site includes frequently asked questions, victim support page, papers of the month, research, and various other files.

Brain Attack/Stroke

Brain Attacks/Strokes
_http://netwellness1.uc.edu/lists/Brain_attack/contents.cfm_
Consumer booklets, electronic books, electronic magazines, journal articles and Internet links.

The Brain Attack Coalition
http://www.stroke-site.org/
Collection of tools for health care professionals to enable the rapid diagnosis and treatment of stroke.

The Brain Matters Stroke Initiative
http://www.strokematters.com/
Devoted to prevention of stroke or brain attack through education and prevention. Provides information on warning signs and high-risk populations.

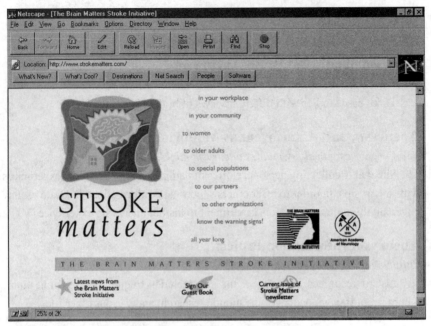

The Brain Matters Stroke Initiative. *http://www.strokematters.com/*

NINDS Stroke Information Guide

http://www.ninds.nih.gov/healinfo/disorder/stroke/strokehp.htm

Information from the National Institute of Neurological Disorders and Stroke includes emergency treatment, risk factors, research, prevention and recovery.

Stroke Support and Information Homepage

http://members.aol.com/scmmlm/main.htm

Support for caregivers and survivors. Free membership.

Virtual Hospital: Stroke and Brain Attack

http://www.vh.org/Providers/ClinGuide/Stroke/Index.html

Hypertext document of stroke basics, resources and clinical treatment guidelines. Some pages available in Spanish.

Coma

Coma Waiting Page
http://www.waiting.com/

A page for those who are waiting while someone they know is in a coma. Offers information on legal issues, intensive care, prognosis, discharge, and other resources and links.

The Persistent Vegetative State
http://www.geocities.com/HotSprings/Oasis/2919/

Provides definition, ethical dilemmas, statistics and links.

Concussion

HealthAnswers: Concussion
http://www.healthanswers.com/adam/top/view.asp?filename=000799.htm&rdir

Information on causes, symptoms, signs, prevention and first-aid treatment of concussions, i.e., significant blows to the head.

The Human Brain Project

The Human Brain Project
http://www-scripps.edu/

Information on this long-term research project focusing on ways to use technology to support research on brain function and behavior, and to create a network sharing brain information and databases. It involves projects at over twenty different facilities, and links to these sites are provided.

The Human Brain Project - Denmark/Images
http://hendrix.ei.dtu.dk/image/imagehome.html

This site uses Java, movies and still images to show MRI, PET and computer graphic images and models of the brain.

Hydrocephalus/Other Neural Tube Defects

See also: Disabilities - Spina Bifida.

Encephalocele Disease Information

http://www.stepstn.com/nord/rdb_sum/867.htm

This is a rare disorder in which a infant is born with a gap in his or her skull. Site offers list of contact organizations, as well as some articles (for a fee).

eSynopsis of Encephalocele of the Brain

http://esynopsis.uchc.edu/S445.htm

Straightforward notes about this disorder.

Hydrocephalus Association Homepage

http://neurosurgery.mgh.harvard.edu/ha/

Hydrocephalus is the abnormal accumulation of cerebrospinal fluid in the brain. Site includes fact sheet, announcements for the hydrocephalus community, and resources. It also provides newsletter articles, links to hydrocephalus information, and a support forum.

Hydrocephalus Brochure

http://www.aans.org/pubpages/patres/hydrobroch.html

Overview of hydrocephalus, including diagnosis, treatment, recovery and frequently asked questions.

Hydrocephalus Center

http://www.patientcenters.com/hydrocephalus/

Information for families with children suffering from this condition, describing hydrocephalus and how to work with the child's doctor. Provides resources, suggested readings, and links to organizations and related Internet sites.

Hydrocephalus Facts and Links

http://members.nova.org/~twinkee/HydroLinks.htm

Includes personal pages, organizations and support networks.

Hydrocephalus Index

http://www.bgsm.edu/bgsm/surg-sci/ns/hyceph.html

Long list of links from Wake Forest University.

Information on Spina Bifida

http://www.fortunecity.com/millenium/plumpton/268/sb.htm

Describes this disorder in layperson's terms.

Living with Spina Bifida

http://www.geocities.com/HotSprings/2474/

Provides information, chat room, resources, facts about spina bifida and hydrocephalus, and Internet links.

Spina Bifida & Hydrocephalus Association of Canada

http://www.sbhac.ca/engl_ind.html

These two disorders often appear together.

Resources

RebPage: The Brain in Health and Disease

http://www.uni-hohenheim.de/~rebhan/rp.html

Information about the understanding, treatment and diagnosis of brain disorders. Contains links, an introduction of the principles that cause brain disorders, selected brain news and a glossary of technical terms.

Shuffle Brain

http://www.indiana.edu/~pietsch/home.html

Popular science articles on the brain and brain transplanting; photographs of brains of humans and other animals; scientific articles, books and miscellaneous items experimenting and contemplating the activity and function of the brain.

Surgery

Brain Surgery Information Center

http://www.brain-surgery.com/

Non-technical information about conditions which require brain surgery. Includes a glossary, information on stroke, brain tumors, and images of surgery.

Gamma Knife Center
http://www.sdgkc.com/

Information about this tool for minimally invasive brain surgery.

History of Brain Surgery
http://brain-surgery.com/history.html

Brain surgery has been taking place since the late Stone Age. Tools from 7000 B.C. have been discovered, as well as evidence showing that such surgeries were often successful.

Neurosurgeon.com: Topics in Neurosurgery
http://neurosurgeon.com/

Search for a neurosurgeon by location.

Neurosurgery://On-Call
http://www.neurosurgery.org/splash.html

Homepage for the American Association of Neurological Surgeons and the Congress of Neurological Surgeons. Public pages describe neurosurgery, allow you to chat with a neurosurgeon and locate one in your area, and provide highlights of neurosurgical news and advancements in treatment. Additional resources for professionals include abstracts, jobs, meetings, and educational opportunities.

Neurosurgery Online
http://www.neurosurgery-online.com/

Official web version of the journal of the Congress of Neurological Surgeons. Complete text of articles available up to December 31, 1998; subscription required to access subsequent editions.

Tumors

ABTA Dictionary for Brain Tumor Patients
http://neurosurgery.mgh.harvard.edu/abta/diction.htm

Defines the many terms a patient with a brain tumor may encounter.

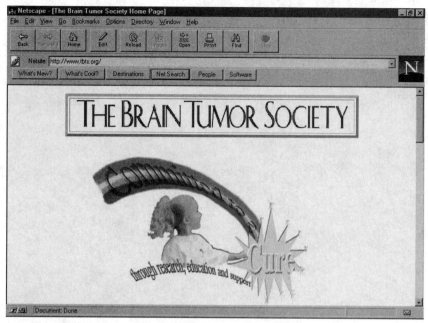

The Brain Tumor Society. *http://www.tbts.org/*

Brain Tumor Society

http://www.tbts.org/

Basic information and resources for patients and health care professionals, bibliography, frequently asked questions, events and conferences.

BRAINTMR Listserv & Bulletin Board

http://tbcnet.com/~jleonard/braintmr/braintmr_hints.htm

To subscribe, send e-mail to *listserv@mitvma.mit.edu* and in the body of the message write "subscribe braintmr *yourfullname*."

Clinical Trials and Noteworthy Treatments for Brain Tumors

http://www.virtualtrials.com/

Browse by tumor type or by treatment: e.g., surgery, radiation, chemotherapy, "less toxics," and immunotherapy. Also find brain tumor news, survivor stories, live chat, newsletter, and many other resources.

Primer of Brain Tumors

http://neurosurgery.mgh.harvard.edu/abta/abta/primer.htm

A manual for patients. Divided into sections, e.g.: *What are brain tumors? Who gets them? What are symptoms? How are they diagnosed?* and *How are they treated?*

CANCER / ONCOLOGY

Bladder Cancer

Bladder Cancer

http://www.mediconsult.com/mc/mcsite.nsf/conditionnav/bladder~section introduction

News updates, cancer basics, bladder cancer information, more.

Bladder Cancer Fact Sheets and Other Information

http://cancernet.nci.nih.gov/wwwprot/minorities/fs_menus/Bladder_cancer.html

Includes risk factors, possible causes, cancer therapy, and rehabilitation.

Bone Marrow Transplantation

See also: Transplantation - Bone Marrow Transplantation.

Blood and Marrow Transplant Newsletter

http://www.bmtnews.org/

For many people diagnosed with leukemia, aplastic anemia and other life-threatening diseases, their only hope for survival is a bone marrow transplant. Chances for a match are very small. This newsletter offers information and support services to bone marrow, peripheral blood stem cell, and cord blood transplant patients and survivors. Written for laypeople.

Bone Marrow Donors Worldwide
http://WWW.BMDW.ORG/

Participants are 42 bone marrow donor registries from 34 countries, and 18 cord blood registries from 12 countries.

The Bone Marrow Foundation
http://www.bonemarrow.org/

Newsletter, patient assistance, frequently asked questions, resources, literature and, with free registration, "Ask the Expert" and "SupportLine" features. Site is for both those wishing to donate and for those in need of donations.

Caitlin Raymond International Registry
http://www.crir.org/

Resource for physicians and patients conducting a search for nonrelated bone marrow and cord blood donors. Accesses information on more than 27,000 international donors annually, not including those participating in the U.S. National Marrow Donor Program.

National Marrow Donor Program
http://www.marrow.org/

This organization maintains a computerized registry of volunteer donors. Visit this site to find out how you can be a donor, find a donor, and how to get financial help.

Virtual Autologous Transplant
http://www.rush.edu/Departments/bmt/AutologousBMT/vabmt.html

Using illustration and text, this site describes the process of autologous bone marrow transplant, where the patient is his or her own marrow donator.

Carcinogens
See also: Environmental Health.

ATSDR Cancer Policy Framework
http://www.atsdr.cdc.gov/cancer.html

Addresses public health concerns relating to carcinogens, from the Agency for Toxic Substances and Disease Registry.

Environmental Tobacco Smoke
http://www.epa.gov/iaq/ets.html

Also called "secondhand smoke." Find out the facts, including risks and prevention. Information from the Environmental Protection Agency.

Huff's Carcinogen Information Page
http://www.mwsc.edu/~dmh1008/

Includes articles, reports and studies of a number of cancer-causing agents, statistics and cancer information.

Report on Carcinogens
http://ntp-server.niehs.nih.gov/Main_pages/NTP_8RoC_pg.html

Includes chemicals that are known to be carcinogens and chemicals that are suspected to be carcinogens. Appendices cover manufacturing processes and conditions that may cause cancer, glossary, acronyms and more.

Chemotherapy

Adjuvant Chemotherapy
http://cancerguide.org/adjuvant.html

This article explains adjuvant chemotherapy, the use of drugs to help treat cancers that have spread beyond their original site.

Chemotherapy
http://www.cancer-info.com/chemo.htm

Includes a listserv for chemotherapy support, and a link to a list and description of the different chemotherapeutic agents used in treating cancer.

Chemotherapy and You:
A Guide to Self-Help During Treatment
http://cancernet.nci.nih.gov/chemotherapy/chemoint.html

This handbook for patients answers questions about what to expect from chemotherapy, how it works, coping with side effects, nutrition and emotional support during the therapy, how to pay for the therapy, and further resources.

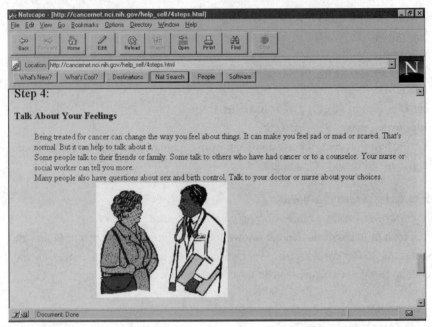

Chemotherapy: How You Can Help. http://cancernet.nci.nih.gov/help_self/4steps.html

Chemotherapy and Your Emotions
http://www0.delphi.com/medsup/chemo.html

Managing the feelings you may have while undergoing chemotherapy.

Chemotherapy: How You Can Help
http://cancernet.nci.nih.gov/help_self/4steps.html

Four steps to follow that can help you in this difficult time.

Colon Cancer

Colon and Rectal Cancers
http://www.meds.com/colon/frameset12.html

Anatomy of the colon and rectum; and classification, symptoms and diagnosis of cancer.

Colon Cancer
http://cancernet.nci.nih.gov/clinpdq/pif/Colon_cancer_Patient.html

Description, stages and treatment information on colon cancer.

Colon Cancer Information Library

http://www.meds.com/colon/colon.html

Articles on colon cancer. The majority of information is for health care professionals, but there are a number of links for patients, too.

Colon Polyps and Colon Cancer

http://www.maxinet.com/mansell/polyp.htm

Common questions and answers, and information about the diagnosis, prognosis and treatment of colon polyps and colon cancer.

Colorectal Cancer At-A-Glance

http://www.cdc.gov/nccdphp/dcpc/colorctl/colorect.htm

The emphasis of this site is on early detection through screening.

Endocrine Cancers

Endocrine Malignancies

http://www.ncl.ac.uk/~nchwww/guides/clinks2e.htm

Information on thyroid, pancreatic, adrenocortical, pituitary, parathyroid and thymus cancers.

Endocrine-Related Cancer

http://journals.endocrinology.org/ERC/erc.htm

Abstracts of articles appearing in this journal of the Society of Endocrinology. Downloadable text of complete articles available in PDF format.

Information for Patients: Endocrine Cancers

http://www.graylab.ac.uk/cancerweb/patients/endocrin.html

Takes you to information from the National Cancer Institute.

OncoLink: Endocrine System Cancers

http://oncolink.upenn.edu/disease/endocrine1/

Provides general information and CancerLit links to articles on the different kinds of endocrine cancers.

Esophageal Cancer

Cathy's Esophageal Cancer Café
http://www.tznet.com/wolfgram/ec/cafe/
   Lots of good information. Discusses the causes of esophageal cancer, treatment options (e.g., alternative therapy, chemotherapy, radiation, experimental therapy and surgery), dietary recommendations and more.

Esophageal Cancer Mailing List
http://www.tznet.com/wolfgram/ec/cafe/articles/subscribe.html-ssi
   To subscribe to this mailing list, send e-mail to: *LISTSERV@LISTSERV. ACOR.ORG* and in the message, write: "Subscribe EC-Group *Firstname Lastname.*"

OncoLink: Esophageal Cancer
http://cancer.med.upenn.edu/disease/esophageal/
   Includes frequently asked questions, journal scan, cancer news and clinical trials search.

Seattle Barrett's Esophagus Program
http://www.fhcrc.org/~barretts/
   Information and research, publications, articles and links.

Kidney Cancer

Kidney Cancer
http://www.uro.com/renalca.htm
   Basic information explaining what kidney cancer (renal cell carcinoma) is, risk factors, symptoms, diagnosis and treatment.

Kidney Cancer Association
http://www.nkca.org/index.stm
   National organization. Provides patient information and support, as well as information on research, clinical trials and advocacy projects.

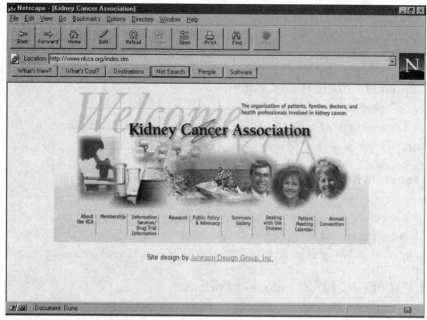

Kidney Cancer Association. *http://www.nkca.org/index.stm*

Renal Cell Cancer

http://cancernet.nci.nih.gov/clinpdq/soa/Renal_cell_cancer_Physician.html

Information that is primarily for physicians and other health care professionals.

Leukemia

Childhood Leukemia Center

http://www.patientcenters.com/leukemia/

For parents and others caring for a child with leukemia. Assistance in coping, communicating with children, preparing them for hospitalization, and more.

GrannyBarb and Art's Leukemia Links

http://www.acor.org/diseases/hematology/Leukemia/leukemia.html

A great deal of information on leukemia and bone marrow transplant, as well as support and resources for leukemia patients, leukemia survivor stories, and more.

Leukaemia Research Fund

http://www.leukaemia.demon.co.uk/patinfo.htm

Online patient information booklets and leaflets.

Leukemia Information Center

http://www.meds.com/leukemia/leukemia.html

Comprehensive library of information on adult myelogenous leukemia (AML) for health care professionals and consumers.

Leukemia Society of America

http://www.leukemia.org/

Leukemia, lymphoma, myeloma and Hodgkin's disease information and statistics, educational pamphlets and booklets; chapter finder, society and member information and events; research, patient services, links, and news and media briefs.

A List of URLs for Leukemia Patients

http://rattler.cameron.edu/leukemia/

Links to leukemia information and support groups on the web.

OncoLink: Adult Leukemias

http://www.oncolink.upenn.edu/disease/leukemia1/

"Bone Marrow Transplant" newsletter and CancerNet updates on acute lymphoblastic leukemia, acute myeloid leukemia, hairy cell leukemia, and much more. Information for physicians and patients.

OncoLink: Pediatric Leukemias

http://www.oncolink.upenn.edu/disease/leukemia/

Frequently asked questions, survival stories, journal scan, and CancerLit search on Hodgkin's disease, non-Hodgkin's disease, chronic myelogenous leukemia, cutaneous T-cell lymphoma, and links.

Yahoo's Diseases and Conditions: Leukemia

http://dir.yahoo.com/Health/Diseases_and_Conditions/Leukemia/

Links to leukemia sites on the Internet.

Lung Cancer

American Cancer Society Lung Cancer Resource Center

http://www3.cancer.org/cancerinfo/res_home.asp?ct=26

The American Cancer Society describes incidence, prevention, signs and symptoms, risk factors, treatment and chances of survival of lung cancer.

Environmental Tobacco Smoke

http://www.epa.gov/iaq/ets.html

Also called "secondhand smoke." Find out the facts, including risks and prevention. Information from the Environmental Protection Agency.

The Lung Cancer and Cigarette Smoking Web Page

http://ourworld.compuserve.com/homepages/LungCancer/

Over 90 percent of lung cancers are caused by cigarette smoking. Site offers information, statistics and links.

Lung Cancer Information Library

http://www.meds.com/lung/lunginfo.html

Information for professionals and patients.

Lung Cancer Online

http://www.lungcanceronline.org/

Gateway to resources on lung cancer. Offers good descriptions and is organized by topic. Includes section on "finding the best care," and medical news updates.

OncoLink: Lung Cancer

http://www.oncolink.com/disease/lung1/

Addresses lung cancer, offering general information about the disease and more specific articles on related topics such as lung cancer screening, prevention, treatment and support, as well as how to quit smoking.

Lymphoma

Cure for Lymphoma Foundation
http://www.cfl.org/
> This foundation supports research and programs to find a cure for lymphoma. Patient information also available at this site.

Glossary of Lymphoma Terms
http://www.lymphomainfo.net/lymphoma/glossary.html
> Easy reference tool to terms a patient suffering from lymphoma may encounter.

Hodgkin's Disease Mail List
http://www.deltronix.com/public/hodgkins/home.htm
> Search their archives and join the list. Information on non-Hodgkin's lymphoma also available.

Hodgkin's Disease Resource Center
http://www3.cancer.org/cancerinfo/res_home.asp?st=wi&ct=20
> Information from the American Cancer Society.

Lymphoma Information Network
http://www.lymphomainfo.net/
> Information on Hodgkin's disease and non-Hodgkin's lymphoma. Written for patients in easy-to-understand and compassionate language. Contains lymphoma support resources.

Lymphoma Research Foundation of America
http://www.lymphoma.org/
> The Foundation supports research, while simultaneously working to educate and support lymphoma patients and their families. Site describes grant process and current research, and hosts a lymphoma helpline, forums, and advocacy.

NHL Cyber Family
http://www.wizard.com/NHL/
> Non-Hodgkin's lymphoma mailing list and links.

Non-Hodgkin's Lymphoma Web Site

http://www.Westvirginia.net/~sigley/NHL_Web_Site.htm

Offers links, treatment information, op/ed pages (under construction at this time), the Human Side (with personal stories), and clinical trial postings.

Melanoma

See also Skin Cancer, later in this chapter.

Checking for Melanoma

http://www.aad.org/ss98/ss98abcd_melanoma.html

As easy as ABCD: check the spot's Assymetry, Border, Color and Diameter.

StopMelanoma.com

http://www.stopmelanoma.com/

Includes a list of links to melanoma sites, patients' stories, melanoma in the media and more.

Melanoma Patients' Information Page

http://www.mpip.org/

Information for patients, abstract search, clinical trials, tools and more.

Melanoma Research Foundation

http://www.melanoma.org/

The Foundation was formed by melanoma patients and survivors to fund melanoma research because there is currently no cure. Newsletter, volunteering, links, memorial page and more.

OncoLink: Melanoma

http://oncolink.upenn.edu/disease/melanoma/index.html

Melonoma research, clinical trials, news, journal briefs and patient information.

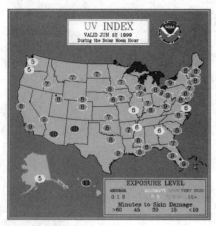

Ultraviolet Index.
http://nic.fb4.noaa.gov:80/products/strato
sphere/uv_index/uvi_map.gif

Skin Cancer: Safe Sun Tips
*http://www.aad.org/SkinCancerNews/
SafeSunTips/index.html*
Sun safety tips for adults and kids.

Sun Protection
http://www.travelhealth.com/sun.htm
Information about how to protect
your skin from harmful ultraviolet rays.

Ultraviolet Index
http://www.nws.noaa.gov/om/uvi.htm
You can find out the day's UV
Index for most major cities around the
country at this site.

Myeloma

Cancer Information Resources
http://myeloma.org/imf_ocir.html
Multiple myeloma is cancer of the bone marrow that results in the uncontrolled
growth of plasma cells. Lots of myeloma resources, and links to leukemia and other
cancer sites.

International Myeloma Foundation
http://myeloma.org/
This site provides good, basic information on myeloma. Information provided
in Spanish as well.

The Multiple Myeloma Research Foundation
http://www.multiplemyeloma.org/
Includes a newsletter for multiple myeloma, patient resources, news and links.

Multiple Myeloma Research Web Server
http://myeloma.med.cornell.edu/
A multitude of information and links for health care practitioners.

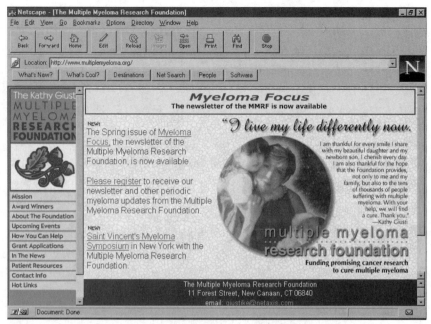

The Multiple Myeloma Research Foundation. http://www.multiplemyeloma.org/

Myeloma Central

http://home.att.net/~vincentvr/index.html

Useful links to myeloma frequently asked questions, resources and cancer-related sites.

Organizations

American Cancer Society

http://www.cancer.org/

Information on ACS programs, which include the Great American Smokeout, Relay for Life, and the Breast Cancer Network. General and specific cancer information (e.g., breast, prostate, colorectal and lung) is available, as well as cancer statistics addressing racial and ethnic patterns, nutrition and diet, environmental risks, etc. Also includes publications, meeting announcements, and links.

International Union Against Cancer

http://www-uicc.who.ch/

There are over 200 member oganizations from 90 countries in this nongovernmental society that works to reduce the mortality and morbidity of cancer.

National Cancer Institute

http://www.nci.nih.gov/

The NCI is the federal government's principal agency for cancer research and training. It coordinates the National Cancer Program and the research efforts of various universities, hospitals and businesses, and it conducts research in its own laboratories and clinics. It also supports education and training, and collects and shares information on cancer. Links can be found to CancerNet and other databases.

Pain Management

American Academy of Pain Management

http://www.aapainmanage.org/index.html

Resources for patients help them to locate a pain management program in their area. Resources for professionals include continuing education and accreditation information, data bank, and discussion group.

Cancer Pain Management

http://www.csccc.com/newslett/art1296.htm

Article for physicians on how to assess and how to manage a cancer patient's chronic pain.

Cancer Pain

http://www.acponline.org/public/h_care/3-pain.htm

Information for patients from the American College of Physicians on cancer pain. Includes how to get help, possible concerns, methods and expectations.

Cancer Pain Page

http://www.mdacc.tmc.edu/~acc/new/home.html

Homepage for the University of Texas, M.D. Anderson Cancer Center's Anesthesiology and Critical Care Department's Pain Program.

The Management of Cancer Pain
http://pain.roxane.com/library/TMOCP/
   Online reprint of article appearing in *CA: A Cancer Journal for Clinicians.*

Managing Cancer Pain: A Consumer's Guide
http://text.nlm.nih.gov/ftrs/tocview
   Downloadable files for this guide from the National Library of Medicine.

Myths about Cancer Pain
http://www-hsc.usc.edu/~dcundiff/mythpain.html
   Six myths about opioids that can interfere with cancer pain management.

Opioid Calculator
http://www.stat.washington.edu/TALARIA/calculatorjava.html
   Helps physicians to determines the proper dosage of pain killer.

Talaria
http://www.statsci.com/talaria/talariahome.html
   Subtitled "The Hypermedia Assistant for Cancer Pain Management," this site for health care professionals addresses issues relating to the management of pain in cancer patients. It includes guidelines, a calculator for drug conversions, links, and movie clips on pain management.

Pancreatic Cancer

Pancreatic Cancer
http://imsdd.meb.uni-bonn.de/cancernet/100046.html
   Information on the classification, treatment and stages of pancreatic cancer, for medical professionals.

Pancreas Cancer Home Page
http://www.path.jhu.edu/pancreas
   Website details research and and clinical advancements in pancreatic cancer, as well as hosts a chat room for patients and their families. Illustrations of pancreatic cancer, frequently asked questions section and much more.

Introduction to Cancer of the Pancreas

http://oncolink.upenn.edu/disease/pancreas/intro_pancreas.html

Incidence, risk factors, clinical manifestations, diagnosis and treatment.

Pathology

Pathology Simplified

http://www.erinet.com/fnadoc/path.htm

Good information for patients about lung cancer, breast cancer, and Pap smear tests. Includes photo archives, and hotlinks.

Prevention

The Cancer Nutrition Center

http://www.cancernutrition.com/

Discusses the connection between cancer and nutrition. Dietary habits are considered as both contributing to and as being a treatment for cancer. This site allows you to access the Cancer Nutrition Handbook and related lectures.

Cancer Preventions Conversations

http://commtechlab.msu.edu/sites/prevention/index.html

Common questions and answers concerning cancer and nutrition, sun exposure, physical activity and tobacco exposure.

Food, Nutrition and the Prevention of Cancer

http://www.aicr.org:80/report2.htm

This report on diet and cancer prevention produced by an expert panel of 15 of the world's leading researchers provides dietary guidelines and public policy recommendations.

Harvard Center for Cancer Prevention

http://www.hsph.harvard.edu/cancer/

Includes cancer prevention brochures, educational materials, cancer prevention guidelines, newsletter and more.

Recipes for Healthier Eating
http://www.aicr.org:80/recipe2.htm

This site is maintained by the American Institute for Cancer Research, and it provides tasty, nutritious, simple, low fat recipes.

Publications

CA: A Cancer Journal for Clinicians
http://www.ca-journal.org/

This is a peer-reviewed online journal from the American Cancer Society. View full text of articles from current and past issues. Searchable.

Cancer Detection and Prevention
http://www.cancerprev.org/

Bimonthly cancer journal of the International Society for Preventive Oncology. Search through abstracts of current and earlier issues.

Cancer Online
http://journals.wiley.com/canceronline/interim.html

View table of contents and read abstracts from current and previous issues of this interdisciplinary international journal published by the American Cancer Society. Full access with paid subscription only.

Journal of Clinical Oncology
http://www.jco.org/

The official journal of the American Society of Clinical Oncology.

Journal of the National Cancer Institute
http://jnci.oupjournals.org/

Published twice a month. Abstracts and news summaries are available online. Subscription required for full text.

Reviews on Cancer Online (ROCO)
http://www1.elsevier.nl/journals/roco/Menu.html

This journal deals with the new developments in cancer investigation at the molecular level. Both subscription and general cancer information can be obtained at this site.

Radiation Therapy

CancerInfo for Patients
http://www.bmi.net/mcaron/cancer.html

Information on radiation therapy and chemotherapy. Includes descriptions, recommended diets, side effects and pain management.

Radiation Oncology Online Journal
http://www.rooj.com/

Radiation oncology information and resources for the public and health care professionals. Information for patients includes description, side effects and treatment of side effects. Information for professionals includes articles, dose calculators, professional organizations, journals, and more.

Radiation Therapy Information Site
http://www.radiation-oncology.com/radonc/html

General information, cancer-specific information, supportive care and resources.

Research

American Institute for Cancer Research Online
http://www.aicr.org:80/

This page discusses the relation of nutrition and diet to cancer. According to this site, researchers estimate that 35% or more of cancer deaths are linked to our dietary choices. Find consumer information and information on AICR grants, as well as links and research news. Includes weekly cooking columns.

International Cancer Alliance for Research and Education
http://icare.org/

Site serves as a cancer information network and includes access to cancer registry, *Cancer Therapy Review* and to research updates. Also includes a cancer newsletter, an area where patients are able to describe their own experiences, a library of cancer and related information, and areas entitled "think tanks" —where small groups of physicians, researchers and patients discuss therapy issues relating to specific forms of cancer.

National Coalition for Cancer Research

http://www.cancercoalition.org/index.html

Congressional lobbyist group promoting cancer research. Site provides information for the public on cancer, cancer research and political action.

Resources

Cancer Directory

http://www.cancerdirectory.com/

For cancer patients and their families. Offers chat groups, directory of community resources including support groups, nonprofit organizations, medical and professional societies. Also has a cancer products shopping mall, a directory of products related to cancer needs (e.g., skin care products, wigs, prosthetics, books) and companies with services such as massage, home care, and financial aid.

Cancer News on the Net

http://www.cancernews.com/quickload.htm

Includes sites of general interest, news and links to information on specific cancer types such as breast cancer, colon cancer, prostate cancer, etc. Also includes information on prevention, clinical trials, cancer support groups and research efforts. In addition, site features a Cancer News e-mail registry, where users can be electronically informed of new cancer developments.

Cancer Related Links

http://seidata.com/~marriage/rcancer.html

Contains links to government servers; education, research and cancer institutes; journals and newletters; disease-specific sites and more.

CancerGuide: Steve Dunn's Cancer Information Page

http://cancerguide.org/

A great place to start, especially if you are investigating a specific type of cancer. Information on rare as well as more common cancers; bone marrow transplantation, treatment and alternative therapies; where to go for more information; and a "How to research medical literature" section.

Cancerhelp UK
http://medweb.bham.ac.uk/cancerhelp/index.html

Information for the general public about cancer and cancer care. Separate window with glossary terms can be open all the time while you negotiate through pages. Separate section for children.

CancerNet
http://cancernet.nci.nih.gov/

This is the National Cancer Institute's cancer information source for patients and the public, health professionals, and basic researchers. The site offers fact sheets, treatment information, support, clinical trial updates, literature search capability, database access, and a page for children.

CancerTrack
http://www.nova.edu/~appu/cancertrack.htm

This site is a good starting place for cancer research, for it offers links to some of the bigger cancer information resources, including scientific literature, biotechnology sites and pharmacology sites.

CancerWEB
http://www.graylab.ac.uk/cancerweb.html

A great source of information for cancer patients and their families and friends, clinicians and other health care professionals. Discusses cancer treatment, research, prevention, screening and support. Links to additional resources and sites.

Guide to Internet Resources for Cancer
http://www.ncl.ac.uk/~nchwww/guides/clinks1.htm

Over 100 pages of links to cancer information for patients and professionals.

Marie Curie Cancer Care
http://www.mariecurie.org.uk/

This British charity provides free home nursing care to patients suffering from cancer.

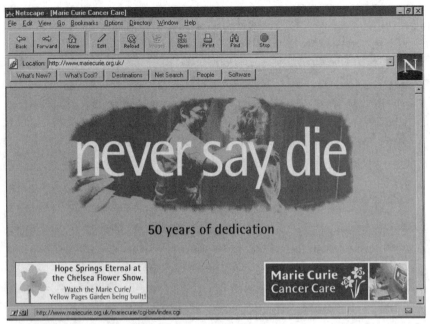

Marie Curie Cancer Care. http://www.mariecurie.org.uk/

OncoLink

http://www.oncolink.upenn.edu/

One of the most comprehensive information sources covering cancer on the web, from the University of Pennsylvania's Cancer Center. Search research literature, link to journals, and get the latest cancer news. There are disease-oriented menus and medical specialty-oriented menus, or else choose from the following: psychosocial support and personal experiences; cancer causes, screening and prevention; clinical trials; global resources; cancer frequently asked questions; symptom management; conferences and meetings; and financial issues for patients.

OncoLink's "Editors' Choice" Awards

http://www.oncolink.upenn.edu/ed_choice

OncoLink's editors have selected Internet resources that, in their opinion, offer the best cancer-related material.

Oncology: From Web Doctor

http://www.gretmar.com/webdoctor/oncology.html

Index of links organized by type of cancer. Also includes caregiver resources, CancerLit link, and journals.

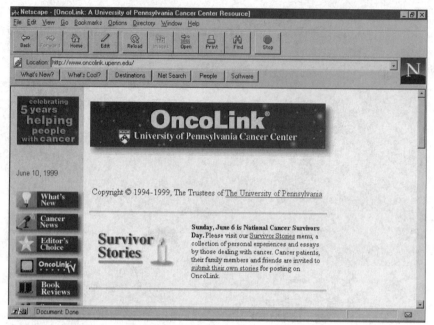

OncoLink. *http://www.oncolink.upenn.edu/*

PDQ: NCI's Comprehensive Cancer Database
http://wwwicic.nci.nih.gov/pdq.htm

PDQ = Physician's Data Query. Use this tool to access peer-reviewed statements on treatment, supportive care, prevention and screening, as well as anti-cancer drugs. These statements are updated monthly. In addition, find a registry of open and closed clinical trials, directories of physicians, organizations and facilities that provide cancer care or cancer screening.

Sarcoma

Kaposi's Sarcoma
http://www.graylab.ac.uk/cancernet/201271.html
Basic information on Kaposi's sarcoma.

Sarcoma Central
http://www.charm.net/~kkdk/sarcoma_html
General information, medical literature searches, treatment options, articles, case studies, and visual images of sarcoma.

Sarcoma Resource Center

http://www3.cancer.org/cancerinfo/res_home.asp?ct=38

Information on adult soft tissue cancer.

Soft-Tissue Sarcoma of the Extremities and Its Mimic

http://rpisun1.mda.uth.tmc.edu/se/sts/index2.html

Magnetic resonance images of sarcoma.

Skin Cancer

See also: Melanoma, earlier in this chapter.

Introduction to Skin Cancer

http://www.maui.net/~southsky/introto.html

Site provides a general introduction to skin cancer and offers links to specific information sources on the Internet. The cause of, description of and risks for skin cancer are addressed, as are diagnosis and treatment information. There is also a daily UV index forecast for 30 cities in the United States.

The Experimental Ultraviolet Index Factsheet

http://www.noaa.gov/uvb/fctsh.html

Explains the UV index to the public and advises on how to use it.

OncoLink: Skin Cancer

http://cancer.med.upenn.edu/disease/skin1/

Information on skin cancer. Includes frequently asked questions.

Skin and Cancer Foundation Australia

http://www.scfa.edu.au/

This site provides basic information and advice on skin cancer and its prevention. Written for teenagers. Information on other skin problems also provided. Special section for specialists and dermatologists.

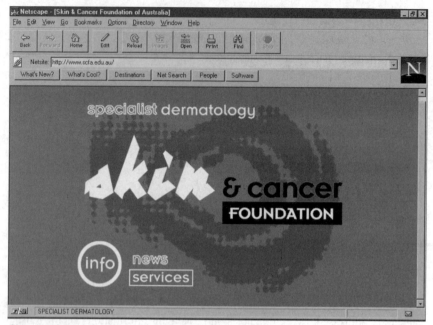

Skin and Cancer Foundation of Australia. http://www.scfa.edu.au/

Skin Cancer

http://www.medinfo.org/nci/cancernet/2/201228.html

The National Cancer Institute has provided these pages containing basic text and information on skin cancer. Includes descriptions of skin cancer, its stages and treatment options.

Skincancerinfo.com

http://skincancerinfo.com/home.html

This site for patients boasts it is "the most informative skin cancer site on the internet." Covers skin basics, pre-cancers, formation and causes of skin cancer, different kinds of skin cancer, atypical moles, spots, melanoma, and much more. For patients.

Tumors of the Skin and Integument

http://www.bioscience.org/atlases/tumpath/skin/resource.htm

Information and resources for both clinicians and patients suffering from tumors of the skin and integument. Includes background on sarcomas, melanomas, and other tumors.

Support for Cancer Patients & Families

The Association of Cancer Online Resources, Inc.
http://www.acor.org/
Hosts over 70 online cancer information and electronic support groups.

Cancer Care, Inc.
http://www.cancercareinc.org/
Find out about different kinds of cancers and services to help cancer patients and their families. Online assistance, contact numbers for support groups, workshops and more.

The Cancer Club
http://www.cancerclub.com/
Humorous site offers helpful products, cartoons and comforting words for those with cancer.

Cancer Information and Support International
http://www.cancer-info.com/
More here than appears at first glance. Find Alternative and Natural Cancer Remedies, books on cancer, news groups, specific cancer information, chat rooms, diet and nutrition, medical symptoms, smoking facts and much more.

Cancer Message Board
http://www.healthboards.com/cancer/
View, post or search the archives of this bulletin board to get your cancer question answered, or to respond to another person's inquiry. Free.

Gilda's Club Home Page
http://www.gildasclub.org/
This is a cancer support community formed in honor of Gilda Radner, the comedian who died of ovarian cancer. The mission is to serve as a place where cancer patients and their family members can share in building social and emotional support. It offers groups, lectures, workshops and social events.

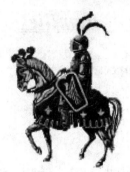

Keepin' the Faith! *http://ktf.org/*

Kcuf Recnac

http://www.kcufrecnac.com/

"This web site is dedicated to causing humorosis in cancer patients." Laughter helps. (Hint: read backwards.)

Keepin' The Faith!

http://ktf.org/

Cancer support for the heart and soul. Includes poems, prayers, jokes, chat groups, personal stories, grief issues and more.

Make-A-Wish Foundation

http://www.wish.org/

Make a wish for yourself or help make the wish of a child who has a life-threatening illness to come true.

OncoChat

http://www.oncochat.org/

Internet relay channel/peer support group for cancer survivors, families and friends. Also has a good list of cancer-related resources, sites and information to be found on the Internet.

OncoLink: Automated E-mail Discussion Group Subscriber

http://oncolink.upenn.edu/forms/listserv.html

Select from more than 75 different listservers covering various cancers.

Shared Experience: Cancer Care and Support

http://www.sharedexperience.org/

Learn from others by reading their experience with cancer and cancer treatments, or add your own story to help other patients, family and friends to understand what it is like.

Treatment/Recovery

See also: Chemotherapy; Radiation Therapy; and Clinical Trials - Cancer.

ACS Alternative and Complementary Therapies

http://www3.cancer.org/cancerinfo/acs_frame.asp?frame=altmeth.html

Lots of information. Includes a general overview, articles and information on specific alternative and complementary therapies.

Alternative Therapies

http://www.cancer-info.com/alt-ther.htm

Some information on alternative cancer therapies, especially essiac, which is used to fight cancer and counter the side effects of chemotherapy.

Cancer Treatment Centers of America

http://www.cancercenter.com/

Covers many different treatment options for cancer. Provides frequently asked questions, information on clinical trials, and more.

CancerAnswers: General Cancer Treatment Information

http://www.canceranswers.com/general.html

Written for the general public. Describes conventional cancer treatments, including surgery, chemotherapy, radiation therapy and hormone therapy, and comments on alternative therapy.

Center for Alternative Medicine Research in Cancer

http://www.sph.uth.tmc.edu/utcam/

Good reviews of alternative cancer therapies, such as different herbs and diets.

Complementary and Alternative Medicine Resources for Cancer Research on the World Wide Web

http://cpmcnet.columbia.edu/dept/rosenthal/Guide6.html

Includes steps for completing a search and suggested resources.

European Organization for Research and Treatment of Cancer

http://www.eortc.be/

This organization seeks to conduct, develop, coordinate, and stimulate research in Europe on the experimental and clinical bases of treatment of cancer.

Home Care Guide for Advanced Cancer

http://www.acponline.org/public/h_care/index.html

Online handbook from the American College of Physicians. Includes a dying person's guide to dying, caregiving advice, cancer pain management, shortness of breath and other topics.

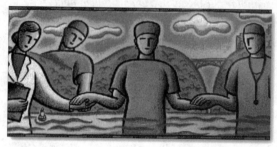

National Comprehensive Cancer Network.
http://www.nccn.org/

National Comprehensive Cancer Network

http://www.nccn.org/

This network is made up of seventeen leading cancer centers across the United States.

Oncology Drug Reviews

http://pharminfo.com:80/pubs/msb/msbonc.html

Updates on drug therapy for cancer treatment as well as links between specific drugs and chemicals and the risk of cancer.

Patient Clinical Trial Information

http://cancernet.nci.nih.gov/p_clinic.htm

Explains what clinical trials are about, and how to find one to participate in.

Rational Approach to the Use of Alternative Medicine in Cancer Therapy

http://www.teleport.com/~ormed/article1.htm

Text of an essay on alternative treatments for cancer.

Q and A About Complementary and Alternative Medicine in Cancer Treatment

http://cancernet.nci.nih.gov/clinpdq/umethods/Q_and_A_About_Complementary_and_Alternative_Medicine_in_Cancer_Treatment.html

Answers basic questions for patients considering complementary or alternative medical treatments of cancer.

State of the Art Oncology in Europe

http://telescan.nki.nl/start/start.html

The objective of this European group is to maintain a concise database on the state-of-the-art treatment of human malignant tumors.

Treatment Information, National Cancer Institute

http://cancernet.nci.nih.gov/h_treat.htm

Cancer treatment summaries, therapy facts, and cancer information by location and type.

CHILDREN'S HEALTH / PEDIATRICS

Covered in this chapter: Adolescents; Asthma; Cancer; Child Development; Child Safety; Chronic Illness; Common Conditions; Dental Health; Diabetes; Diet & Nutrition; Disabled Children; Heart (Cardiology); HIV/AIDS; Immunizations; Infant Care; Neonatology; Neurosurgery; Organizations; Orthopedics; Pain Management; Parenting; Pathology; Radiology; Resources; Single Parents; Sudden Infant Death Syndrome; Surgery; Teen Parents.

Related chapters: Drugs/Pharmacology - Children; Pregnancy & Childbirth.

Adolescents

See also: HIV/AIDS and Teen Parents, later in this chapter.

Acne Agony

http://www.fda.gov/opacom/catalog/ots_acne.html

What causes acne and how it can be treated. Online article is part of the Food and Drug Administration's "On the Teen Scene."

ADOL: Adolescence Directory On Line

http://education.indiana.edu/cas/adol/adol.html

Includes resources on conflict and violence, mental health and physical health; as well as counselor resources and a section entitled "For Teens Only."

Adolescent Health Articles

http://www.ama-assn.org/insight/ h_focus/adl_hlth/teen/teen.htm

Site provides information for teens on violence, peer pressure, family issues, personal health issues, sexual health, and alcohol and drugs.

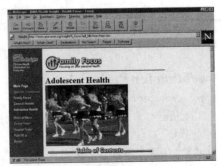

Adolescent Health Articles.
http://www.ama-assn.org/insight/h_focus/ adl_hlth/teen/teen.htm

165

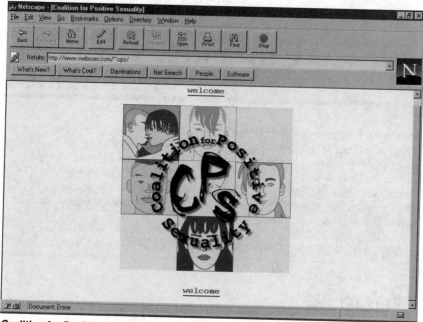

Coalition for Positive Sexuality. *http://www.webcom.com/~cps/*

The AIDS Handbook

http://www.westnet.com/~rickd/AIDS/AIDS1.html

Written by middle school kids for middle school kids to provide a better understanding of AIDS prevention, transmission, symptoms, treatment and how the immune system fights disease. Links.

CAPS Hot Topic: Adolescents

http://www.epibiostat.ucsf.edu/capsweb/hotteens.html

Chat-line and information on youth programs, fact sheets and opinions, articles and research on sexuality, HIV infection and adolescents.

Coalition for Positive Sexuality

http://www.webcom.com/~cps/

Information about sexuality for teenagers.

Does Your Friend Have a Drug Or Alcohol Problem?

http://www.health.org/pubs/guidteen.htm

What teens can do to help their friends who they think may have a substance abuse problem.

Girl Power! Get Body Wise!

http://www.health.org/gpower/girlarea/bodywise/

Information for teenage girls on healthy eating and fitness habits, body image and more.

Puberty 101

http://www.virtualkid.com/p101/p101_menu.shtml

A place for teens to go to find honest answers to their questions about puberty and the changes they are experiencing.

YouthHIV.com

http://www.youthHIV.org/

News, features, links, roundtable and HIV fact sheets and information for teenagers.

YOUTHINFO

http://youth.os.dhhs.gov/

The Department of Health and Human Services provides information about America's adolescents. Includes a profile of America's youth, parental resources, reports and publications on substance abuse, teen pregnancy, violence and other health topics; links and more.

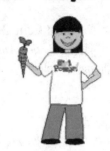

Eating Right the Girl Power! Way

Girl Power! Get Body Wise!
http://www.health.org/gpower/girlarea/bodywise/

Asthma

See also: Allergy & Immunology; Lungs/Respiratory & Pulmonary.

Asthma

http://galen.med.virginia.edu/~smb4v/tutorials/asthma/asthma1.html

Multimedia asthma tutorial for kids and their parents. Audio and images discuss what is asthma, why it occurs, what are the symptoms of asthma, and how it is treated.

Asthma Information Page

http://www.allergy-clinic.com/ASTHMA.HTM

Information on what an asthma attack is, how to control and prevent an asthma attack, eliminating asthma triggers, asthma and exercise and more.

Being a Sport with Exercise-Induced Asthma
http://www.fda.gov/opacom/catalog/ots_asth.html
Online article from the FDA is part of "On the Teen Scene."

Your Asthma Can Be Controlled
http://www.nhlbi.nih.gov/nhlbi/lung/asthma/gp/asthma.htm
Online pamphlet discusses what you can do to gain control of your asthma.

Cancer
See also: Cancer/Oncology.

Candlelighters Childhood Cancer Foundation
http://www.candlelighters.org/
Nonprofit agency for parents of children with cancer provides support, advocacy and information.

Childhood Cancer
http://kidshealth.org/parent/healthy/cancer.html
Article provides basic information on childhood cancers, including leukemia, lymphoma and osteosarcoma.

Emory University Pediatric Oncology Resources
http://www.emory.edu/PEDS/onc.htm
Lots of links to online resources about pediatric cancer or oncology in general.

Guide to Internet Resources for Childhood Cancer
http://www.ncl.ac.uk/~nchwww/guides/guide2.htm
Provides an index to some of the key cancer-related sites. Many links to online resources about pediatric cancer. Includes a menu for disease-specific information.

Jule's Home Page for CancerKids
http://www.geocities.com/Broadway/2616/
Page was created by a teenager who suffered from leukemia to show how cancer may have changed her but did not take her over. Information and resources on leukemia and other cancers.

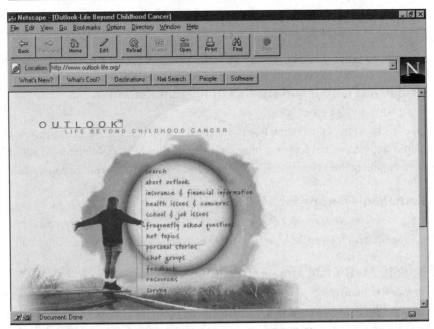

Outlook: Life Beyond Childhood Cancer. *http://www.outlook-life.org*

Kid's Home at NCI

http://wwwicic.nci.nih.gov/occdocs/KidsHome.html

This site of the National Cancer Institute site provides pictures and stories by and for kids who are receiving treatment for cancer; and information for parents.

Melinda's Page for Cancer Kids

http://www.monkey-boy.com/melinda/

Created by a 15-year-old cancer patient. Information, contacts and games.

National Childhood Cancer Foundation/Children's Cancer Group

http://www.nccf.org/

The NCCF supports pediatric cancer and treatment projects. The Children's Cancer Group is a network of 2800 cancer specialists. This site includes fact sheets, information, news, resources, personal stories, and NCCF and CCG background.

Outlook: Life Beyond Pediatric Cancer

http://www.outlook-life.org/

Addresses the needs of survivors of childhood cancer and their families. Includes insurance, job and financial information, chat room and more.

Pediatric Oncology Group Web Site

http://www.pog.ufl.edu/

Research and clinical trials to fight childhood and adolescent cancers.

Pediatrics: Childhood Brain Tumor Foundation

http://www.mnsinc.com/cbtf/

The mission of the Foundation is to raise funds for research efforts, to increase public awareness, and improve prognosis and quality of life of those who suffer from childhood brain tumors. Site contains articles, links, and Foundation news.

Radiation Therapy for Pediatric Cancer

http://www.oncolink.upenn.edu/specialty/ped_onc/radiation/pedschap/index.html

Online article from the University of Pennsylvania Cancer Center's OncoLink.

Ronald McDonald House Charities

http://www.rmhc.com/

The Ronald McDonald Houses are temporary lodging facilities where families of children being treated for cancer or other serious illnesses may stay while the child receives medical care at a nearby hospital. This site describes the program's start, its philosophy, and how to get involved. There are now more than 197 Ronald McDonald Houses in 16 different countries.

Child Development

ABC of ECD

http://www.worldbank.org/children/

Describes what early child development (ECD) is and provides information for program supervisors of all kinds to help them in their efforts to promote the growth and development of children from birth to age eight.

American Academy of Child and Adolescent Psychiatry Homepage

http://www.aacap.org/

This is a public service site that offers *Facts for Families*, a series of pamphlets for parents on issues that affect children, such as depression, parental divorce, abuse and violence. Related topics are clinical practice, public health and managed care. Also find publications, research papers, meeting and legislative updates.

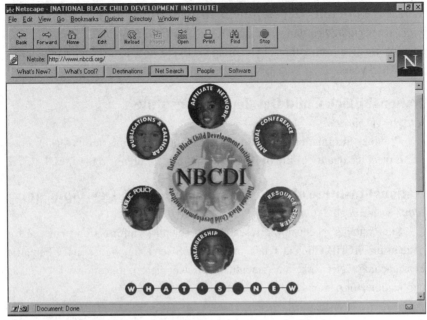

National Black Child Development Institute. *http://www.nbcdi.org/*

Behavior OnLine
http://www.behavior.net/index.html

For mental health professionals and applied behavioral scientists. Primarily contains ongoing discussions and editorials.

Child Development
http://laf.cioe.com/~mrshawn/Welcome.html

Tips for parents and teachers on child and infant behavior, finding child care, book reviews, checklist for child development, age-appropriate activities and more.

The Child Development Website
http://idealist.com/children/

Learn about different development theories, chat, or sign up for a free newsletter. Information for parents and those who work in childhood education or childhood development.

Child Health and Development Information
http://www.public.health.wa.gov.au/PAGES/SUPCHILD.html

Information from asthma, to learning to talk, to worms, for parents of children ages 0 to 5 years.

National Black Child Development Institute
http://www.nbcdi.org/

Provides information about this organization whose mission is "to improve and protect the quality of life of African American children and families."

National Institute of Child Health and Human Development
http://www.nih.gov:80/nichd/

Site contains recent news, research and scientific information; material for patients on NICHD Clinical Trials, the Back to Sleep Campaign, and the Pediatric Pharmacology Network; and scientific and technical publications, as well as publications for patients and the general public.

Child Safety

Children's Safety Network
http://www.edc.org/HHD/csn/

Provides resources and technical assistance to maternal and child health agencies and other organizations seeking to reduce unintentional injuries and violence to children and adolescents.

ChildSecure
http://www.childsecure.com/

Children's health and safety advice, "Ask the Doctor" e-mail action, discussion groups, online shopping for child health and safety products, pediatric news, consumer alerts, book reviews, parents' page and links to interesting sites.

Injury Control Resource Information Network
http://www.injurycontrol.com/icrin/

Connects you to Internet resources on injury control. Main sections include government agencies, injury data and statistics, publications and bibliographies, references, education and training, safety products, discussion groups, professional groups, injury-specific sites (drowning, transportation, etc.) and much more.

Introduction to Baby Proofing

http://poolfence.com/intro.htm

A room-by-room guide. Includes latches, kitchen, food safety, bedroom, bath, garage and swimming pool safety tips.

National SAFE KIDS Campaign

http://www.safekids.org/

This organization is devoted solely to the prevention of unintentional childhood injuries. It includes helpful fact sheets, frequently asked questions, a checklist of family safety, links and an online quiz.

The Parent's Guide to the Internet

http://www.geocities.com/EnchantedForest/Tower/4241/

Information for adults about the Internet and how to keep children safe online.

Protect Your Children on the Internet

http://www.med.jhu.edu/peds/neonatology/protect.html#protect

A number of links to articles, discussions, sites and computer software addressing safety on the Internet.

Safensoundkids Children's Safety Products

http://www.safensoundkids.com/

All sorts of child safety products online.

U.S. Consumer Product Safety Commission

http://www.cpsc.gov/

Includes a number of pamphlets related to child safety; for example, children's furniture and toy safety, child drowning prevention, poison prevention, and more. Also includes an area where items that have been recalled are announced.

Chronic Illness

Band-Aides And Blackboards

http://funrsc.fairfield.edu/~jfleitas/contents.html

Describes what it is like to grow up with a serious illness. Separate parts for children, teens and adults. Stories, activities, tips on coping and much more.

Children's Life Link, Inc.
http://pages.prodigy.com/cllin/home.htm

Site describes this organization which helps seriously ill children by aiding in their transportation expenses. Links.

Rare Genetic Diseases in Children
http://mcrcr2.med.nyu.edu/murphp01/homenew.htm

This support resources directory is for parents whose children suffer from rare genetic disorders, and it offers links to hospice groups, death and dying support sites, parent-to-parent groups, respite care information, mailing lists, newsgroups and bulletin boards. Find both disease-specific and more general support links.

Common Conditions

Common Cold
http://KidsHealth.org/parent/common/cold.html

Signs and symptoms, treatment and when to consult a pediatrician.

Dr. Koop's Book of Home Remedies for Children
http://www.healthyideas.com/children/remedies/

Natural, common-sense remedies for dozens of conditions or problem behaviors (e.g., from aggressiveness to warts).

Kids Doctor
http://www.kidsdoctor.com/

Advice and information for parents on common childhood dilemmas or conditions.

Dental Health

American Academy of Pediatric Dentistry
http://www.aapd.org/

Information for parents, teachers, nurses and kids. Includes links and a service to locate a local pediatric dentist.

Health: Childrens Dental
http://parentsplace.com/health/kidsdent/
Practical advice on tooth care for children.

Pediatric Dental Health
http://pages.ivillage.com/ps/kidsdental/index.html
Information on dental care for infants and children.

Yo, It's Time for Braces
http://tqjunior.advanced.org/5029/
This page was written by fifth graders and provides information for their peers to helps them understand what having braces and other orthodontic devices is like.

Diabetes

Children with Diabetes
http://www.childrenwithdiabetes.com/
Diabetes basics and diabetes product information for parents, kids and friends. Includes chat rooms and surveys, news, links and a search engine. Read the personal stories of a number of diabetic children.

DFAN Kids Diabetes Page
http://pages.prodigy.net/dfan/kiddm.htm
Information for children with diabetes. Includes interviews and stories of kids with diabetes. Definitions, "graffiti wall" for kids' comments, and much more.

Juvenile Diabetes Foundation
http://www.jdf.org/index.html
Non-governmental international organization that funds research to find a cure for juvenile diabetes and its complications.

Kids Learn About Diabetes
http://www.geocities.com/HotSprings/6935/index.html
Tutorial for kids covering diabetes basics, and links to other diabetes sites.

Diet & Nutrition

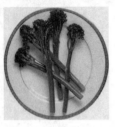

The Broccolini Splash Page. At:
http://www.broccoli.com

Broccoli Town, U.S.A.
http://www.broccoli.com/

Everything you could possibly want to know about broccoli. Includes recipes and a "kids club."

Children's Nutrition Research Center
http://www.bcm.tmc.edu/cnrc/

Includes the newsletter "Nutrition and Your Child," as well as research overviews, news items and links.

Chow Club!
http://www.cspinet.org/kids/

Recipes and healthy eating tips for parents and kids. Includes the ten best and the ten worst foods for kids, and kitchen fun for 7- to 12-year-old cooks.

Kids Can Make a Difference
http://www.kids.maine.org/

This site educates children about hunger and poverty issues. It provides activities, presents hunger facts, and allows children to express their thoughts on the subject.

Kids Food CyberClub
http://www.kidsfood.org/

Includes recipes, activities, food facts and discussion about nutrition, diet and other food-related issues. Section for adults.

Mylifepath: Children's Nutrition
http://www.mylifepath.com/topic/childnutrition

Includes a section for adolescents on weight reduction.

Nutrition Café
http://www.exhibits.pacsci.org/nutrition/

Colorful site presents games that teach children about nutrition.

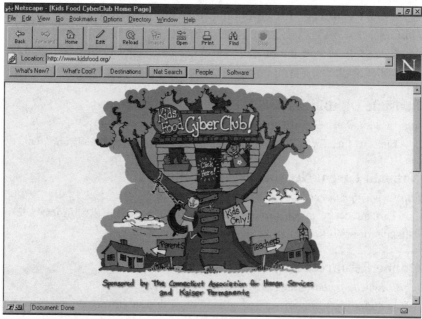

Kids Food CyberClub. http://www.kidsfood.org/

Disabled Children

See also Disabilities.

Children with Disabilities
http://codi.buffalo.edu/children-text.htm

Links to sites on the web for special kids, their parents, teachers and health care professionals.

Great Art Ideas for Special Artists
http://www.edbydesign.com/specneedsres/specialart/index.html

Self-expression and the pleasure of creating are just as relevant and enjoyable for children with disabilities as they are for those without disabilities. Site provides some creative suggestions.

Helpful Links for Kids with Learning Disabilities
http://apelslice.com/kidlinks.htm

Links to magazines, newspapers, references, libraries and homework aids on the web.

Internet Resources for Special Children

http://www.irsc.org/

Lots of links and information for children with many different kinds of disabilities or illnesses. Well-organized and easy to use.

Invisible Disabilities

http://www1.shore.net/~dmoisan/disability/kids.html

Links to sites for children whose disabilities aren't immediately apparent.

National Parent Network on Disabilities

http://www.npnd.org/

This advocacy group provides a voice for those with disabilities. Site is valuable for providing important legislative updates and news.

Online Resources for Kids with Disabilities

http://www.lib.pg.bc.ca/docs_graphics/kid_disab.htm

Includes links to homeschooling children with disabilities, and resources for parents and teachers of blind children.

Our-Kids

http://www.our-kids.org/

Devoted to raising children with special physical and/or mental disabilities or delays. This site provides an archive and information about the Our-Kids mailing list, as well as a reading list, nutrition list, newsgroup, and links to adaptive technology, toy and organization sites.

Special Olympics International

http://www.specialolympics.org/

Information on this sporting event for the mentally retarded. Competitions in acquatics, basketball, soccer, figure skating and many other sports.

Yoga for the Special Child

http://www.specialyoga.com/

Information about yoga techniques for children with Down syndrome, cerebral palsy, attention deficit disorder and learning disabilities.

Heart (Cardiology)

Cardiac Disease in Children

http://www.amhrt.org/Heart_and_Stroke_A_Z_Guide/cardk.html

Statistics on heart disease in children from the American Heart Association, and information on cholesterol and children, heart transplants in infants, and many other pediatric cardiac conditions.

Cardiac Kids

http://www.strata.ca/~plittle/pdheart/kids.html

Support group for kids with congenital heart defects. Click on a kid's name and learn his or her personal story, or add your own story.

Families with Heart

http://www.ntrnet.net/~hhbc1/fwh/fwh.html

This group of parents of children with heart disease offers information, support, and encouragement to others in the same situation.

March of Dimes: Congenital Heart Defects

http://www.noah.cuny.edu/pregnancy/march_of_dimes/birth_defects/Rcongnitl .html

Public health information sheets.

Pediatric Cardiology

http://www.cardio-info.com/linkpeds.htm

A long list of links for patients, their families and professionals.

PediHeart

http://www.pediheart.org/

This site is divided into three sections: one section for kids with heart problems, another for their families, and a third for their medical practitioners. Kids and adults can learn about the heart and common defects, and can locate resources and links.

Special Hearts Online

http://www.sentex.net/~s_hearts/

Support and information for families of children with heart problems, cardio/apnea monitors, and pacers. Features general information, e-mail contacts and support.

HIV/AIDS

Be a Force For Change
http://www.thebody.com/aawh/force/aawh14.html

This quiz for young people reveals how much they know about HIV/AIDS.

CAPS Hot Topic: Adolescents & AIDS Prevention
http://www.epibiostat.ucsf.edu/capsweb/hotteens.html

Chat-line and youth programs, descriptions, fact sheets and opinions, articles and research.

Children with AIDS Project
http://www.aidskids.org/

This organization matches families who wish to adopt, with children or infants who either have HIV or who have been orphaned by AIDS. It also provides AIDS education and advocacy.

Elizabeth Glaser Pediatric AIDS Foundation
http://www.pedaids.org/

In their own words, the Foundation is "dedicated to identifying, funding and conducting basic pediatric HIV/AIDS research. The Foundation's goals include reducing HIV transmission from an HIV-infected mother to her newborn, prolonging and improving the lives of children living with HIV, eliminating HIV in infected children and promoting awareness and compassion about HIV/AIDS world-wide." Site provides information about pediatric AIDS and describes the Foundation's activities to combat it.

HIV/AIDS Info from Children's Animated Television
http://www.qcfurball.com/cat/aids.html

There is a lot of information here, and links to dozens of resources for everyone.

Information for Young People about HIV & AIDS
http://www.avert.org/yngindx.htm

Provides basic and frank information on HIV/AIDS, its transmission, and other issues. Sections on contraception, puberty, and sexual feelings, as well as information about homosexuality for young men.

Living with AIDS

http://desires.com/1.4/Sex/Docs/aids.html

HIV-positive teens tell their stories.

Mothers' Voices United to End AIDS

http://www.mvoices.org/

This nonprofit organization uses mothers as educators, and it advocates for the prevention, research, treatment and cure of AIDS. Site describes their efforts and shows how others can join in.

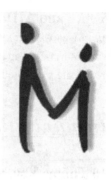

Mothers' Voices United to End AIDS.
http://www.aidskids.org

National Pediatric AIDS Network

http://www.npan.org/

A resource for information on children and adolescents with HIV/AIDS. It provides access to material on treatment, clinical trials, services for children and youth, conferences, publications, and educational resources.

National Pediatric & Family HIV Resource Center

http://www.pedhivaids.org/

There is a great deal of information at this site for health professionals caring for children and youth with HIV and their families. Includes various fact sheets, educational materials, questions and answers, links and much more.

Pediatric AIDS Clinical Trials

http://cancernet.nci.nih.gov/proto/pedaids.html

From the National Institutes of Health, this site describes on-going trials of drugs for the treatment of HIV/AIDS.

The Pediatric AIDS Clinical Trials Group

http://pactg.s-3.com/

Seeks to evaluate treatment for HIV-infected children and adolescents, and to provide ways to interrupt the vertical transmission of HIV from mother to infant.

Research on AIDS & HIV in Children

http://www.thebody.com/treat/ped_research.html

Collection of articles from different news and research sources.

Youth and AIDS Project.

http://www.peds.umn.edu/Centers/YAP/

Information on AIDS transmission among the youth population can be found at this site sponsored by the University of Minnesota.

Immunizations

10 Things You Need to Know about Immunizations

http://www.cdc.gov/nip/vacsafe/fs/q10vac.htm

Answers to basic questions parents may have about immunizations.

Ask NOAH About: Childhood Immunization

http://noah.cuny.edu/wellness/healthyliving/ushc/childimmuniz.html

Information and immunization schedule.

Health OnLine: Immunizing Your Child

http://www.smtmoves.com/HOL/immuniz6.html

Includes an immunization schedule and online booklet addressing questions and concerns consumers may have about immunization, such as why it is important, when not to immunize, and more.

National Immunization Program

http://www.cdc.gov/nip/

A part of the Centers for Disease Control and Prevention, NIP plans, coordinates and conducts immunization programs nationwide. Site offers access to resources, publications and data.

Parent's Guide to Childhood Immunization

http://www.hoptechno.com/book42.htm

Basic text from the U.S. Department of Health and Human Services.

Vaccines/Immunization Information

http://wchd.neobright.net/wc_immunize.html

Links to many sites.

What Parents Need to Know About Immunizations and Childhood Disease

http://www.aap.org/family/vaccine.htm

Guidelines for parents from the American Academy of Pediatrics.

Infant Care

Baby Booklet

http://members.aol.com/allianceMD/booklet.html

Online information for new parents: "Your Newborn: a Guided Tour."

Baby Place

http://www.baby-place.com/

A starting point for information on pregnancy, birth, babies and parenting. Lots of links.

Babyhood

http://www.babyhood.com/

Information for parents on infant care (from birth to 24 months).

Babysoon.Com

http://Babysoon.com/

Articles and information for expectant parents.

Infant Development

http://www.ecsu.ctstateu.edu/depts/edu/textbooks/infantdev.html

An electronic textbook that teaches what to expect from infants in their first year. It includes their physical, social, emotional and intellectual development.

Infant Life Saving Basics

http://www.baby-care.com/lifesaving.htm

How to help a choking infant, and how to apply CPR on an infant.

Postnatal Care Issues

http://obgyn.uihc.uiowa.edu/Patinfo/pstnatal.htm

Main topics include infant care, breast and bottle feeding, immunizations and more.

Neonatology

See also: Pregnancy & Childbirth - Neonatology.

Neonatology Network

http://www.neonatology-net.com/

The purpose of this site is to stimulate international cooperation in the field of neonatology, by providing the global neonatology community with the facilities to publish and search for information, and to exchange knowledge and maintain relations on a global scale.

Neonatology on the Web

http://www.neonatology.org/

Various resources for neonatology professionals. Includes a job directory, literature citation, and classic papers in neonatology.

Neurosurgery

See also: Neurological Disorders.

Child Neurology Society

http://www1.umn.edu/cns/index.htm

Meeting information and links of interest.

Pediatric (Developmental) Neurosurgery Unit

http://neurosurgery.mgh.harvard.edu:80/pedi-hp.htm

Massachusetts General Hospital/Harvard Medical School specializes in the surgical treatment of pediatric brain and spine tumors, and surgery of developmental anomalies.

Pediatric Neurosurgery

http://cpmcnet.columbia.edu/dept/nsg/PNS/

This page from Columbia-Presbyterian Medical Center was written for parents and friends looking for answers to common pediatric neurosurgical questions. It is organized in text files and covers the most common conditions. Links to resources and support groups are also provided.

Pediatric Neurosurgery Journal

http://www.karger.com/journals/pne/

Sample issue available, and free access to table of contents.

Organizations

American Academy of Child & Adolescent Psychiatry

http://www.aacap.org/

Assists parents in understanding developmental, behavioral, emotional and mental disorders that may affect young people and children. Find information on child and adolescent psychiatry, fact sheets for parents and caregivers, AACAP membership, current research, practice guidelines and managed care information.

American Academy of Pediatrics

http://www.aap.org/

Membership information, publications, family and professional resources, advocacy and research.

Canadian Paediatric Society

http://www.cps.ca/

Professional development, publications and research.

Cards for Kids

http://www.cardsforkids.com/

Volunteer organization that sends homemade cards to children who face life-threatening illnesses.

List of Children's Health Organizations

http://www.sdkids.com/parents/hc_prov/pediatri.htm

Links to a few dozen organizations.

Save the Children

http://www.savethechildren.org/

International nonprofit organization supporting health and nutrition, education, economic and emergency programs that help children in poverty, illness or other critical situations. Site provides information about the agency and how people can help.

WHO Child Health and Development
http://www.who.int/chd/
The World Health Organization has programs to fight acute respiratory infection, diarrheal diseases, cholera and other childhood illnesses world-wide.

Orthopedics

Guide to Pediatric Orthopedics for Family Members
http://www.orthoindustry.com/patientpediatric.htm
List of websites dealing with orthopedic problems in children.

Jeni Drake Scoliosis Support
http://www.geocities.com/HotSprings/8095/
Links, personal stories, and chat.

Pediatric Orthopedics
http://www.mliles.com/pedortho/index.shtml
An index of some websites.

Scoliosis Support Page
http://users.csionline.net/~cbuckle/supportpg.html
Contact others who have scoliosis and learn their stories.

Pain Management

All in Their Heads? When Your Child Has a Headache
http://kidshealth.org/parent/healthy/headache.html
What to do, and when you should be concerned about your child's headache.

Pain, Pain, Go Away
http://is.dal.ca/~pedpain/ppga-ti.htm
What is pain, how to measure and manage it in children, and where to go for advice.

Pediatric Pain and Health Resources

http://www.painandhealth.org/pediatric-links.html

Links to articles and related sites.

Pediatric Pain: Science Helping Children

http://is.dal.ca/%7Epedpain/pedpain.html

Professional, research and self-help resources. Lots of links.

Pediatric Pain Links

http://neurosurgery.mgh.harvard.edu:80/lnkpedi.htm#Pain

Includes an e-mail discussion group and several other links.

Parenting

National Parent Information Network

http://npin.org/

Provides news and resources for parents and those who work with parents. Includes a bimonthly magazine, a question-answer service available through "Parents Ask ERIC," and PARENTING-L, an electronic e-mail discussion group.

Parent News

http://parent.net/

Weekly online e-zine that contains a few articles, health tips, news, resources and family facts. Particularly geared to parents of school-aged children.

Parent Time!

http://www.pathfinder.com/ParentTime/homepage/homepage.all.html

Ask an expert (choose from several), and learn about child behavior and development, education, nutrition, pregnancy and more. For parents of children who are from 0 to 6 years old.

ParenthoodWeb

http://www.parenthoodweb.com/

Formatted like a newsletter. There are numerous subjects dealing directly and indirectly with parenting. Some major topic titles are: shopping, pregnancy, names, recipes, chat, and sleep. Product recall information, feature articles, children's book reviews, and much more are also found.

Parenting of Multiples
http://multiples.about.com/
Health and parenting issues for parents of twins and multiples.

Parenting Questions and Answers
http://www.parenting-qa.com/
Answers to your parenting questions. Browse through archive by topic, age or keyword, or submit your own question.

Parent's Place
http://www.parentsplace.com/
Chat rooms on different parenting issues: "From pregnancy to baby to parenting parents."

Positive Parenting On-line
http://www.positiveparenting.com/
Features the Positive Parenting newsletter, with articles like "9 Things to Do Instead of Spanking," "What is Normal Development?" and "Children's Feelings."

Stepmoms.Net
http://www.stepmoms.net/
Support for those involved in a stepfamily.

Pathology

Pediatric Pathology and Laboratory Medicine
http://path.upmc.edu/spp/pubs/pplm.htm
Professional publication for scientists and physicians with an interest in pediatric pathology.

Radiology

Paediapedia: An Imaging Encyclopedia of Pediatric Diseases
http://vh.radiology.uiowa.edu/Providers/TeachingFiles/PAP/PAPHome.html
Handbook of basic pediatric radiology.

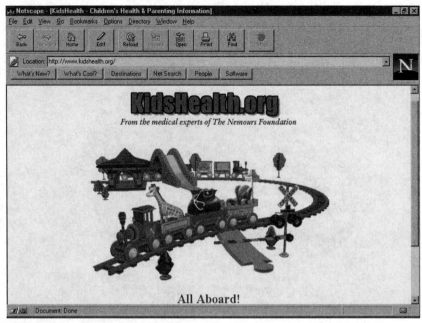

KidsHealth. http://www.kidshealth.org/

Resources

The Best of the Pediatric Internet

http://www.aap.org/bpi/

Sites are selected by the American Academy of Pediatrics, for pediatricians.

Facts for Families

http://www.aacap.org/factsfam/index.htm

Information for children, teenagers and their families from the American Academy of Child and Adolescent Psychiatry. Articles are available in English, Spanish, German and French, and range from bedwetting to teen suicide.

Family Web Home Page

http://www.familyweb.com/

Comprehensive information on pregnancy and child-rearing.

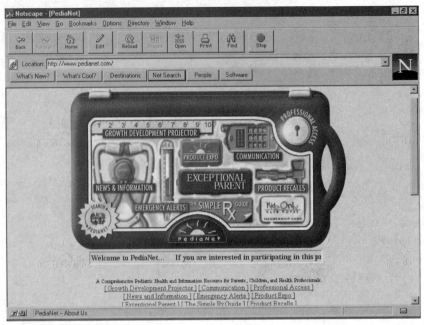

PediaNet. *http://www.pedianet.com*

KidsHealth

http://www.kidshealth.org

Information sorted for kids, teenagers and parents on infections, behavior & emotions, food and fitness, and growing up healthy.

Mount Sinai Department of Pediatrics

http://www.mssm.edu/peds/www_peds.html

Features links to selected children's health Internet sites.

PediaNet

http://www.pedianet.com

A comprehensive pediatric health and information resource for parents, children, and health professionals. Includes emergency alerts, growth projector, resources, product recalls, guide to prescriptions and nutrition information.

Pediatric Points of Interest

http://www.med.jhu.edu/peds/neonatology/poi.html

As selected by the Johns Hopkins Hospital Virtual Children's Center.

PEDINFO
http://www.pedinfo.org/

Information for pediatricians and others interested in children's health issues. Site offers a great deal of material on disease-specific conditions, health education, subspecialties and related issues. A convenient subject search engine is also provided.

Vanderbilt Pediatric Interactive Digital Library
http://www.mc.Vanderbilt.Edu/peds/pidl/index.htm

Information for professionals. The table of contents includes developmental pediatrics, acute illnesses, genetic and metabolic disorders, neonatology, adolescent issues, allergy and immunology, and various other specialties.

Virtual Children's Hospital
http://www.vh.org/VCH/

Information for patients, children and health care providers.

Single Parents

Parents Without Partners, Inc.
http://www.parentswithoutpartners.org/

International organization for single parents of all kinds. Site provides help in the way of discussions, professional speakers, study groups, publications and suggestions on social activities for families and adults.

Single Parents World
http://www.nucleus.com/~jlassali/

For all types of single parents.

Sudden Infant Death Syndrome

American Sudden Infant Death Syndrome Institute

http://www.sids.org/

This organization promotes research, clinical services, family support and professional and community education. Information about Sudden Infant Death Syndrome (SIDS) and links.

Back to Sleep Campaign

http://www.nih.gov/nichd/news/SIDS_HP_2/home1B.html

A national campaign to reduce the risk of SIDS. The theme is that parents should always place their infants on their backs to sleep.

Information for Sudden Infant Death Syndrome

http://www.thelastplanet.com/bbsudden.htm

Recommended links to SIDS sites on the web.

National SIDS Resource Center

http://www.circsol.com/sids/

Information sheets, bibliographies and references to promote an understanding of SIDS and related topics, and to provide comfort for SIDS families.

SIDS Alliance

http://www.sidsalliance.org/

National, nonprofit organization dedicated to the support of SIDS families, SIDS education and research. Site offers SIDS facts, questions and answers, public policy information and more.

SIDS FAQ Archive

http://www.cis.ohio-state.edu/hypertext/faq/usenet/misc-kids/sids/faq.html

Answers some basic information about what SIDS is and what it isn't.

SIDS Network

http://www.sids-network.org/

Includes resources and advice for parents and siblings, and frequently asked questions about SIDS. A large amount of information.

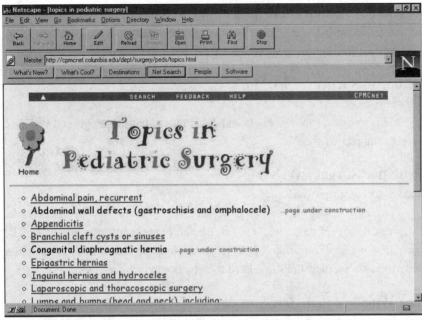

Topics in Pediatric Surgery at Columbia-Presbyterian Medical Center.
http://cpmcnet.columbia.edu/dept/surgery/peds/topics.html

SIDS Ring

http://www.webring.org/cgi-bin/webring?ring=sidsring;list

Numerous links to SIDS information and resources, and to sites memorializing infants who have died.

Surgery

American Pediatric Surgical Association

http://ped-surg.org/

Contains organization information, as well as PEDSURG-L, the International Pediatric Surgery Listserver.

Columbia-Presbyterian Medical Center Pediatric Surgery

http://cpmcnet.columbia.edu/dept/surgery/peds/

As well as information about this facility, you can find frequently asked questions about pediatric surgery, information on common problems that may require pediatric surgery, links, research and advice on how to assess surgeons.

Journal of Pediatric Surgery

http://www.wbsaunders.com/catalog/wbs-prod.pl?0022-3468

Information on how to subscribe.

Pediatric Surgery, MedMark

http://members.iworld.net/medmark/peds/

Links to associations, schools and departments, consumer, general pediatric surgery and related sites.

Pediatric Surgery Web Site

http://pedsurg.surgery.uab.edu/

For pediatric surgeons and other health care professionals with an interest in the surgical care of children. This site provides access to news and editorials, continuing medical education (CME) programs, meeting information, case studies and surveys, as well as links to related listservers and websites.

The World of Pediatric Surgery

http://pediatricsurgery.gen.com/

Site emphasizes pediatric laparoscopic surgery. Information on clinics, research and links.

Teen Parents

Parenting Help for Teens Online!

http://members.tripod.com/xila/teens.html

Links, advice, helpful hints and chat for teen parents.

The Teen Pregnancy and Parenting Place

http://hometown.aol.com/mnn1121/index.html

Advice and support for pregnant teens and teen parents. Share your story, find a penpal, learn about pregnancy and parenting.

Teen Pregnancy Ring

http://nav.webring.com/cgi-bin/navcgi?ring=teenpreg;list

Links to nearly 50 sites on the web about teen pregnancy.

CHIROPRACTICS

Discussion Groups

Chiro-List
http://www.chiro.org/chat/chiro-list.html

Site provides instructions on how to participate in this unmoderated, popular discussion group. There is also a "best of" section.

Parcelus
http://www.mbnet.mb.ca/~jwiens/paracel.txt

Mailing list for "eclectic" health care professionals, including chiropractors.

History

The History of Chiropractics
http://www.strose.edu/facstaff/cis/Avitabile/cis111/Kipp/kipp1.htm

Interesting facts about the start of chiropractics.

YourSpine
http://www.yourspine.com/history/modern1.htm

Modern and ancient history of chiropractic medicine.

Organizations

American Chiropractic Association
http://www.amerchiro.org/

You can use this site to find a chiropractor near you. Member information, publications, research and legislative updates.

International Chiropractors Association
http://www.chiropractic.org/

This international organization aids in the professional growth of its members, as well as in public advocacy, research and education. Consumer and professional information on posture, legislative updates, and information for parents.

National Association for Chiropractic Medicine
http://www.chiromed.org/

A consumer advocacy association.

Products & Insurance

Directory of Chiropractic and Bodyworker Suppliers
http://www.makura.com/dir1/dir_top.html

Locates products and resources for chiropractors, acupuncturists, and others who deal with bodywork. Find by product or company name.

ChiroNet: Managed Chiropractic Care
http://www.chiro-net.com/

A provider group that contracts with insurance carriers and managed health care organizations to provide chiropractic benefits.

Publications

Chiropractic Online Today
http://www.Chiro-Online.com/

Includes discussion and chat group, links, advertising and referral pages.

Chiropractic Research Journal
http://lifenet.life.edu/newlife/crj/crj.html
A semi-annual journal dedicated to subluxation-related research.

The Journal of Chiropractic Humanities
http://www.chiro.edu/humanities/
Scholarly publication with articles online.

In Touch Newsletter
http://www.chirousa.com/education/intouch.asp
Online newsletter.

Radiology

Chiropractic Radiology WebPage
http://web.idirect.com/~xray/chiro.html
Review cases online and submit your diagnosis via e-mail.

Resources

Chiro-Web
http://pages.prodigy.com/CT/doc/doc.html
Chiropractic resources on the Internet, including chiropractic research, education, networking, licensure, associations, products and services.

Chiropractic America
http://www.chirousa.com/
News, education, products, resources and doctors.

Chiropractic Glossary
http://www.bworks.com/chiro/gloss.htm
Definitions to some of the terms you might encounter in a chiropractic visit.

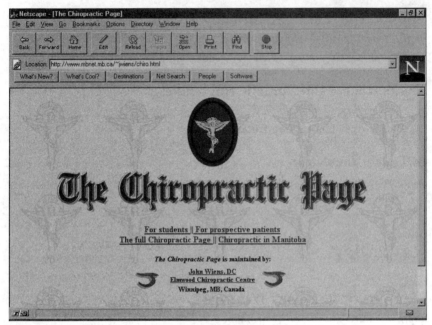

The Chiropractic Page. *http://www.mbnet.mb.ca/~jwiens/chiro.html*

Chiropractic Page

http://www.mbnet.mb.ca/~jwiens/chiro.html

Information for students and patients, including links to colleges, organizations, research sites, mailing lists, and bulletin boards.

The Chiropractic Resource Page

http://www.chiro.org/

This site is for chiropractors. Register for free. Sections on politics, starting out, the Internet, research, referrals and more.

Chiroweb

http://www.chiroweb.com/

Information on and for chiropractors. Includes discussion forums, chat rooms, patient and consumer information, meetings, classified ads, and pages for chiropractic students.

Schools

Chiropractic Colleges
http://www.bworks.com/chiro/college.htm
> Mailing addresses, phone numbers and, where applicable, website addresses.

Chiropractic School Links
http://www.geocities.com/CollegePark/Library/9886/chiro2.htm
> Links to school in the U.S., Canada, and several other countries.

Life University Home Page
http://www.life.edu/
> Four-year academic university that teaches chiropractics.

CLINICAL TRIALS

Covered in this chapter: *Cancer; HIV/AIDS; Other Diseases.*

Cancer

Cancer Trials
http://cancertrials.nci.nih.gov/
Clinical trials resource from the National Cancer Institute. Learn what clinical trials are and how to choose one to participate in. Search NCI's Trials Database.

CancerWEB Clinical Trials
http://www.graylab.ac.uk/cancerweb/trials.html
Information and links.

Clinical Trials and Noteworthy Treatments for Brain Tumors
http://www.virtualtrials.com/
Browse by new listing, tumor type, treatment, or keyword. Also offers a brain tumor virtual tour, and information about different brain tumor treatments.

Clinical Trials: Cancer
http://cancer.med.upenn.edu/clinical_trials/
Part of the services of OncoLink, from the University of Pennsylvania.

Finding Cancer Clinical Trials on the Internet
http://cancerguide.org/internet_trials.html
Leads you to several databases to search for a clinical trial.

National Alliance of Breast Cancer Organizations
http://www.nabco.org:80/trials/
Learn about clinical trials and look through the breast cancer trial directory.

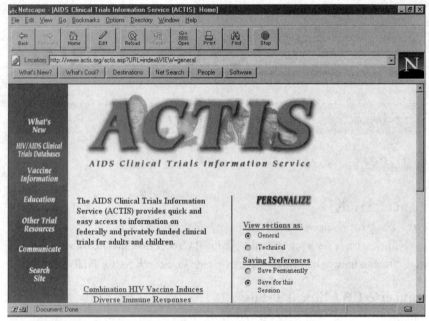

AIDS Clinical Trials Information Service. *http://www.actis.org/*

Southwest Oncology Group Clinical Trials

http://www.swog.saci.org/

> You can download the open protocols for the many kinds of cancer tests.

HIV/AIDS

The Adult AIDS Clinical Trials Group

http://aactg.s-3.com/

Helps set standards of care for HIV infection and opportunistic diseases related to HIV/AIDS.

AIDS Clinical Trials

http://www.critpath.org/trials.htm

Features the full text of the open protocols for major HIV/AIDS clinical trials networks.

AIDS Clinical Trials Information Service

http://www.actis.org/

Current information on federal and privately-sponsored clinical trials for people with AIDS or HIV infection.

Canadian HIV Trials Network

http://www.hivnet.ubc.ca/ctn.html

Information on clinical trials for treatments, vaccines and cures for HIV/AIDS in Canada.

Pediatric AIDS Clinical Trials Group

http://pactg.s-3.com/

Evaluates treatment for HIV-infected children and adolescents and develops preventive measures for mother-infant HIV transmission.

Other Diseases

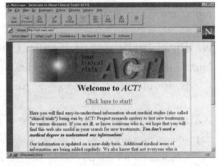

About Clinical Trials!

http://act.musc.edu/

For non-professionals. Offers a listing of clinical trials, as well as tutorials.

About Clinical Trials! *http://act.musc.edu/*

Applied Clinical Trials Online

http://www.actmagazine.com/

Magazine covering clinical trials topics. Complimentary subscriptions available for those who fit their audience demographics.

CenterWatch Clinical Trials Listing Service

http://www.centerwatch.com/

Site describes clinical trials currently being undertaken and provides a patient notification service of when new clinical trials are begun. Also describes newly approved drug therapies, provides background information on clinical research, and offers links to industry providers.

Clinical Trials Discussion Group

http://pharminfo.com/conference/clntrl.html

E-mail discussion group for professionals engaged in clinical trials.

ClinicalTrials.Com

http://www.clinicaltrials.com/

Attractive site offering support services, clinical trials posting, patient registry, frequently asked questions and updates on newly approved drugs.

drkoop.com: Clinical Trials

http://www.drkoop.com/hcr/trials/

Includes articles about clinical trials, and allows you to browse through listing of active therapeutic clinical trials.

MDAdvice: Clinical Trials

http://www.mdadvice.com/resources/clinical_trials/index.html

Provides information on clinical trials, drug testing, and understanding research and how it works. Links.

National Institutes of Health Clinical Trials Databases

http://www.nih.gov/health/trials/index.htm

Boasts of "one-stop shopping" for clinical trials information.

National Library of Medicine Clinical Alerts

http://www.nlm.nih.gov/databases/alerts/clinical_alerts.html

Clinical alerts are posted to release important findings from the NIH-funded clinical trials where such release could significantly affect morbidity and mortality.

Rare Diseases Clinical Trials Database

http://rarediseases.info.nih.gov/ord/wwwprot/index.shtml

Search this database from the Office of Rare Diseases at the National Institutes of Health.

Society for Clinical Trials Home Page

http://www.sctweb.org/

International professional organization to develop and disseminate information about clinical trials.

CONSUMER HEALTH

Covered in this chapter: *Expert Advice & Consultation; Gateways; Handbooks & Guides; Health News; Internet Use; Links; Organizations; Physician Search & Background Checks; Publications; Support Groups; Surgery.*

Note: These are some of the gest general health sites or "starting places" for basic consumer health information. Please check Medical References and other chapters for resources on specific conditions, systems and specialties.

Expert Advice & Consultation

Caution: Medical advice you receive on the Internet is not a substitute for a consultation with your own physician. Please consider it only as supplementary information.

Ask the Experts

http://www.ama-assn.org/insight/spec_con/crossrds/tabtoc.htm

The American Medical Association gives you the opportunity to submit health questions to a nationally-known medical expert.

Diagnostic Doc

http://diagnosticdoc.com/

Free medical information service. Includes ability to enter your symptoms and receive a possible diagnosis.

On Call Online

http://www.muhealth.org/~oncall/

Send a question to be answered via e-mail or posted anonymously.

Talk with the Experts

http://www.mayohealth.org/mayo/common/htm/talk.htm

A Mayo Clinic physician will answer questions on a wide range of diseases and conditions; or a Mayo Clinic dietition can address your diet and nutrition concerns.

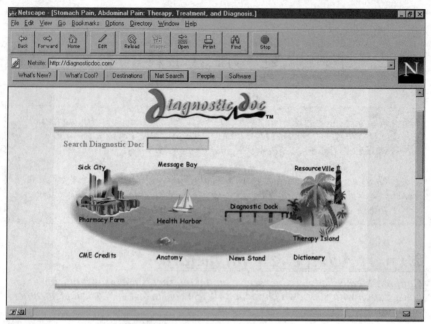

Diagnostic Doc. http://diagnosticdoc.com/

Pharmaceutical Care Associates

http://www.wnwcorp.com/pharmca/

Type in personal information such as allergies, diagnoses, current medications, and a description of your medical history and condition to receive medical advice via the Internet.

Gateways

AMA Health Insight

http://www.ama-assn.org/consumer.htm

American Medical Association health information for consumers. Nicely organized website lets you find information based on specific conditions, general health information, and family member/age. Also has interactive health pages that you can use to assess your risk for heart disease and skin cancer; forms to keep track of the your personal and family health history; and consultations about your diet and exercise regimes. Site also provides medical news, as well as a hospital and a doctor finder.

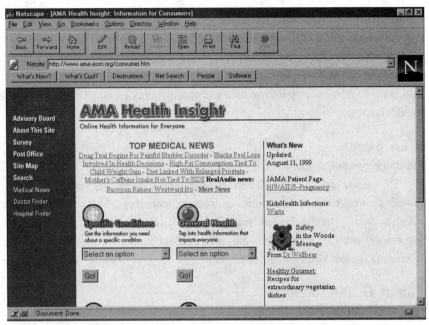

AMA Health Insight. http://www.ama-assn.org/consumer.htm

AmericasDoctor.com

http://www.americasdoctor.com/

Information, chat rooms, and health news for consumers. Includes frequently asked questions on various health topics, and "Ask the Doc," where you can consult with a doctor on non-emergency health questions directly.

Ask NOAH About: Health Topics and Resources

http://www.noah.cuny.edu/qksearch.html

Great information and links on a large variety of health topics. Part of New York Online Access to Health.

Ask Your Family Doctor

http://familydoctor.org/

Information, questions and answers from the American Academy of Family Physicians. Arranged by body system and common condition, or search for specific terms.

Cyberspace Telemedical Office

http://www.telemedical.com/Telemedical

Medical library, product shopping and home care consultations. Free registration allows you to store up to 3 megabytes of personal health care information and to look up information and products. Paying members have access to additional services.

drkoop.com

http://drkoop.com/

The former U.S. Surgeon General has given his name to this health site which provides a wealth of information for consumers, including health news briefs and articles, family health issues, nutrition and fitness information, resources (drugstore, drug checker, personal insurance center, clinical trials listing), interactive communities and much more.

Family Health Radio

http://www.fhradio.org/

Daily series of 2-1/2 minute long audio programs for a general audience. Answers most of the frequently asked health and medical-related questions, from information on anoxia, to jet lag, to vaccinations.

GlobalMedic

http://www.globalmedic.com/

Self-help health information and tools for physical health, mental health and pregnancy. Includes health quiz and check-up for kids, for women, and for men; encyclopedia of medicine, drug book, and first aid reference. Site also promotes the Health & Wellness Companion, a health care benefit that companies can consider offering to their employees.

Health Answers

http://www.healthanswers.com/index.htm

Free membership includes customized health page, newsletter, drug database and medical reference book. Health subjects range from addiction, to women's health; with daily health news briefs and indexes for drugs, injuries, diseases, surgical procedures, poisons, symptoms, tests, extended care facilities, and home care assistance.

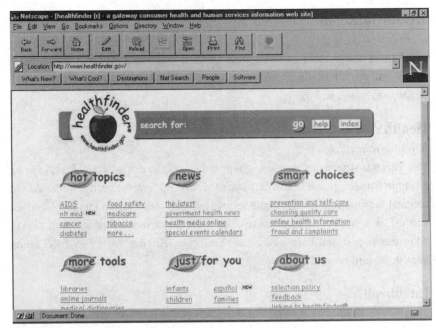

Healthfinder. *http://www.healthfinder.gov/*

The Health Connection
http://www.thehealthconnection.com/

Disease center, bookstore, and drug guide.

Healthfinder
http://www.healthfinder.gov/

This is a free gateway to consumer health and human services information developed by the U.S. Department of Health and Human Services. It directs browsers to selected online publications, clearinghouses, databases, websites, and support and self-help groups, as well as to government agencies and not-for-profit organizations that produce reliable information for the public. Major features include search capabilities, hot topics featuring 20 key areas, news, smart choices (i.e., self-care), links and tools (such as medical dictionaries), databases, online journals, foreign language resources, support groups and libraries. Area entitled "Just for You" targets special needs of infants, teens, elderly, men, women, minorities, and others with specific health concerns.

HealthGate.com
http://bewell.com/

Patient and consumer information. Contains a number of webzines on health issues, such as alternative health, healthy man, healthy parenting, healthy mind, healthy sexuality, and more.

HealthWorld Online
http://www.healthy.net/

This site stresses its mission is to promote "self-managed care." It seeks to be a comprehensive global health network providing integrative health, wellness, and medical information, products and services. It provides links to medical libraries, and offers a marketplace, alternative medicine, nutrition, fitness, professional, educational and self-care resources. You can also find a health food store, bookstore, forums, and more.

Intelihealth
http://www.intelihealth.com/IH/ihtIH

Find health information from Johns Hopkins. A great deal of information, including drug search, condition center, newsletter, healthy living, men's and women's health topics. Information also provided on general health subjects such as allergy, weight management, headache, pregnancy and more.

Mayo Clinic's Health O@sis
http://www.mayohealth.org/

Information for health care consumers, including access to an online library, cancer center, and heart center. Also offers resources on diet and nutrition, pregnancy, children's health care, and other health topics. You can submit your own question directly to a physician, via e-mail.

MedExplorer
http://www.medexplorer.com/

Browse or search through long list of categories, check out discussion forums, chat with others, or ask a doctor your medical question online.

MedicineNet
http://www.medicinenet.com/Script/Main/hp.asp

"Doctor-produced" medical information. Covers diseases, procedures, treatments, first aid, medical dictionary and more.

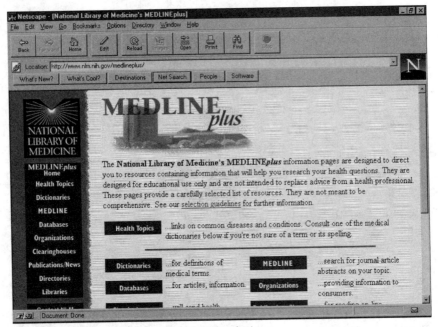

MEDLINEplus. *http://www.nlm.nih.gov/medlineplus/*

Mediconsult.com

http://www.mediconsult.com/

Newly-revised site will provide access to over 60 medical conditions, health centers, articles, reports and summaries, as well as community information, support groups, polls and surveys.

MEDLINE*plus*

http://www.nlm.nih.gov/medlineplus/

Health information for consumers from the National Library of Medicine. As well as access to MEDLINE, includes health topic breakdowns, medical dictionaries, databases, organizations, clearinghouses, publications/news, directories and libraries.

NetWellness

http://www.netwellness.org/

Web-based consumer health information from the University of Cincinnati Medical Center.

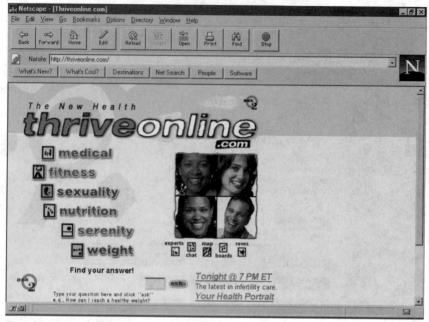

ThriveOnline. *http://www.thriveonline.com*

OnHealth.Com

http://www.onhealth.com

Daily briefs and in-depth reports from the consumer's perspective. Conditions A-Z, herbal index, drug database, expert questions and answers, and more.

Prevention Online

http://www.healthyideas.com/index.html

Preventive medicine and health maintenance articles and resources.

ThriveOnline

http://thriveonline.com/

Healthy lifestyle information and advice. Major topics include medical, fitness, sexuality, nutrition, serenity, and weight. Look up comprehensive information from experts, check out bulletin boards or chat online.

Wellness Health Care Information Resources

http://www-hsl.mcmaster.ca/tomflem/consumer.html

Links to consumer health sites on the Internet.

WellnessWeb: The Patient's Network

http://www.wellweb.com/

WellnessWeb is collaboration of patients, health care professionals and other caregivers who seek to provide the most appropriate medical information and support available. This site covers both conventional and alternative medicine. Information on clinical trials, community health, drug dosages and compliance, treatment and health options, research, and how to select a health care provider is provided. It reports on dozens of illnesses and conditions, and offers tips about healthy life styles.

Handbooks & Guides

Complete Home Medical Guide

http://cpmcnet.columbia.edu/texts/guide/toc/all.html

From the Columbia University College of Physicians and Surgeons. Discusses how to use the health system, basics of good health, symptoms and diseases, first aid and safety, treatment and prevention of diseases, and proper use of medications.

Emedicine

http://emedicine.com/

Free online medical textbooks for physicians, veterinarians, medical students, physician assistants, nurse practitioners, nurses and the public. Currently, the only finished project is emergency medicine (and it is extensive), but textbooks on dermatology, surgery, neurology, ophthalmology, otolaryngology, pediatrics and plastic surgery are all in progress and due to be completed early in 2000.

Prescription Medicines and You

http://www.ahcpr.gov/consumer/ncpiebro.htm

Advice on how to get involved in your treatment decisions and avoid medication errors.

University of Iowa Family Practice Handbook

http://www.vh.org/Providers/ClinRef/FPHandbook/FPContents.html

Electronic clinical reference source that places an emphasis on the diagnosis and treatment of common medical illnesses. Chapters study different medical specialties, with a special section on AIDS.

Health News

CNN Health Pages
http://www.cnn.com/HEALTH/#top
Health-related news articles.

Health News Online
http://www.healthfinder.gov/news/netmedia.htm
Long list of sites providing health news and headlines.

News Parents Can Use
http://www.kidshealth.org/News/news.cgi
The latest scoop on children's health issues, updated weekly. Searchable article database.

NPR Online
http://www.npr.org/news/healthsci/
The day's health and science news reports from National Public Radio. Audio available, as well as archives.

ReutersHealth
http://www.reutershealth.com/
Medical news and article archive, drug database and access to MEDLINE.

Internet Use

Health Information on the Internet: How to Get the Right Stuff
http://www.noah.cuny.edu/eval.html
Advice on evaluating websites and newsgroups, and their medical content.

A Patient's Guide to Healthcare on the Internet
http://www3.bc.sympatico.ca/me/patientsguide/
Provides medical terminology, reference sites, support groups, informational databases and links to featured sites.

HealthWWWeb: Choices for Health

http://www.healthwwweb.com/index.html

Presents educational and networking services to patients, practitioners, and others. Professional and consumer resources, health information, tools and news items are offered. The site is sponsored by the Integrative Medical Arts Group, and provides links to a variety of alternative medicine sites.

Your Health and the Internet

http://www.medinfo.ufl.edu/other/health/

A series of slides with key points for patients on how to use the Internet as a tool for obtaining health information. Good overview, suggestions and hints.

Links

BioSites

http://www.library.ucsf.edu/biosites/

Selected Internet resources covering the biomedical sciences.

Consumer Health Information

http://alabanza.com/kabacoff/Inter-Links/health/consumer.html

Consumer Internet resources that were chosen selectively.

Consumer Health Resources

http://www.ornl.gov/Library/medicine.html

Links to good general, government-sponsored, drug, cancer, and AIDS health sites for consumers.

Health Mall

http://www.hlthmall.com/

Links to sites of companies that sell health, fitness, nutrition and personal development natural products. Includes classified ads, find a health food store, resource center and links.

Health Links

http://www.hslib.washington.edu/

Information and references about basic sciences, diseases and common illnesses, health care practice and health care specialties. Includes links to journals and legislative updates, as well as databases, tutorials and news links. From the University of Washington Health Science Library.

InsideHealthCare

http://www.InsideHealthCare.com/ihcmagic.html

Hundreds of links to health-related sites. Main topics include: news, directories, organizations, publications, government sites, vendors, clinical and consumer resources, pediatric and family health, medical law, education, insurance, managed care, Medicaid, Medicare, mental health, substance abuse, minority health, nursing, public health, rural health, technology, and even health care humor.

MEDguide

http://www.medguide.net/

Guide to medicine and health care links and news on the Internet.

Medical Matrix

http://www.medmatrix.org/

Offers in-depth searches for high-quality medical resources. Sites listed are approved by an editorial board, and rated. Registration is required, but free.

Medinex

http://www.medinex.com/

Specialty search engine searches a database of thousands of health sites and gives priority to "certified" sites that have agreed to follow the Medinex Code of Ethics.

Organizations

Agency for Health Care Policy and Research

http://www.ahcpr.gov/

The lead federal agency charged with supporting research designed to improve the quality of health care, reduce its cost, and broaden access to essential services. AHCPR's broad programs of research bring practical, science-based information to medical practitioners and to consumers and other health care purchasers. Site describes the Agency and its programs, and provides information on health issues.

American Council on Science and Health

http://www.acsh.org/medical/index.html

Varied collection of press releases, news articles, publications, magazine feature articles, editorials, and offsite links discussing consumer medical care issues, some of them controversial.

The Health Consumer Alliance

http://healthconsumer.org/

The Alliance is an effort of eight legal services and health policy agencies to address the health problems of low-income consumers. "Cheat sheets" provide condensed description of topics. Material especially relevant to California.

National Institutes of Health

http://www.nih.gov/

Site is the federal focus for biomedical research in the United States. It supports and conducts research, and provides grants for research efforts.

U.S. Department of Health and Human Services

http://www.os.dhhs.gov/

The Department is responsible for more than 300 national health programs and research efforts. Site provides you an overview of these programs, and a gateway to reach the many different agencies it oversees.

U.S. National Library of Medicine

http://www.nlm.nih.gov/

Access to the world's largest medical library, and the creator of MEDLINE.

Physician Search & Background Checks

AMA Physician Select

http://www.ama-assn.org/aps/amahg.htm

Provides information on virtually every licensed physician in the United States, including more than 650,000 doctors of medicine (MD) and doctors of osteopathy or osteopathic medicine (DO). Search for doctor by name or specialty.

Folio Associates

http://www.foliomed.com/

For a fee, you can access their up-to-date database of physicians and health care facilities found in the Northeastern U.S. It shows names, practice location, medical school information, certification status, and other relevant information.

Medi-Net

http://www.askmedi.com/

Receive background information on every physician licensed to practice medicine in the United States. Service tells medical school, year of graduation, residency, medical specialty certifications, licensure data, and records of sanctions or disciplinary actions taken against a physician. The cost is $14.75 (e-mail queries) or $24.99 (phone or fax queries).

MedSeek

http://medseek.com/specsear.stm

Physician directory. Search by specialty and state.

Your Doctor's Credentials

http://www.tese.com/cas/

Physician credential search. Site was being reorganized at the time of this verification, but service supposed to check medical school, board certification, licensing, disciplinary action, and more.

Publications

Consumer Information Center Health Catalog

http://www.pueblo.gsa.gov/health.htm

Describes various publications and pamphlets, many of which are available for free from the government.

Consumer Reports Online Health and Foods

http://www.consumerreports.org/Categories/FoodHealth/index.html

Browse through online issues of *Consumer Reports*. Requires registration.

Core Bibliography of Consumer Health Books

http://www3.uchc.edu/~uchclib/departm/hnet/corelist.html

Assembled by the Connecticut Consumer Health Information Network, these books are recommended for consumer libraries.

Health Gazette

http://www.freenet.scri.fsu.edu/HealthGazette/gazette.html

New articles on family health topics appear quarterly, or look at previous editions. The treatment of acne, domestic violence, St. John's wort, and melatonin were some subjects covered in earlier gazettes. Written by a family physician.

Healthcare Publications for Consumers

http://www.ihr.com/publcons.html

Information about both online and hardcopy newsletters, magazines, and books with practical health care information for consumers.

NIH Consumer Health Information

http://www.nih.gov/health/consumer/conicd.htm

List of consumer titles published by each National Institute of Health.

Support Groups

Disease and Disorder Support Groups

http://www.noah.cuny.edu/support.html

It's easy to use to locate the support group of interest to you.

Health/Fitness Forums About

http://home.about.com/health/boards.htm?COB=home&PID=

Main topic areas for forums include: alternative medicine, medicine, disabilities, diseases/conditions, mental health, fitness, mental health and women's health.

Lycos Directory: Health Consumer Support Groups

http://dir.lycos.com/Health/Consumer_Support_Groups/

Connect to clubs, chats, and message boards for over 64 health disorders and issues, everything from AIDS/HIV to heart disease to thyroid disorders.

Self-Help Sourcebook Online

http://www.cmhc.com/selfhelp/

Starting point for locating real-life support groups and networks that are available throughout the world and in your community. The organizations listed can help you find and/or start a support group in your area.

Support

http://www3.bc.sympatico.ca/me/patientsguide/support.htm

Explains different forms of support groups on line, e.g., Usenet, mailing lists, newsgroups, web forums, and IRC (Internet Relay Chat), and provides links to indices of mail lists.

Support and Self-Help Groups

http://www.healthfinder.gov/moretools/support.htm

Alphabetical list.

Yahoo! Health Communities

http://health.yahoo.com/health/community.html

Message boards, clubs and net events on alternative medicine, mental health, children's health, nutrition, diseases and conditions, stress, fitness, weight issues, medicine, men's health and women's health.

Surgery

Be Informed: Questions to Ask Your Doctor Before You Have Surgery

http://www.ahcpr.gov/consumer/surgery.htm

Suggestions from the Agency for Health Care Policy and Research.

Pain Control after Surgery

http://www.nyssa-pg.org/HANYS/auth/AHCPRGuidelines/apmptoc.html

Online pamphlet for patients.

DEATH & DYING

Cemeteries & Memorials

Arlington National Cemetery
http://www.arlingtoncemetery.com/homepage.htm
> Photographs, map, epitaphs and information.

Cemeteries, Graveyards, Burying Grounds
http://www.potifos.com/cemeteries.html
> Everything you could possibly want to know about cemeteries. Directories, history, etiquette and more.

Virtual Memorials
http://virtual-memorials.com/
> A place to celebrate the lives of those those who have passed away.

Children and Death

Kidsaid
http://griefnet.org/KIDSAID/welcome.html
> A place for children to share and help each other deal with grief and loss.

A Parent's Guide to Helping Children Understand
http://hospice-cares.com/hands/library/pt_care/children.html
> Things a parent can do to help a child when someone is ill or has died.

Cryonics

Alcor Foundation and Cryonics

http://www.alcor.org/

According to this site, approximately 100 people have been placed in cryonic suspension since 1967, and another 1000 have signed up. No humans have yet been thawed out. Links and information about the process.

American Cryonics Society, Inc.

http://www.jps.net/cryonics/

Text also available in Spanish, Portuguese, French, Italian and German.

CryoCare: Human Cryopreservation Services

http://www.cryocare.org/

Information on cryonics, overview of company and description of services and costs.

CryoNet Home Page

http://cryonet.org/

Cryonics is defined as an experimental procedure for select patients who cannot be kept alive with today's medical abilities. Patients are are preserved at low temperatures with the hope that medical treatment will be available in the future. Site provides links to many online cryonics resources, including organizations and institutions that offer the service.

Cryonics

http://merkle.com/merkleDir/cryo.html

Links and commentary.

Life Extension Society

http://www.clark.net/pub/kfl/les/les.html

Information on this association and links. This group publishes a newletter.

Prometheus Project

http://www.prometheus-project.org/prometheus/

Suspended animation.

"Dark" Humor

Darwin Awards
http://www.DarwinAwards.com/
All of you with e-mail friends are aware what these are...
True stories often about ironic and ridiculous ways people
have died.

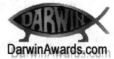

The Death Clock
http://www.deathclock.com/
Plug in your info to find your expected-date-of-death.

The Political Graveyard
http://www.politicalgraveyard.com/
Find out where dead politicians are buried. Humorous? You decide.

To Die For
http://www.2diefor.com/
"Celebrating cemetaries and the lighter side of death."

Yahoo's Tasteless Death Humor
http://dir.yahoo.com/Entertainment/Humor__Jokes__and_Fun/
Tasteless_Humor/Death/
Lots of links to humorous sites about death.

You're Outta Here!
http://www.cjnetworks.com/~roryb/outta.html
Obituaries of famous people.

Definition of Death

Biology, Consciousness and the Definition of Death
http://www.puaf.umd.edu/ippp/winter98/biology_consciousness.htm
Report from the Institute for Philosophy and Public Policy that presents a
biological perspective and the "person-based" perspective.

Brain Injury and Brain Death Resources
http://changesurfer.com/BD/Brain.html
Includes articles on, "Are the brain dead really dead?"

International Network for the Definition of Death
http://www.changesurfer.com/BD/Network.html
Medical, philosophical and psychological definitions of death.

Doctors and Death

Doctors Cry, Too
http://dr-boehm.com/dr_cry.htm
A collection of essays on how death affects doctors.

Essay on Dealing with Death
http://www.med.harvard.edu/publications/Focus/May12_1995/On_Becoming_A_Doctor.html
A medical student grapples with the human and physical aspects of death.

Euthanasia
See also: Biomedical Ethics - Advance Directives/Do Not Resuscitate

Doctor-Assisted Suicide: A Guide to WEB Sites and the Literature
http://web.lwc.edu/administrative/library/suic.htm
Varied points of view on physician-assisted suicide. Includes journal and newspaper articles, books, web resources, television programs, and legal decisions.

Euthanasia Definition
http://www.utm.edu/research/iep/e/euthanas.htm
Includes a discussion of the euthanasia controversy.

Euthanasia and End-of-Life Decisions
http://ethics.acusd.edu/euthanasia.html
Coverage from *Ethics Updates*.

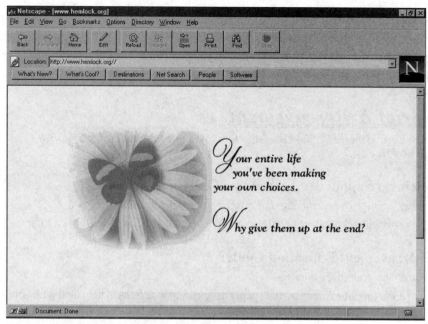

The Hemlock Society & Foundation. *http://www.hemlock.org//l*

Euthanasia and Physician Assisted Suicide

http://www.religioustolerance.org/euthanas.htm

Basic information on both sides of the issue, with essays and links. Seems especially concerned with religious viewpoints on the issue.

Euthanasia World Directory

http://www.finalexit.org/index.shtml

Includes a list of Right-to-Die societies, frequently asked questions, glossary, and laws. Also features news developments, statistics about euthanasia and suicide, book previews and other information.

The Hemlock Foundation and Hemlock Society

http://www.hemlock.org//

Information about the Society, which advocates the right to end one's life, and about the Foundation, which provides information on end-of-life issues.

Not Dead Yet!

http://acils.com/NotDeadYet/

This group fights euthanasia, especially when the disabled are involved.

Suicide Machine
http://www.freep.com/suicide/index.htm

Six-part article on Dr. Kevorkian; as published in the Detroit Free Press.

Grief & Bereavement

See also: Mental Health - Grief and Bereavement; Pregnancy & Childbirth - Miscarriages.

Being a Supportive Friend to a Grieving Persons
http://hospice-cares.com/hands/library/pt_care/gfriend.html

Advice and pointers to help someone you care about who suffered a loss.

Bereavement Education Center
http://www.bereavement.org/

Find brochure reprints, newspaper articles and web links to help deal with your own bereavement and grief, or the bereavement of children and friends. Includes information on outreach, funerals, palliative care, and suicide. Special section for helping men who have suffered a loss.

Crisis, Grief and Healing
http://www.webhealing.com/

Includes an honor page, where people write of their grief and healing process, as well as columns, discussion groups, links and a search engine.

Death, Dying and Grief
http://www.emanon.net/~kcabell/death.html

Bereavement resources, grief and loss support, and related web links.

GriefNet
http://rivendell.org/

A collection of resources valuable to those who are experiencing loss and grief. Includes a list of Usenet and mailing list support groups.

Suicide Loss
http://www.geocities.com/Heartland/Hills/8416/Poem.html

Support and help for suicide survivors.

Willowgreen

http://www.willowgreen.com/

Advice and books, audiotapes and videotapes that are designed to help with death and dying, loss and grief, healthy caregiving, life transitions and related topics.

Webster's Death, Dying and Grief Guide

http://www.katsden.com/death/index.html

Support and information on grief and dying.

Living Wills

See also: Biomedical Ethics - Advance Directives/Euthanasia.

Choice in Dying

http://www.choices.org/

This nonprofit organization originally created the idea for living wills. It provides advance directives, counsels patients and families, trains professionals, advocates for improved laws, and offers a range of publications and services.

Living Wills and Durable Powers of Attorney

http://www.wellweb.com/SENIORS/SRWILLS.HTM

Description of these legal documents and example of a living will.

Living Wills Registry (Canada)

http://www.sentex.net/~lwr/

Describes a living will, decisions you need to make, and how to order one.

Wills and Estate Planning

http://www.nolo.com/ChunkEP/EP.index.html

Includes information on estate planning, living trusts, taxes, funeral planning, living wills and powers of attorney.

U.S. Living Will Registry

http://www.uslivingwillregistry.com/

Stores wills electronically and keeps them available for hospital recall.

Organ Donation

See also: Transplantation.

American Association of Tissue Banks

http://www.aatb.org/

Facts about organ and tissue donation.

National Organ and Tissue Donation Initiative

http://www.hhs.gov/news/press/1999pres/990416.html

Fact sheet from the U.S. Department of Health and Human Services on efforts to encourage organ and tissue donations.

Organ Donation

http://www.organdonor.gov/

Frequently asked questions and links to organ donation and organ procurement organizations, transplant networks and government agencies.

United Network for Organ Sharing

http://www.unos.org/frame_Default.asp

How to give the gift of life. Resources and more.

Reflecting on Death

End of Life: Exploring Death in America

http://www.npr.org/programs/death/

Contains a transcript of this National Public Radio feature series, as well as resources, bibliography, and the opportunity to share your story.

Sociology of Death and Dying

http://www.trinity.edu/~mkearl/death.html

A comprehensive sociological study of death, with lots of links and hypertext.

Transhumanist Resources

http://www.aleph.se/Trans/

Transhumanists believe humans can strive to higher physical, mental & social levels, and they encourage research into life extension, cryonics & nanotechnology.

Resources

Borrowed Time
http://members.aol.com/BorrowTyme/death.html
Contains a collection of sites dealing with death in an informative or entertaining manner.

Death and Dying
http://dying.about.com/
Feature and news articles, and other resources on different aspects of death, from autopsy to teen grief.

Death Related Web Sites
http://www.stolaf.edu/people/leming/ death.html
Contains links and information on understanding death, especially social, religious and philosophical perspectives.

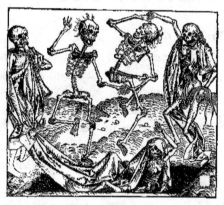

Death/Tod
http://www.totentanz.de/
Lots of links to all kinds of sites related to death, some in German.

Death Related Web Sites.
http://www.stolaf.edu/people/leming/death.html

DeathNET: Advancing the Art and Science of Dying Well
http://www.rights.org/deathnet/open.html
Award-winning site specializes in end-of-life issues.

E-Books on Death and Dying
http://www.buddhanet.net/r_booksd.htm
Buddhist perspectives.

End of Life Resources
http://ccme-mac4.bsd.uchicago.edu/CCMEDocs/Death
Information on all perspectives regarding the end of life, including euthanasia, do-not-resuscitate (DNR) orders, advanced directives, body donation, life extension, religious beliefs, etc. Site has related essays and web links.

Growth House
http://www.growthhouse.org/default.html
Guide to death, dying, grieving and end-of-life resources.

Quotes & Epitaphs

Death Quotes
http://members.aol.com/BorrowTyme/quote.html
"Quotations about abortion, assassination, death, dying, funerals, graves, killing, murder, suicide, and other pleasantly morbid topics."

Famous Quotes at Near Death
http://www.near-death.com/quotes.html
"I'm not afraid of death. It's just that I don't want to be there when it happens." - Woody Allen (and more).

Gravestone Quotes
http://members.aol.com/WordPlays/graves.html
Famous people's epitaphs.

Terminal Illness

Guide throught the Journey of Death
http://www.teleport.com/~hospice/states/oregon/hopewell/journey.htm
Online booklet to help survivors deal with the terminal illness of a loved one.

Help for the Dying
http://dying.miningco.com/msub9.htm
Words to comfort and help those who are terminally ill.

Last Acts

http://www.lastacts.org/

Discusses end-of-life issues and pursues efforts to find better ways to care for our dying.

Preparing for Approaching Death

http://hospice-cares.com/hands/library/pt_care/signs.html

Physical and mental signs and symptoms that one is preparing for death.

Widowhood

How to Cope with Being Widowed

http://www.seniors-site.com/widow/coping.html

Lots of good advice for dealing with the loss of a spouse.

Single Again

http://www.singleagain.com/

An online magazine for those who are divorced, separated or widowed.

Widow Net

http://www.fortnet.org/widownet/

Information and self-help resources for widows and widowers.

DENTISTRY

Bad Breath

American Breath Specialists
http://www.breath-care.com/
> How to treat bad breath, and/or hook up with a bad-breath treatment center.

Fresh Breath Resource Center
http://www.fresh-breath.com/
> Site is dedicated to helping people do something about bad breath.

Halitosis
http://www.betterhealth.com/childrens/dental/0,4264,1645,00.html
> Information for parents about children and bad breath.

Help for Halitosis?
http://cgi.pathfinder.com/drweil/archiveqa/0,2283,263,00.html
> Basic advice from Dr. Weil, at Pathfinder.

OnHealth: Checking Up on Halitosis
http://www.onhealth.com/ch1/columnist/item,40706.asp
> Information about bad breath.

Career Resources

See also: Health Care Careers and Education - Dentistry.

Careers in Dentistry

http://www.dent.unc.edu/careers/cidtoc.htm

Describes different career opportunities, their advantages, disadvantages, job opportunities, preparation, salary, licensure and more.

DDS-Online

http://www.dds-online.com/

Continuing dental education.

Dental Career Brochures

http://www.ada.org/prac/careers/br-dent.html

Brochures and fact sheets on becoming a dentist, dental hygienist, dental assistant, or dental laboratory technologist.

Dentist Tree

http://www.dentisttree.com/

Employment opportunities for dental professionals. View classified ads or resumés, or post your own information.

Children's Dentistry

Baby Teething

http://www.thelastplanet.com/bbteethi.htm

Information and web resources on teething infants.

Children's Dentistry: Making Dentists, Dentistry and Dental Education Fun

http://www.dentalreview.com/kids/

Kids can learn about bacteria, tooth care, and the proper way to brush their teeth at this site which features the character Stinky Tooth.

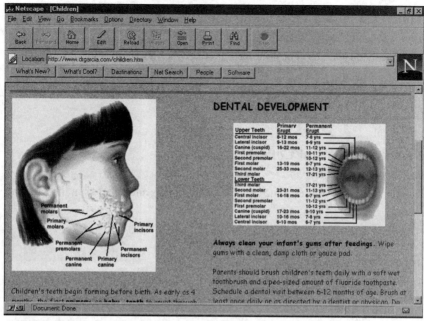

Children's Teeth. *http://www.drgarcia.com/children.htm*

Children's Teeth

http://www.drgarcia.com/children.htm

Dental development and dental care for infants.

Healthy Teeth and Gums

http://www.healthyteeth.org/teeth.html

Tooth growth and development.

How to Get Your Child to Brush

http://www.saveyoursmile.com/parents/dzgettingkidstobrush.html

Some hints to encourage your child to brush his or her teeth.

Tooth Fairy Online

http://www.toothfairy.org/

Dental information and tooth fairy adventures.

Wisdom Tooth Home Page

http://www.umanitoba.ca/outreach/wisdomtooth/

A page primarily for children that includes frequently asked questions (FAQs) and tips on proper oral health care. Offers a special section for parents.

Your Child's Teeth: A Guide for Parents
http://www.aafp.org/patientinfo/teeth.html

Questions and answers from the American Academy of Family Physicians.

Dental Schools

Dental Schools and Colleges
http://www.vh.org/Beyond/Dentistry/colleges.html

Links to the websites of dozens of dental schools and colleges in the U.S. and Canada.

Fear of Dentists

Beyond Fear
http://www.beyondfear.org/

A dental phobia self-help page with lots of information, support and suggestions.

Conquer Your Fear of the Dentist
http://saveyoursmile.com/healtharticles/dzdentalanxiety.html

Tips for overcoming dental phobia/dental anxiety.

Dental Phobia and Anxiety
http://www.dentalfear.org/

Comments for those who suffer from dental phobia and suggestions on what can be done to help it.

Holistic Dentistry

Holistic Dental Association
http://www.holisticdental.org:80/

Complementary and alternative dentistry.

Holistic Networker: Dentistry
http://holisticnetworker.com:80/listings/holisticdentistry.html
Listing of several holistic dentists and their contact information.

Implants

Dental Implant Home Page
http://www.dental-implants.com/
Patient treatment about dental implants, published articles, frequently asked questions, seminars, study group and more.

Oral Implantology
http://www.personal.u-net.com/~implants/
Basic information about oral implants as well as an implantology course for dentists and links to other implant websites.

Dental Implants: Are They Right For You?
http://www.dentistryinfo.com/dentalimplants.htm
Answers basic questions regarding dental implants.

Organizations

Academy of General Dentistry
http://www.agd.org/
Articles, archive and Academy information.

American Association of Pediatric Dentistry Online
http://aapd.org/
This page provides parent, media and member information on pediatric dentistry, including Internet links and publications, as well as links to kids' pages and to an online dental-themed coloring book.

American Dental Association Online
http://www.ada.org/

Find information for both consumers and professionals about dental care products and services, as well as news updates and links to related Internet sites.

Dental Society Internet Sites and E-mail Addresses
http://www.ada.org/sites/ass-soc.html

State-specific dental society contact information.

National Institute of Dental and Craniofacial Research
http://www.nidr.nih.gov/

Research, news, publications, funding and health information relating to oral and dental health. Part of the National Institutes of Health.

Orthodontistry

Braceface
http://www.braceface.com/

Information for kids and their parents about braces. Includes before and after photographs.

The Orthodontic CYBERjournal
http://www.oc-j.com/

Contains a lot of articles of interest to orthodontic professionals. Meetings and continuing education also offered.

Orthodontic Information Page
http://www.bracesinfo.com/

Information about braces for children and adults. Includes jokes, costs, general dental information, products, and links to other orthodontic sites.

Orthodontics Online!
http://www.aaortho.org/

The American Association of Orthodontists homepage offers consumer information regarding braces as well as organizational information for members.

Pets

Dental Care for Cats
http://newschannel5.webpoint.com/pets/dental.htm
    Suggestions on how to introduce tooth-brushing to your cat.

Dogs and Other Pets and Animals Dental Care Regime
http://www.planetpets.simplenet.com/subject3.htm
    Site says that 80 percent of dogs and 70 percent of cats show signs of gum disease by the age of 3. Learn to care for your pet's teeth.

Pets Need Dental Care, Too
http://www.petdental.com/
    Information on how to brush your pet's teeth.

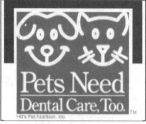

Pets Need Dental Care, Too.
http://www.petdental.com

Publications

@Dentistry
http://dentalxchange.com/@dentistry/index.htm
    Online journal of clinical and managerial dental issues.

The Blue Book
http://www.dentalbluebook.com/
    The "blue book" is a handbook of over-the-counter and prescription drugs used in treating dental patients. Drug monographs are available showing indications, dosage, description, interactions and more.

Dentistry Tomorrow
http://dentistry.mal.it/dentistry/index.html
    This international dental journal is available online in English and Italian. Read articles from the current issue or draw from the archives.

Dentists' Practice Publication Page

http://www.dentistpractice.com/publicat.htm
Links to a number of dental journals and publications.

Resources

Dental Consumer Advisor

http://www.toothinfo.com/
This site is intended for the public and includes advice on how to find a good dentist and what kind of dental benefits are practical. Also includes dental health basics, fact sheets, dental terminology, dental images and diagrams. Links to related Internet sites.

Dental Cyberweb

http://www.netsville.com/dental-web/
World-wide exchange of dentistry-related information for patients and dentists.

Dental Directory Service

http://www.teeth.com/
Find a dentist or a dental-related company online.

Dental Disease Prevention and Resources

http://www.holisticmed.com/dental/
Articles and links, from the Holistic Healing Home Page.

Dental Globe

http://dentalglobe.com/public.html
Site advises on how to find a dentist and provides definitions of dental terminology and information about dental insurance. In addition, it offers opportunities for online chat time with a dentist and links to dental websites written in Spanish.

Dental Icon

http://www.dentalicon.com/
Dental services, products and dealers, classified advertising, and an area devoted to professional education.

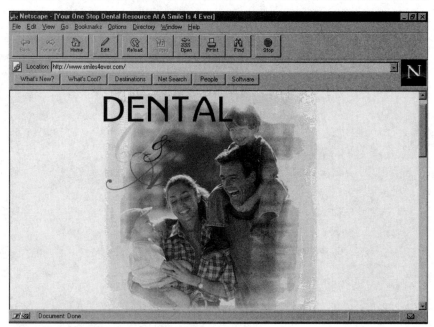

Dental Q & A. http://www.smiles4ever.com/

Dental Q and A
http://www.smiles4ever.com/

Contains not only frequently asked questions, but also an "Ask the Doc" service, information on child dentistry, cosmetic dentistry, tooth whitening and more.

Dental Related Internet Resources
http://www.dental-resources.com/

Topics include education, insurance, mail lists, and more.

Dental Site
http://www.dentalsite.com/

Provides links of interest to dental patients, dentists, dental assistants, dental hygienists, dental technicians, and vendors.

Dental X Change
http://dentalxchange.com/

Information for the public and for dental professionals. Includes products and discussion forums, as well as a directory of dentists.

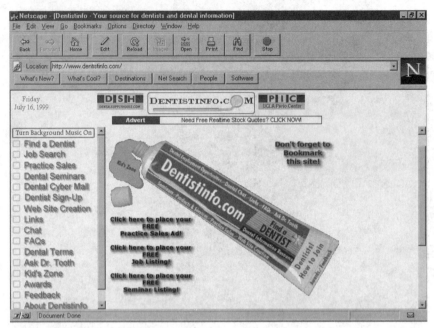

Dentistinfo. *http://www.dentistinfo.com/*

Dentistinfo

http://www.dentistinfo.com/

Everything from finding a dentist or dental seminar, to frequently asked questions, chat, and an area for kids.

Dentistry

http://www.mic.ki.se:80/Diseases/e6.html

Links from the Karolinska Institute. Primarily for dental professionals.

HSLS Dentistry Internet Resources

http://www.hsls.pitt.edu/intres/health/dental.html

Links to Internet metasites, web pages, reference resources, dictionaries, discussion groups, organizations, schools and patient information for the dental profession.

Galaxy's Dentistry (Health Occupations)

http://www.galaxy.com/galaxy/Medicine/Health-Occupations/Dentistry.html

Lots of links to dental sites on the web. Includes schools, articles, image collections, directories, organizations and periodicals.

Internet Dentistry Resources

http://www.vh.org/Beyond/Dentistry/sites.html

Links to dental colleges, organizations and journals, as well as dental education pages and commercial/dental vendor homepages.

"Virtual" Dental Center

http://www-sci.lib.uci.edu/HSG/Dental.html

Resources include medical and dental dictionaries and glossaries, journals, a dental anatomy browser, teaching files and tutorials, and dental images.

WHO Oral Health Country Profile Programme

http://www.whocollab.od.mah.se/index.html

Presents information on dental diseases and oral health services, by country.

DIABETES

Blood Sugar

Do Your Level Best: Start Controlling Your Blood Sugar Today

http://www.niddk.nih.gov/health/diabetes/dylb/home.htm

Online pamphlet from the National Institute of Diabetes and Digestive and Kidney Diseases.

Goals for Blood Sugar Control

http://www.joslin.harvard.edu/education/library/wbggoal.html

Brief article and chart that outlines the usual blood sugar ranges for a person who does not have diabetes.

How to Estimate Your Blood Sugar Level

http://www.insulin-pumpers.org/howto/HOWTO-estimate-BIR.shtml#toc2

Hints and information on how to check that your blood sugar to insulin, carbo to insulin, and blood sugar to carbo ratios are appropriate.

Diet

Diabetes and a Vegetarian Diet

http://www.envirolink.org/arrs/VRG/diabetes.html

Online article presents diabetes basics, the goals of the diabetic diet, good sources for fiber, and effects of alcohol. The main idea is to limit (or eliminate) animal fat, control blood lipid and weight, and keep carbohydrate and fiber intake high.

Diabetes Diet

http://www.diabetesdiet.com/diabetesdiet.htm

Basic guidelines and information about diabetes and diet.

Diabetes Library: Recipes

http://www.vmmc.org/diabetes/l/l-recipes.html

Main dishes, desserts, salads, soups and sauces from the Diabetes Café.

Diabetic Gourmet Magazine

http://diabeticgourmet.com/dgrcp2.shtml

Gourmet recipes for diabetics.

Nutrition

http://www.diabetes.org/nutrition/

Column on nutrition and diabetes, frequently asked questions and a recipe of the day (and archive) for diabetics. From the American Diabetes Association.

Discussion Groups

Diabetic Mailing List Home Page

http://www.lehigh.edu/lists/diabetic/

Subscription information, frequently asked questions (FAQs), and archives. To subscribe, send e-mail to: *listserv@lehigh.edu* and in the message type: "SUBSCRIBE DIABETIC *Yourname.*"

Joslin Diabetes Center Discussion Groups

http://www.joslin.org/managing/discussion.html

There are three different discussion groups here. One is for nutrition concerns, another is for those having trouble staying motivated in diabetes care, and the third provides support for family members of those with diabetes.

USENET FAQ's on Diabetes

http://www.cis.ohio-state.edu/hypertext/faq/usenet/diabetes/top.html

Frequently asked questions are sorted into sections: e.g., general, blood glucose monitoring, treatment, sources and research topics. There are also links to two discussion groups.

Eye Care

Diabetes and Your Eyes

http://www.jdfcure.com/brch14.htm

Brochure that explains why your eyes need special attention if you have diabetes.

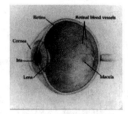

Don't Lose Sight of Diabetic Eye Disease

http://www.nei.nih.gov/publications/diabeye.htm

Don't Lose Sight of Diabetic Eye Disease. *http://www.nei.nih.gov/ publications/diabeye.htm*

It's possible to prevent vision loss due to diabetic eye disease. Important questions and answers.

Eye Problems for Diabetics

http://daily-apple.com/level3/ds3/diabetes/dehmdd3.htm

Signs of diabetic eye disease and how someone who is diabetic can protect his or her sight.

Foot Care

Amputation Prevention Global Resource Center

http://www.diabetesresource.org/

By following a few simple foot care tips, people with diabetes can reduce their chances of having foot problems like sores, cuts and bruises that may lead to amputation. Site offers clinical, educational and research information for patients and health care professionals.

Foot Care for Diabetes

http://www.niddk.nih.gov/health/diabetes/feet/feet.htm

Diabetes is the leading cause of leg and foot amputation. Good foot care is essential to managing the disease.

Footcare Direct: Diabetes

http://www.footcaredirect.com/diabetes.html

Explains the link between diabetics and foot ulcers, and the necessity of good foot care.

Organizations

American Association of Diabetes Educators

http://www.aadenet.org/

This association is made up of health professionals who teach people with diabetes. The site describes continuing education, research and meeting information.

American Diabetes Foundation

http://www.diabetes.org/

The mission of the ADF is to prevent and cure diabetes and to improve the lives of all people affected by the disease. This site provides information for people with diabetes types I and II, as well as for their families, teachers, child-care providers and health professionals. "Living with Diabetes" addresses issues of sex, pregnancy, parenting, complications and nutrition. ADF's research programs and grant support are also described. Legislation news and updates are offered in the form of a newsletter, "Diabetes Advocate." The monthly publication, *Diabetes Forecast*, presents the latest diabetes research and treatment news as well as day-to-day coping issues. Browse current and past issues, or subscribe. Links to related sites.

International Diabetes Foundation

http://www.idf.org/

Non-governmental, world-wide alliance of over 115 different diabetes organizations. Seeks to be a united voice for diabetes patients around the world.

International Diabetic Athletes Association

http://www.diabetes-exercise.org/

Having diabetes doesn't mean a person can't be physically active, this association proves.

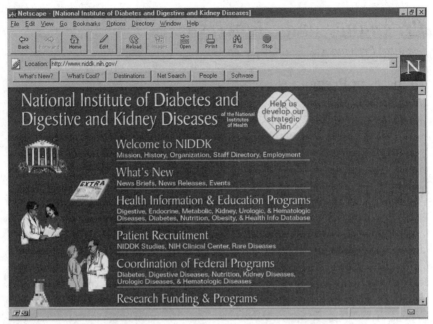

National Institute of Diabetes and Digestive and Kidney Disease.
http://www.niddk.nih/gov/

National Institute of Diabetes and Digestive and Kidney Diseases

http://www.niddk.nih.gov/

This site provides health information for the public about diabetes, digestive diseases, endocrine and metabolic diseases, hematological and kidney diseases, nutrition and obesity, and urologic diseases. In addition, it offers clinical information and databases, news, and funding resources for health professionals.

Organizations Offering (Diabetes) Support

http://www.demon.co.uk/diabetic/orgs.html

Organizations are listed geographically, by country.

Pregnancy and Diabetes

See also: Pregnancy & Childbirth - Diabetes.

Diabetes in Pregnancy

http://www.noah.cuny.edu/pregnancy/march_of_dimes/pregnancy.illness/
diabetes.html

A Public Health Information Fact Sheet includes fetal risks, pregnancy complications, screening, diet, exercise and other related topics.

Pregnancy and Diabetes

http://www.jdfcure.com/brch8.htm

Information about gestational diabetes, planning a pregnancy if you have diabetes, monitoring your blood glucose levels, fetal health and more.

Publications

Bob's Good Stuff List of Diabetes Magazines

http://goodstuff.orphanage.com/Diabetes/Magazines/index.html

Provides a link and description to approximately ten different diabetes magazines available on the web.

Diabetes Interview World

http://www.diabetesworld.com

Publication comes out every two months. Subscription information and articles are available at this website.

Diabetes Monitor

http://www.diabetesmonitor.com/mdcc.htm

Monitors diabetes happenings in cyberspace. Includes over 260 websites and 2700 links.

Research

Diabetes Action Research and Education Foundation

http://www.daref.org/

Include information and tips for those with diabetes. The Foundation funds grants to medical experts and researchers, and advocates for public diabetes health promotion. It also helps to provide equipment and programs to the needy.

Diabetes Education and Research Center

http://www.libertynet.org/~diabetes/

Includes frequently asked questions (FAQs), tips for individuals with the disease, and a diabetes chat area.

The National Diabetes Education Initiative

http://www.ndei.org

Offers educational programs for endocrinologists, diabetologists, primary care physicians, and other health care professionals. Includes "Literature Alert" providing diabetes research abstracts (and full text with subscription), diabetes news items, and "Physician's Focus," which offers quarterly newsletter, discussion, meeting highlights and data sharing.

Resources

Ask a Question about Diabetes

http://www.allexperts.com/medical/diabetes.shtml

Submit a question to a volunteer expert or browse through archives.

Bob's Good Stuff: Diabetes

http://goodstuff.orphanage.com/Diabetes/index.html

A great source of links to diabetes-related websites. Includes associations, coping, events, food, magazines, research, news, drugs and commercial sites, and provides a description and rating of each link.

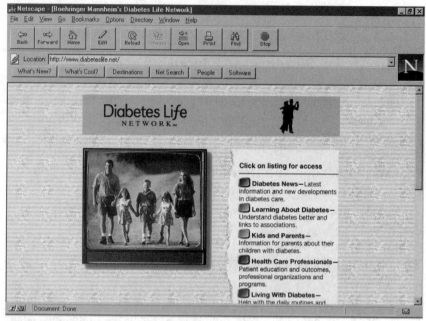

Diabetes Life Network. http://www.diabeteslife.net/

CDC's Diabetes and Public Health Resources
http://www.cdc.gov/nccdphp/ddt/ddthome.htm

Diabetes basics and advice from the Centers for Disease Control. It "translates scientific research findings into health promotion, disease prevention, and treatment strategies."

Complications of Diabetes Mellitus
http://aepo-xdv-www.epo.cdc.gov/wonder/prevguid/p0000063/body0002.htm

Starting page of online brochure for practitioners regarding the complications of diabetes mellitus. Follow the document sequence to progress in the publication.

Diabetes and Other Endocrine Disorders
http://cpmcnet.columbia.edu/texts/guide/toc/toc21.html

Information from Columbia University College of Physicians and Surgeons.

Diabetes Home Page
http://www.wvhealth.wvu.edu/clinical/diabetes/diagprev.htm

Good information on diabetes, including types, treatments, complications and prevention.

Diabetes Information Page
http://www.geocities.com/Athens/Forum/5769/diabete.html
Describes the different kinds of diabetes and presents diabetes statistics.

Diabetes Insipidus and Related Disorders Network
http://members.aol.com/ruudh/dipage1.htm
Information, practical hints, support and more on diabetes insipidus.

Diabetes Life Network
http://www.diabeteslife.net/
Provides patients and families with current diabetes news, education and health tips. Basic information.

Diabetes Mall
http://www.diabetesnet.com/
Diabetic products and publications, information and links.

Diabetes Mellitus Tutorial
http://www-medlib.med.utah.edu/WebPath/TUTORIAL/DIABETES/DIABETES.html
Information on diabetes mellitus and its complications.

Diabetes.com
http://www.diabetes.com/site/
Great information for adult patients with diabetes. Contains information and resources on diet, exercise, sexual intimacy, risk factors and prevention, and a section for the newly diagnosed.

Diabetic Data Centre
http://www.demon.co.uk/diabetic/index.html
Good information, news, frequently asked questions and pages for children.

Doctor's Guide to the Internet: Diabetes Information and Resources
http://www.pslgroup.com/DIABETES.htm
Lots of medical news and alerts. Information on diabetes for patient education and for health care professionals.

Facts about Diabetes
http://www.novo.dk/backgrou/backgrou/badia1uk.htm
Good, basic information in a very readable format.

Family's Guide to Diabetes
http://diabetes.cbyc.com/
A guide for diabetic kids and their families, based on experience. Includes feature articles, diabetes discussion and chats, information on the disease and resources.

Joslin's Online Diabetes Library
http://www.joslin.harvard.edu/education/library/index.html
Site is organized into diabetes information, and information on diabetes monitoring, insulin, oral medications, nutrition and exercise and disease complications. Also contains the *Beginner's Guide to Diabetes*.

Managing Your Diabetes
http://www.lilly.com/diabetes/
For health care professionals, patients and consumers in the United States.

The National Diabetes Information Clearinghouse
http://www.niddk.nih.gov/health/diabetes/ndic.htm
The Clearinghouse publishes the *Diabetes Dictionary*, an illustrated glossary of diabetes-related terms; publications online, which is made up of online brochures and fact sheets for patients; and an online database which describes numerous diabetes resources and provides their reference information.

Online Diabetes Resources
http://www.cruzio.com/~mendosa/faq.htm
Lists websites with substantive information about diabetes, as well as general diabetes information, organizations, universities, publications, medications and much more.

Patient Information on Diabetes
http://www.niddk.nih.gov/health/diabetes/diabetes.htm
Lots of information about diabetes, diabetes control, complications, kidney diseases, support and research information.

Rick Mendosa's Diabetes Directory

http://www.mendosa.com/diabetes.htm

A great deal of links to articles and websites about diabetes, written by Rick Mendosa, a freelance journalist.

Ten Facts about Diabetes and Kidney Disease

http://www.kidney.org/general/news/diabetes.cfm

From the National Kidney Foundation.

Risks & Symptoms

ADA African American Program

http://www.diabetes.org/africanamerican

More and more African-Americans are at risk for diabetes, but it can be controlled.

Diabetes Risk Test

http://www.diabetes.org/ada/risktest.asp

Sixteen million Americans have diabetes, yet one in three isn't aware of it.

Sepa Las Señales de Advertencia de La Diabetes

http://www.jdfcure.org/spanfact.htm

Diabetes warning signs in Spanish.

DIET & NUTRITION

Celiac Diet

See also: Digestive Disorders - Celiac Disease.

Celiac Disease On-Line Support Group

http://www.geocities.com/HotSprings/Spa/4003/delphi.html

Support for this auto-immune digestive disease. Moderated and unmoderated chats, message board, products and links.

Celiac Support Page

http://www.celiac.com/

Celiac disease is gluten or wheat intolerance. This site provides frequently asked questions, overview of the disease, and support, as well as lists of similar diseases, recipes and cooking tips, and doctors who specialize in its treatment.

The Gluten Free Page

http://www.panix.com/~donwiss/

Lots of links to educational, journal, association and commercial sites, as well as cookbooks, mailing lists and much more. With brief descriptions.

Gluten-Free Pantry Recipes

http://www.glutenfree.com/recipes.html

Free, downloadable wheat-free recipes.

Fasting & Detoxification

Detoxification Techniques
http://www.holisticmed.com/detox/detox.html
> Online book discusses detoxification techniques, tips, and ways to cleanse systems of the body.

Fasting
http://www.healthy.net/library/books/haas/detox/fasting.htm
> Duscusess the benefits and hazards of fasting and how to do it.

Health Facts about Fasting
http://www.freez.com/cinque/facts.html
> Eleven pointers to the benefits of occasional fasting.

Fat Acceptance

Big Folks Health FAQ
http://www.cis.ohio-state.edu/hypertext/faq/usenet/fat-acceptance-faq/health/faq.html
> Frequently asked questions about health issues for fat people.

Fat-Acceptance FAQs
http://www.cs.ruu.nl/wais/html/na-dir/fat-acceptance-faq/.html
> This site leads you to over a dozen different frequently asked questions concerning fat acceptance, and health and lifestyle for "big folks."

Fat Friendly Health Professionals List
http://www.bayarea.net/~stef/Fat/ffp.html
> Alphabetical list (by country, state and city) of health professionals that some fat people have deemed fat-friendly or who have declared themselves fat-friendly.

Fat Person's Home Page
http://www.io.com/~joeobrin/fat.html
> As the author of this site says, "Fat is not a four letter word. If it were, then it would be fate."

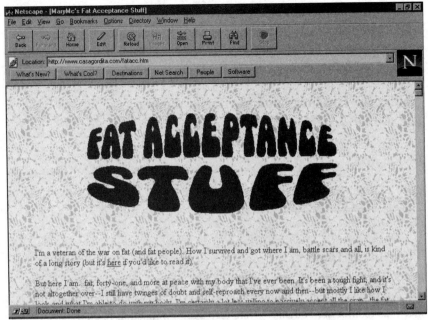

MaryMc's Fat Acceptance Stuff.   http://www.casagordita.com/fatacc.htm

Fat! So?

http://www.fatso.com/

Web-zine for individuals who are not ashamed of their weight.

Largesse: The Network for Size Esteem

http://www.fatso.com/fatgirl/largesse/

Site is described as a resource center and clearinghouse for "size diversity empowerment."

Lee Martindale's Rump Parliament

http://web2.airmail.net/lmartin/

E-zine by a veteran size rights advocate.

MaryMc's Fat Acceptance Stuff

http://www.casagordita.com/fatacc.htm

Links and commentary about size acceptance. Includes links to fat art and fat artists, as well as clothing for larger people.

National Association to Advance Fat Acceptance
http://www.naafa.org/
Nonprofit human rights organization dedicated to eliminating discrimination based on body size and improving the quality of life of fat people.

Radiance: The Magazine for Large Women
http://www.radiancemagazine.com/
Read back issues and get subscription information.

Food Allergies
See also: Allergies/Immunology.

The Allergy Center
http://www.onlineallergycenter.com/
It is estimated that 35 million Americans suffer from upper respiratory allergic reactions to airborne pollen.This site offers an introduction to allergies and their symptoms, as well as specifics regarding food allergy, airborne allergy and "hormone" allergy. Diagnosis, treatment and resources are also provided.

The Food Allergy Network
http://www.foodallergy.org/
Provides information for consumers and health professionals about food allergies, FAN activities, product alerts and daily tips.

Food Allergy Sites - Suite 101.com
http://206.186.163.160/linkcategory.cfm/allergies/4132
Links, discription and rating.

Mastering Food Allergies
http://www.nidlink.com/~mastent/
Contains allergy information, allergen-free recipes and a resource page.

Food Safety

See also: Public Health.

Facts about Food Irradiation

http://www.dainet.de/bfe/english/thmliste.htm

Includes frequently asked questions, links and bibliography.

International Food Information Council

http://ificinfo.health.org/

Food safety and nutritional information, including facts about food labeling and food allergies. The purpose of the IFCC is to provide sound and scientific information on food safety and nutrition for journalists, health professionals, educators, government officials and consumers.

Food Safety Consortium

http://www.uark.edu/depts/fsc/

The Consortium is a group of university researchers who conduct extensive investigation into all areas of poultry, beef and pork meat production, from the farm to the consumer's table.

FoodLaw

http://www.ift.org/divisions/food_law/

Cites specific food laws and regulations.

Institute of Food Technologists

http://www.ift.org/

The Institute for Food Technologists has a website that offers career information, publications and scientific communications, as well as meetings, membership and employment news. Food scientists study food and principles underlying food processing, while food technologists study methods of preserving and processing foods in healthful ways.

National Center for Food Safety and Technology

http://www.iit.edu/~ncfs/

This is a consortium of academic, industry and government groups that seek to protect food safety in light of the emerging food technologies.

National Food Safety Database

http://www.foodsafety.org/

Food safety materials for consumers, the food industry, and educators, along with coverage of critical issues in food safety.

General Nutrition

AHA: Diet and Nutrition

http://www.americanheart.org/catalog/Health_catpage4.html

Dietary Recommendations from the American Heart Association. Also find sample recipes and nutrition facts.

American Dietetic Association

http://www.eatright.org/

Nutrition resources and facts for consumers and professionals. Includes marketplace of ADA publications, news updates, classified ads, and a searchable database of dietitians.

Arbor Nutrition Guide

http://www.arborcom.com/

A huge number of links regarding clinical nutrition (physician, diseases, deficiencies, diets, sports nutrition, toxicology), applied nutrition (commercial, dietitians, dietary guidelines, journals, patient information), food (food industry, cooking, cultural nutrition, ancient diets) and food science (i.e., food composition, genetic engineering, food law, food safety).

Blonz Guide to Nutrition, Food Science and Health

http://blonz.com/

Site offers a large number of resources on nutrition, food and fitness resources and associations; food resources, companies and associations; health and medical resources and associations; online newspapers, magazines and networks; government resources, U.S. and other; food and nutrition discussion groups; health, medical and wellness publications; nutrition resources; as well as agriculture and sustainable agriculture and gardening resources.

CyberDiet

http://www.cyberdiet.com/

Nutritional profile and self-assessment, tips on diet and nutrition, exercise and fitness, weight loss, seven-day vegetarian and nonvegetarian diets, and more.

Dietetics Online

http://www.dietetics.com/

Information and newsletter on nutrition and the dietetic profession.

Dole 5-a-Day Homepage

http://www.dole5aday.com/

Dole sponsors this site for children, to remind them to eat five servings of fruit and vegetables every day. According to research, the health benefits of eating fruit and vegetables are indisputable, but Americans average only half of the recommended five servings. Along with some basic information, the site offers fun stuff for kids, using cartoon characters to tell details about asparagus, apples, bananas, blueberries, broccoli, cauliflower, carrots and other fruits and veggies.

Food Pyramid Guide

http://www.ganesa.com/food/index.html

Click on a food group to get a brief description of what is included as well as recommended serving suggestions.

Full USDA Nutrient Database Listings

http://www.fatfree.com/usda/all.shtml

Huge database which provides nutrient information (vitamin, energy, minerals etc.) for many food products.

Grand Style Women's Club and Spa

http://www.grandstyle.com/spa.htm

Promotes a healthy lifestyle, no matter what you weigh.

Internet FDA

http://www.fda.gov/

Information about the U.S. Food and Drug Administration and product alerts. Major areas covered are food, drugs, animal drugs and cosmetics.

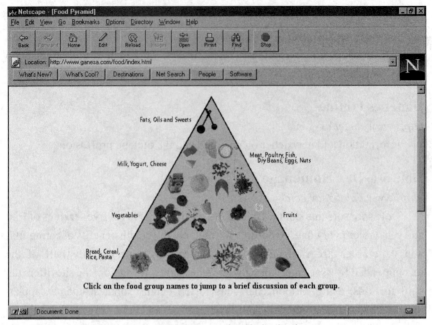

Food Pyramid Guide. *http://www.ganesa.com/food/index.html*

Krispin Komments on Nutrition and Health
http://www.krispin.com/

This site provides information on magnesium, potassium and protein and the sources from which they can be derived. Also find information on thyroid disease and an article linking abuse and nutrition.

My Virtual Encyclopedia: Health and Nutrition
http://www.refdesk.com/health.html

This site alphabetically lists an enormous number of health and nutrition web pages.

Nutritional and Metabolic Diseases
http://www.mic.ki.se/Diseases/c18.html

The Karolinska Institute's comprehensive list of links to sites involving nutritional and metabolic diseases.

Penn State Nutrition
http://nutrition.hhdev.psu.edu/

Graduate and undergraduate programs in nutrition.

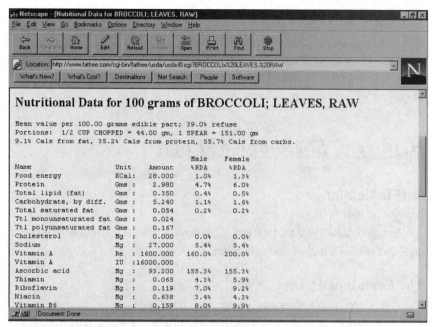

*Sample page showing the nutritional content of broccoli from the: **Full USDA Nutrient Database Listing**. Start at: http://www.fatfree.com/usda/all.shtml*

People's Place

http://www.peopleplace.com/

Offers listings for personal and environmental healthy living in the form of products, services, resources and self-education, as well as a forum for interaction with product and service providers. Main topics include healthy eating, personal growth, professional growth, yoga and meditation, and "other nice places."

Professor Geoff Skurray's Food, Nutrition and Health Information Page

http://www.hawkesbury.uws.edu.au/~skurrayg/

Includes adult RDA dietary guidelines, a free dietetic simulation program and information on the food pyramid. Describes courses from the Centre for Advanced Food Research and provides exam questions.

Sound Nutrition: An International Appeal

http://www.fcs.uga.edu/~selbon/apple/guides/

Based on a display at the 1996 summer Olympics in Georgia, this site includes guidelines on nutrition and accompanying graphics from approximately 20 countries.

"Virtual" Nutrition Center
http://www-sci.lib.uci.edu/HSG/Nutrition.html

This site has a good section on nutritional calculations, including body mass index, calories, heart rate and longevity. Also features courses and tutorials, links, news, journals and anatomy information.

History & Sociology of Food

EatEthnic.com
http://www.EatEthnic.com/

Everything about ethnic food and ingredients, international holidays, religious diets and customs, recipes and cultural nutrition resources.

The Evolutionary Diet
http://www.sccs.swarthmore.edu/~aaron/nutrition2.html

Author seeks to explain how our current diet is not suited to the foods that natural selection best allows us to digest and seeks to examine present-day health and eating habits from a Darwinian perspective.

The Paleolithic Diet Page
http://www.panix.com/%7epaleodiet/

Links to what our ancient ancestors ate.

SANE: Sociological Approaches to Nutrition and Eating
http://www.newcastle.edu.au/department/so/tasa/tasa16.htm

Discusses the social context of food with conferences, databases and associations, books and journal links.

World Food Habits
http://www.ilstu.edu/class/anth273-foodways/foodbib.html

Resources for the anthropological study of food. Select a region or select a topic.

Lactose Intolerance

Lactose Intolerance
http://www.niddk.nih.gov/health/digest/pubs/lactose/lactose.htm
What lactose intolerance is, how it is diagnosed and treated.

Milk Allergy and Lactose Intolerance
http://www.adelaide.net.au/~ndk/no_milk.htm
Information and support group.

No Milk Page
http://www.panix.com/~nomilk/
Lactose maldigestion, milk allergies, and casein intolerance: definitions, information and resources on the web.

Steve Carper's Lactose Intolerance Clearinghouse
http://ourworld.compuserve.com/homepages/stevecarper/welcome.htm
Lactose news, research, basic dairy facts, questions and answers, and products.

Why Does Milk Bother Me?
http://www.niddk.nih.gov/health/digest/pubs/whymilk/index.htm
Very simple facts about lactose intolerance and what can be done about it.

Macrobiotic Diet

Carbondale Center for Macrobiotic Studies
http://www.macrobiotic.org/
Includes a monthly column, macrobiotic booklist, and questions and answers about the macrobiotic diet and philosophy.

Macrobiotics Internet Resources
http://www.holisticmed.com/www/macrobiotics.html
Links to macrobiotics sites on the web.

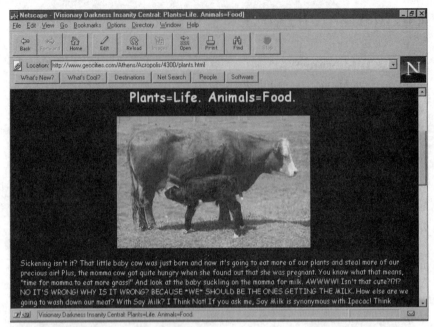

Plants=Life. Animals=Food.

Sickening isn't it? That little baby cow was just born and now it's going to eat more of our plants and steal more of our precious air! Plus, the momma cow got quite hungry when she found out that she was pregnant. You know what that means, "time for momma to eat more grass!" And look at the baby suckling on the momma for milk. AWWWW! Isn't that cute?!?!? NO IT'S WRONG! WHY IS IT WRONG? BECAUSE *WE* SHOULD BE THE ONES GETTING THE MILK. How else are we going to wash down our meat? With Soy Milk? I Think Not! If you ask me, Soy Milk is synonymous with Ipecac! Think

The Official Meatatarian Homepage.
http://www.geocities.com/Athens/Acropolis/4300/meat.html

Macrobiotics Online

http://www.macrobiotics.org/

The macrobiotic way of life is a holistic approach to health and diet. Site describes the macrobiotic diet, including its principles and philosophy, guidelines and recipes, recommendations, frequently asked questions and health information.

MacroNews

http://www.macronews.com/

Includes links to publications.

Health Recovery Pages

http://www.macrobiotics.org/recovery1.html

Information and stories about curing illness through macrobiotics.

Meatatarian Diet

Official Meatatarian Homepage
http://www.geocities.com/Athens/Acropolis/4300/meat.html
Humorous page for meat-eaters.

Recipes

Berry Recipes
http://www.hursts-berry.com/recipes.html
Things you can do with blackberries, rasberries, currants, loganberries, blueberries and more-berries.

FATFREE: The Low-Fat Vegetarian Archive
http://www.fatfree.com/
Contains 2,541 fat free and low fat recipes and information on low fat, vegetarian diets.

Great Vegetarian Recipes
http://www.webvalue.net/recipes/
Particular emphasis on Chinese and American vegetarian recipes.

HealthGate Healthy Eating
http://www.healthgate.com/healthy/eating/index.shtml
Lots of information on food, recipes and healthy eating.

The Healthy Kitchen
http://www.healthykitchen.com/
Healthy recipes using foods that are in season.

Paleolithic Eating Support Recipe Archives
http://www.panix.com/~paleodiet/list/
All recipes are grain-free, dairy-free and bean-free.

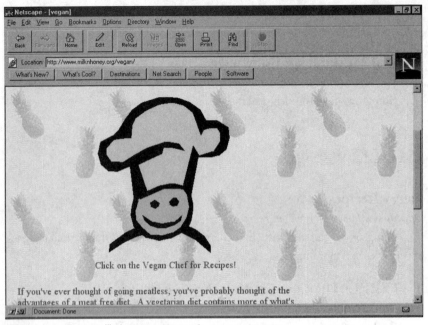

Vegan. *http://www.milknhoney.org/vegan/*

Research

Purdue University Food Science

http://www.foodsci.purdue.edu/

Describes faculty research, publications, outreach programs, and the graduate and undergraduate programs. Also provides web links.

Rutgers University Department of Food Science

http://foodsci.rutgers.edu/

Food scientists study the physical, microbiological and chemical make-up of food, and develop ways to process, preserve, package and store food safely. This site describes Rutgers' program and the work of a food scientist. Fact sheets on safe food preparation, handling and storage are provided, along with frequently asked questions and web links.

Vegan Diet

Essays on Vegan Living
http://www.vegsource.com/joanne/essays.htm
Being vegan, sowing seeds of compassion, and feeding the heart.

Vegan
http://www.milknhoney.org/vegan/
Recipes for a non-dairy, egg- and animal-product free way of cooking.

Vegan Action
http://www.vegan.org/
A nonprofit organization formed to enhance public awareness of the benefits of a vegan lifestyle and to improve the availability of vegan food. Site provides information on veganism, a catalog of products and books, news alerts, campaign information and activist opportunities.

Vegan Awakening
http://www.vegan.org/awakening/
News, recipes, quotes, articles, information and a picture gallery of animals, all supporting a vegan lifestyle.

Vegan Biker's Domain
http://www.nildram.co.uk/veganmc/
Links to vegan and motorcyclist sites on the web.

Vegan Outreach
http://www.vegsource.com/vo/
Arguments for veganism from healthy, ecological, theological and ethical perspectives. Newsletter and resources.

Vegetarian Diet

Mega Index to Vegetarian Information
http://www.veg.org/veg/Docs/vegindex.html
Tool for finding information on vegetarianism drawn from a variety of resources.

North American Vegetarian Society
http://www.cyberveg.org/navs/
Offers *Vegetarian Voice Magazine* and membership information.

Vegetarian Nutrition: Frequently Asked Questions
http://members.aol.com/sauromalus/vegnutr.htm
Information on vegetarian and vegan nutrition that is based on the most recent scientific research.

Vegetarian Pages
http://www.veg.org/veg/
Guide to the Internet for vegetarians, vegans and others.

Vegetarian Resource Group
http://www.vrg.org/
Includes information on vegetarianism, lifestyle and travel guides, nutrition and recipes, as well as a catalog of vegetarian products.

Vegetarian Society of the United Kingdom
http://www.vegsoc.org/
Many links and good information.

Very Vegetarian Sites
http://www.cyber-kitchen.com/index/html/gp35.html
Comprehensive list of web resources for vegetarians.

World Guide to Vegetarianism
http://www.veg.org/veg/Guide/index.html
Site lists vegetarian and vegetarian-friendly restaurants, stores, organization and services by country, state, county and city. In addition, it lists chain restaurants that offer vegetarian and vegetarian-friendly products.

The World of Tofu

http://www.tofu.com/

Recipes, information and arguments for vegetarianism.

Vitamins

Dr. Duke's Phytochemical and Ethnobotanical Databases

http://www.ars-grin.gov/duke/index.html

You can find the chemical content of particular plants, find out which plants have highest concentrations of a particular chemical, and/or learn about the ethnobotanical uses of plants.

MN-NET Home Care

http://www.idrc.ca/mi/mnnet.htm

Micronutrient malnutrition information.

Nutrient Data Laboratory Food Composition Data

http://www.nal.usda.gov/fnic/foodcomp/

Gives the nutritional content of numerous food products. Input food and it will supply you with the composition into water, energy, protein, lipid, fiber, carbohydrate and other proximates, then further into lipid type, amino acid, fats, vitamins and minerals. Includes frequently asked questions, glossary and links.

Office of Dietary Supplements

http://odp.od.nih.gov/ods/databases/ibids.html

Database of published, international, scientific literature on dietary supplements, including vitamins, minerals, and botanicals.

Prevention's Vitamin Dispenser

http://www.healthyideas.com/healing/vitamin/

Select from a number of health problems and receive information on vitamins recommended to help treat the condition.

Reference Guide for Vitamins
http://www.realtime.net/anr/vitamins.html

Briefly describes the importance of a number of items (including vitamins A, B-1, B-2, B-6, B-12, niacin, pantothenic acid and others), and presents deficiency symptoms.

Vitamin Buzz
http://www.vitaminbuzz.com/

More than simply vitamins are discussed here. This site answers questions about nutritional supplements, herbal remedies, homeopathic treatments, as well as indicates drug interactions and explains diet and treatment therapies.

Vitamin Update
http://bookman.com.au/vitamins/

The latest developments in vitamin and mineral research. Includes news briefs, links and information on micronutrients.

Vitamins
http://www.doitnow.com/~gillick/ph05000.html

Brief information on the different vitamins and their functions and uses.

Weight Loss

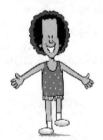

At Home with Richard Simmons. *http://www. richardsimmons.com/*

At Home with Richard Simmons
http://www.richardsimmons.com/

Includes club and chat rooms, information on exercise, diet and recipes, as well as enthusiastic support.

Body Fat Calculator
http://top.monad.net/~vsi/java/bfc.html

Body fat calculations for men and women.

Burn Barometer
http://homearts.com/helpers/calculators/burnf1.htm

Enter the amount of time you spent doing an activity to learn the approximate number of calories you have expended.

Circle of Hope

http://www.swlink.net/~colonel/coh.html

Support group open to anyone with a desire to lose weight and who is 100 or more pounds overweight.

Diet and Weight Loss/Fitness Home Page

http://www1.mhv.net/~donn/diet.html

Diet and weight loss tips and resources.

Diet Doc

http://www.mweb.co.za/health/diet/dietdoc.html

Includes the DietDoc expert forum, with talkback, and questions and answer opportunities on weekly topics.

Dieter's Guide to Weight Loss During Sex

http://www.maui.net/~jms/weight.html

Not everything good for you is a chore.

Diettalk

http://www.diettalk.com/index.shtml

Many diet links. Includes nutrition calculators, diet products, information on eating disorders and obesity, fitness, recipes, personal homepages, journals, magazines, support groups and more.

Health Information about Fatness

http://www.cs.stir.ac.uk/~scu/BF/Inf/main.html

Links to articles and research relating fatness to diseases.

Medical Information on Obesity and Weight Control

http://www.weight.com/

Objective information from an M.D. Includes specific current topics, general information on obesity and weight control, information on obesity-related medical conditions, and facts about eating disorders.

The Science of Obesity and Weight Control

http://www.loop.com/~bkrentzman/

Includes news and information on medications, weight control, alternative therapy, nutrition, exercise, and a section for physicians.

Starting Your Weight-Loss Journal
http://homearts.com/gh/health/1196opb3.htm

Advice on creating a weightloss journal that you write in two times a day for the first three months of your diet.

Yeast (Candida)

Candid Candida
http://dspace.dial.pipex.com/town/park/gcn23/candida/

Candida is linked to chronic fatigue syndrome and many other reactions. Site contains description, treatment, diets, support and links.

Candida Page
http://www.panix.com/~candida/

Many links to *Candida albicans* and candidiasis websites.

Yeast Connection
http//www.yeastconnection.com/

Information about yeast-connected (candida) disorders.

Yeast Syndrome
http://www.healthy.net/LIBRARY/Books/Haas/medtreat/YEASTSYN.HTM

Factors common to patients with yeast syndrome, how to treat it, and how to avoid it.

Yeast Virtual Library
http://genome-www.stanford.edu/Saccharomyces/VL-yeast.html

Explains what yeasts are and provides links to numerous research and educational sites about candida and other kinds of yeasts, many used in lab experiments.

DIGESTIVE DISORDERS / GASTROENTEROLOGY

Celiac Disease

See also: Diet & Nutrition - Celiac Diet.

Celiac Disease

http://www.icondata.com/health/pedbase/files/CELIACDI.HTM

Clinical information on celiac disease, the inability to digest gluten or wheat.

Celiac Disease and Gluten Sensitivity

http://cpmcnet.cpmc.columbia.edu/dept/gi/celiac.html

Includes a description of celiac sprue, its symptoms, treatment and contact organizations.

What Is Celiac Disease and Dermatitis Herpetiformis?

http://www.wwwebguides.com/nutrition/diets/glutenfree/faq.html

The Celiac Action Line fact sheet.

Colon and Bowel

See also: Cancer/Oncology - Colon Cancer.

AfraidToAsk.com's Bowel Movement Guide

http://www.afraidtoask.com/bowel/

"All things bowel." Find information on digestive diseases, the GI tract, normal bowel movement appearance and regularity, bowel hygiene and gas.

The Colon Health Network
http://colonhealth.net/index.htm

The focus of this site is on alternative medical treatments for colon problems. It also includes a therapist search, links and a series of free health reports.

The Health Connection: Bowel
http://www.crha-health.ab.ca/hlthconn/topics/bowel.htm

Covers Crohn's Disease, laxatives, spastic colon and ulcerative colitis.

IBS PAGE: Irritable Bowel Syndrome Web Sites
http://www.panix.com/~ibs/

Links to and descriptions of websites about irritable bowel syndrome. Includes sites by individuals, organizations, alternative medicine and pharmaceutical sites, newsgroups and more.

Irritable Bowel Syndrome Self Help Group
http://www.ibsgroup.org/

Contains a lot of information on IBS and membership to this group. Includes a medication listing, information on studies, a bulletin board and discussion group.

Spastic Colon
http://www.plgrm.com/health/S/Spastic_Colon.HTM

Provides searches on several search engines and directories, as well as direct links to spastic colon news, pictures, resources and discussion.

Crohn's Disease

Crohn's and Colitis Foundation of America
http://www.ccfa.org/

Information on inflammatory bowel disease. This organization sponsors clinical research, provides education for public and professionals, and support for those who suffer from the disease.

Crohn's Disease Site
http://www.angelfire.com/ga/crohns/

Great information describing Crohn's; for patients.

Crohn's Disease Support & Information

http://web3.foxinternet.net/samphire/

Medications, news, related links, alternative medicine, mailing list and Crohn's disease club.

Crohn's Disease Web Page

http://members.aol.com/bospol/homepage/crohns.htm

General information, illustrations, articles, frequently asked questions and other resources.

Crohn's Disease/Ulcerative Colitis/Inflammatory Bowel Disease Pages

http://qurlyjoe.bu.edu/cduchome.html

Contains FAQs, links to other medical institutions, pharmaceutical companies, government agencies, commercial sites, support groups, mail lists and more.

Facts about Crohn's Disease and Ulcerative Colitis

http://www.ccfc.ca/facts.html

Information from the Crohn's and Colitis Foundation of Canada, presented in English and French.

Teens with Crohn's Disease

http://pages.prodigy.net/mattgreen/

Experience, stories and advice for teens from teens diagnosed with Crohn's disease. Also offers recipes and links.

Constipation

Chronic Constipation and Encopresis in Children

http://www.med.virginia.edu/cmc/tutorials/constipation/symptoms.htm

What these two conditions are, why they happen to children, and how they can be treated.

Constipation

http://www.gastro.com/cnstipa.htm

Misconceptions regarding constipation, as well as common causes, diagnosis, treatment and information on laxatives.

Constipation: HealthWorld Online

http://www.healthy.net/clinic/dandc/constipa/

Articles discuss herbal, integrative and nutritional approaches to this condition.

Esophagus

See also: Cancer/Oncology - Esophageal Cancer.

Dysphagia Resource Center

http://dysphagia.com/

Resources for swallowing and swallowing disorders.

GERD: Gastroesophageal Reflux Disease

http://www.pathcom.com/~minaise/gerd.html

Cause, signs and symptoms, treatment, diagnosis and treatment options for GERD, which is linked to hiatal hernias and esophageal cancer.

GERD Information Resource Center

http://www.gerd.com/

Contains an introduction to GERD, GERD frequently asked questions, and an articles archive.

Heartburn, Reflux and Esophagitis (Some Things You Should Know)

http://www.cyberstreet.com/swfrmc/GI-HEART.HTM

What is heartburn? What drugs are used to treat it? Information for patients.

Seattle Barrett's Esophagus Program

http://www.fhcrc.org/~barretts/

People who develop Barrett's esophagus may have symptoms of heartburn, indigestion, difficulty swallowing solid foods, or nocturnal regurgitation.

Gallstones

Dieting and Gallstones
http://wellweb.com/nutri/dieting_and_gallstones.htm
During periods of rapid weight loss, an individual's risk of developing gallstones is increased.

Gallstones
http://www.healthtouch.com/level1/leaflets/nddic/nddic080.htm
Describes gallstones, their cause, symptoms, diagnosis and treatment.

Gallstones: A National Health Problem
http://gi.ucsf.edu/alf/info/infogallstones.html
Describes who is at greatest risk of developing gallstones and how to treat and prevent gallstones.

Infoseek: Gallstones
http://infoseek.go.com/WebDir/Health/Diseases_and_ailments/Gallstones?
Links to several rated sites about gallstones and gallbladder disease.

Laparoscopic Cholecystectomy
http://www.anesthesia.org/public/guides/lap_chole.html
Online booklet with general information on gallbladders and laparoscopic cholecystectomy, which is the removal of your gallbladder in a closed procedure.

Types of Gallstones
http://websurg.uth.tmc.edu/digestive/gallstone/gall6.html
Photographs and description of gallstones.

Gastritis and Ulcers

CURE: The Center for Ulcer Research and Education
http://www.med.ucla.edu/Cure/
Although this Center began with a focus on ulcer research, it has evolved to adress all kinds of digestive disorders.

Helicobacter Foundation

http://www.helico.com/

All about *Helicobacter pylori*, its diagnosis, treatment and clinical correlations. Site includes frequently asked questions, discussion group, helicobacter movie, history and pathogenesis. *Helicobacter pylori* are the bacteria which cause gastritis, which may lead to ulcers and other digestive complaints.

Treatment for Helicobacter Pylori

http://www.vianet.net.au/~bjmrshll/table1.htm

This is a table for physicians to consult when using medications to treat patients with this bacteria.

Helicobacter Pylori in Peptic Ulcer

http://text.nlm.nih.gov/nih/cdc/www/94cvr.html

Full text of a National Institutes of Health Development Conference consensus statement from 1994.

Helicobacter Pylori and Peptic Ulcer Disease

http://www.cdc.gov/ncidod/dbmd/hpylori.htm

Fact sheets from the Centers for Disease Control and Prevention; in both English and Spanish.

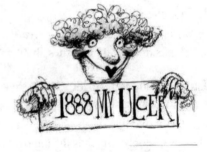

H. Pylori and Peptic Ulcers

http://www.niddk.nih.gov/health/digest/pubs/hpylori/hpylori.htm

Call this number for information on ulcers and H. Pylori. Site: **Helicobacter Pylori and Peptic Ulcer Disease.**
http://www.cdc.gov/ncidod/dbmd/hpylori.htm

For patients from the National Digestive Diseases Information Clearinghouse.

Stomach and Duodenal Ulcers

http://www.gastro.com/ulcers.htm

Describes ulcers, their cause (lifestyle, smoking, caffeine, alcohol, stress, acid and pepsin), diagnosis, treatment and much more.

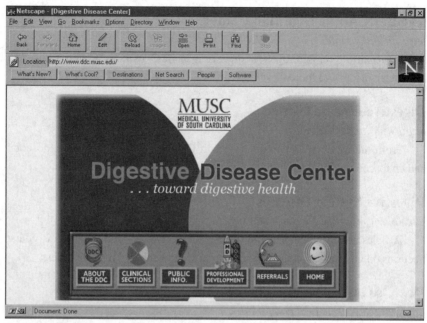

Digestive Disease Center of the Medical University of South Carolina.
http://www.ddc.musc.edu/

General Resources

Atlas of Digestive Endoscopy
http://www.zulia.com/gastro/i_index.html

English version of a Spanish language site that includes a collection of endoscopic images of the esophagus, stomach, duodenum and colon.

Atlas of Gastrointestinal Endoscopy
http://www.atl.mindspring.com/~dmmmd/index.html

Endoscopic images of the stomach, esophagus, duodenum, colon and more.

Columbia University Gastroenterology Web
http://cpmcnet.columbia.edu/dept/gi/

Information about the faculty and department specialties, as well as information and links on specific digestive diseases. Includes links to academic gastroenterology sites, organizations, pathology, radiology, and endoscopy.

The Daily Apple Digestion Center
http://thedailyapple.com/Level2/kd-hm3.htm
Information on kidney and digestion topics, such as Crohn's disease, heartburn, ulcers and food allergies.

Digestive Disease Center
http://www.ddc.musc.edu/
From the Medical University of South Carolina, information on endoscopy and endoscopic-related techniques, liver diseases, and digestive diseases.

Digestive System Diseases
http://www.mic.ki.se/Diseases/c6.html
Articles about the digestive system, gastroenterology and specific disorders. Sections on gastric, esophageal, biliary tract, pancreatic and liver disorders.

Dr. K's Gastrointestinal Diseases Web Page
http://www.cybermedical.com/drk/drk.html
Professionals and patients alike can find up-to-date information on diseases of the gastrointestinal tract and liver.

"Everything You Ever Wanted to Know about Gastroenterology" Page
http://www.cyberstreet.com/swfrmc/GI-PAGE.HTM
General information about gastroenterology and fact sheets on disorders of the digestive tract. From Barrett's esophagus, ulcers and swallowing disorders, to treatment and examinations such as colonoscopy and ambulatory pH monitoring.

Gastroenterology Consultants
http://www.gastro.com/
Provides information on gastroenterology and liver diseases; for patients.

Gastroenterology Resources
http://cait.cpmc.columbia.edu/dept/gi/elsewhere.html
Many links to academic and research facilities, organizations and other sources dealing in some way with gastroenterology, liver disease, or nutrition.

HealthWeb: Gastroenterology Disease Resources
http://www.medlib.iupui.edu/hw/gastro/
Disease, career and educational resources for health care professionals.

National Digestive Diseases Information Clearinghouse

http://www.niddk.nih.gov/health/digest/nddic.htm

Responds to requests for information; provides online publications, professional and patient education and other information from NIDDK.

NIDDK Health Information: Digestive Diseases

http://www.niddk.nih.gov/health/digest/digest.htm

Includes the digestive diseases dictionary, and information on appendicitis, bleeding in the digestive tract, celiac disease, cirrhosis, constipation, Crohn's disease, diarrhea, gallstones, gas, ulcer, heartburn, hemorrhoids, hernia, iritable bowel syndrom, pancreatitis, Whipple's disease, and many other disorders of the digestive system. Literature available in Spanish as well.

PharmInfoNet's Digestive Disease Center

http://pharminfo.com/disease/gastro.html

This site offers links to patient information and frequently asked questions (FAQs), sorted by organ and by disease.

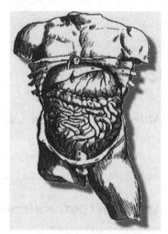

Texas Virtual Clinic

http://websurg.uth.tmc.edu/digestive/index.shtml

Both actual and virtual patients are presented in a way in which viewers are able to appreciate and understand common gastrointestinal problems and the steps taken to solve them. Provides disease overviews, case presentations and photographs.

PharmInfoNet's Digestive Disease Center. *http://pharminfo. com/disease/gastro.html*

UNC Division of Digestive Diseases and Nutrition

http://www.med.unc.edu/medicine/gi/

Contains resources for patients and for the staff.

Hemorrhoids

Health Answers: Hemorrhoids
http://www.healthanswers.com/adam/top/view.asp?filename=000292.htm&rdir
Definition, causes, symptoms, treatment, complications and more.

Hemorrhoids
http://www.niddk.nih.gov/health/digest/pubs/hems/hemords.htm
Information from the National Institute of Diabetes and Digestive and Kidney Diseases. What hemorrhoids are, how they are diagnosed, and how they are treated.

Hemorrhoids Forum
http://www.MedicineNet.com/Script/Main/Forum.asp?ArticleKey=383
The forum is a compilation of articles related to hemorrhoids.

Organizations

American College of Gastroenterology
http://www.acg.gi.org/
This professional organization recognizes common GI problems, offers digestive health tips, and suggests how to choose a GI physician.

American Gastroenterological Association
http://www.gastro.org/
American Gastroenterological Association news, meetings, clinical policy statements, publications and message board.

American Society for Gastrointestinal Endoscopy
http://www.asge.org/
Organization news, clinical and patient information, publications, products, news, resources, and "Find an Endoscopist" capability.

Directory of Digestive Diseases Organizations for Patients
http://www.niddk.nih.gov/health/digest/pubs/ddorgpat/ddorgpat.htm
Voluntary and private organizations offering educational materials and services about digestive diseases.

Publications

Gastroenterology

http://www.gastrojournal.org/

Subscription information and abstracts of published articles.

Digestive Health and Nutrition Magazine

http://www.gastro.org/digest/index.html

Practical, up-to-date news, tips and treatment information for sufferers of digestive disorders. Site provides sample articles and subscription information.

GastroNews Online

http://www.gastronews.com/

The online journal of digestive health.

Scope

http://www.kitsap.net/health/ccl/scope.html

Newsletter by and for people with inflammatory bowel disease.

Disabilities

Adaptive Technology & Accessibility

See also: Aging/Gerontology - Housing & Home Modification.

Access Media

http://www.human.com/mkt/access/index.html

Access Media is a nonprofit organization that works to acquire important documents for individuals with disabilities, in forms that are usable to them (e.g., braille, audio).

The Adaptive Technology Resource Centre's Web Resources

http://www.utoronto.ca/atrc/reference/web.html

This page provides links to resources on web accessibility, disability accessibility, adaptive technology vendors, disability organizations as well as to resources arranged by disability (e.g., visual, hearing, motor and learning impairments).

Alliance for Technology Access

http://www.ataccess.org/

ATA is a network of resource centers dedicated to providing information and support services to the disabled, and increasing their use of standard assistive and information technologies. Provides list of vendors, frequently asked questions (FAQs), and links to other assistive technology resources.

291

Apple Disability Resources

http://www.apple.com/education/k12/disability/

Personal computer products for the disabled.

Assistive/Adaptive Technologies

http://www.nchrtm.okstate.edu/webfiles/Assistive_Technology.html

Links to different sites from the National Clearinghouse of Rehabilitation Training Materials.

AZtech, A to Z Assistive Technology

http://cosmos.ot.buffalo.edu/

AZtech, Inc., is a nonprofit, community based enterprise that helps vendors and manufacturers develop assistive technology.

Designing a More Usable World

http://trace.wisc.edu/world/

Discusses design principles and guidelines for making technology and structures more accessible to the disabled. Numerous web links are offered on subjects such as computers, telecommunications, ATMs, and recreation facilities.

Equal Access to Software and Information

http://www.isc.rit.edu/~easi/

Information and guidance in the area of access-to-information technologies for the disabled. Contains lists of adaptive technology resources and publications, including libraries without walls.

James Stanfield Publishing Company

http://www.stanfield.com/

Books, videos and other media programs for students with cognitive challenges and those who teach them. Includes programs on teaching assertiveness, sexuality, social and working skills.

Macintosh Disability Shareware and Freeware

http://www.ECNet.Net/users/gnorris/place.shtml

Survey of the shareware and freeware available for disabled Macintosh computer users. Site is maintained by Scott Norris, a disabled computer user.

References on Web Accessibility
http://www.w3.org/WAI/References/

This site is devoted to the developments and issues as they relate to implementing accessibility to the web for people with disabilities. It offers links to news and disability resources, guidelines and specifications, research projects and white papers, utilities, tools, conferences, news and events information.

WebABLE!
http://www.yuri.org/webable/

Lists hundreds of websites that deal with accessibility issues.

Asperger's Syndrome

Asperger's Syndrome
http://www.autism-society.org/packages/aspergers.html

Description of Asperger's syndrome and how it differs from autism; links.

O.A.S.I.S.: On-Line Asperger's Syndrome Information and Support
http://www.udel.edu/bkirby/asperger/

Asperger's syndrome is a disorder similar to mild autism. This site describes research and educational projects; and lists conferences, mailing lists and support groups. Included is a section of personal accounts and poetry written by individuals with AS. Part of the Asperger's syndrome web ring.

Ataxia

About Hereditary Ataxias and Euro-Ataxia
http://www.vsn.nl/euroatax/index.htm

Ataxia is a degenerative neurological disease that results in the loss of muscle coordination. This site describes and classifies the different kinds of ataxias, tells about the activities of Euro-Ataxia and provides links to related sites.

International Ataxia Friends Mailing List

http://132.183.145.103/neurowebforum/ChildNeurologyArticles/JoinourATAXI Amailinglist.html

To subscribe, send e-mail to: *Majordomo@citi.doc.ca* and in the body write: "Subscribe INTERNAF" or, to receive a digest version, in the body type: "Subscribe INTERNAF-DIGEST."

National Ataxia Foundation

http://www.nwwin.com/houston/mall-a/ataxia.htm

Basic information about NAF and its fight against the various kinds of ataxias. Hereditary ataxia is said to affect an estimated 150,000 people in the United States alone.

Attention Deficit Disorder

A.D.D. WareHouse

http://www.addwarehouse.com/

Site describes products for Attention Deficit/Hyperactivity Disorder and related problems.

Attention Deficit Hyperactivity Disorder

http://home.health-center.com/english/brain/adhd/

Written for non-professionals, this site addresses ADHD, its effects and treatment approaches. It describes symptoms and the biology of the brain.

Attention-Deficit Hyperactivity Disorder

http://www.mentalhealth.com/dis/p20-ch01.html

Description, diagnosis, treatment, research, online booklets, magazine articles, links and web pages.

CH.A.D.D.: Children and Adults with Attention Deficit Disorders

http://www.chadd.org/

CH.A.D.D. is a nonprofit, parent-based organization that offers family support and advocacy, public and professional education, and research support. Links to *Attention!* a magazine for individuals dealing with ADHD, general information on ADD and how to treat or parent individuals with ADHD.

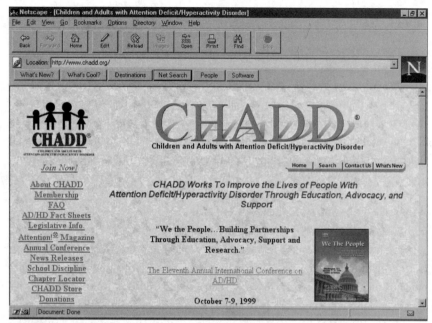

CHADD: Children and Adults with Attention Deficit Hyperactivity Disorder.
http://www.chadd.org/

Online Attention Deficit Disorder Test

http://www.med.nyu.edu/Psych/addc/addscr.htm

A 12-question, preliminary screening test for symptoms of ADD. Note: this test should not serve as a psychiatric or medical evaluation.

About.com: Attention Deficit Disorder

http://add.miningco.com/mbody.htm

Lots of articles and links regarding attention deficit disorder. Includes general information, advocacy, medication, myths, frequently asked questions, nutrition information and parenting links.

Does Food Change Behavior?

http://www.vegsource.com/attwood/add.htm

Article provides an overview of ADD and possible causes. It also includes a questionnaire for parents and teachers to use to evaluate the possibility that a child has ADD.

Autism

#Autism Channel

http://www.autism.clarityconnect.com/

All about proper procedure and etiquette for interacting with others through the Autism Channel, an Internet Relay Channel (IRC) or real-time forum where parents and family, educators and health care professionals can talk about autism, sharing personal stories and support, and discussing treatment options and other issues.

Autism Frequently Asked Questions

http://web.syr.edu/~jmwobus/autism/autism.faq.html

In addition to answers to frequently asked questions, this site provides mailing list information, a glossary, information on coping with autism, educational methods and advice for parents, as well as a list of well-known individuals with autism or those who have family members with autism. To subscribe, send e-mail to: *LISTSERV@MAELSTROM.STJOHNS.EDU* with the message: "subscribe autism *Firstname Lastname.*"

Autism Resources

http://autism-resources.com/

Links to websites around the world having anything to do with autism. Broken down by topic, including general information, online discussion, news, books, articles, treatment methods, academic and research programs, organizations and resources by language, and support for parents.

Autism Society of America

http://www.autism-society.org/asa_home.html

What is autism? This site has an autism checklist, and describes the activities and mission of the Autism Society of America.

Autism/PDD Resources Network

http://www.autism-pdd.net/

Great information for parents and others covering autism and autism-related disorders. Includes diagnosis, treatment, average development schedule, autism by country and language, and an autism forum. Communicate with other people affected by autism.

Indiana Resource Center for Autism

http://www.isdd.indiana.edu/~irca/

The IRCA focuses on strategies to empower communities to support individuals with autism in typical work, school and community activities.

Cerebral Palsy

Cerebral Palsy: A Guide for Care

http://gait.aidi.udel.edu/res695/homepage/pd_ortho/clinics/c_palsy/cpweb.htm

Good information on cerebral palsy and overview of a book by the same name.

Cerebral Palsy: A Multimedia Tutorial

http://galen.med.virginia.edu/~smb4v/tutorials/cp/cp.htm

For children and their parents.

Cerebral Palsy Fact Sheet

http://weber.u.washington.edu/~wscchap/NoMoreLabels/palsy.html

Basic information about cerebral palsy.

Cerebral Palsy Info Central (CPIC)

http://www.geocities.com/HotSprings/Sauna/4441/CPIC.html

Learn about cerebral palsy, new treatment, links to CP and aging issues, organizations, mailing lists and more.

The Cerebral Palsy Network

http://www.geocities.com/Heartland/Plains/8950/

The Network links parents of children with cerebral palsy around the world.

Links2Go: Cerebral Palsy

http://www.links2go.com/topic/Cerebral_Palsy

This site offers a long list of links to Internet CP resources.

Susie's Cerebral Palsy Homepage

http://www.susiecphome.com/home.html

Personal account, inspiration and resources for those with cerebral palsy, their parents, students and health care professionals. Susie, the web page author, is very inspiring.

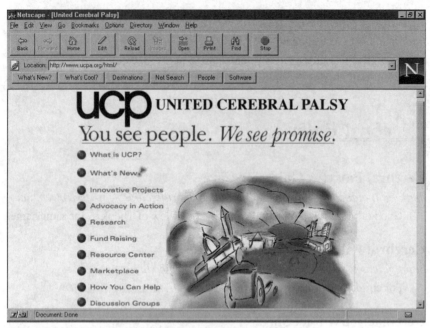

United Cerebral Palsy Association. http://www.ucpa.org

United Cerebral Palsy Association
http://www.ucpa.org/

This charity seeks to advance the independence, productivity and full citizenship of people with cerebral palsy and other disabilities. It serves as an information source and advocacy group. Resources, research, projects and discussion groups are available.

Communication/Speech Disorders

Aha! American Hyperlexia Association Home Page
http://www.hyperlexia.org/

Information about hyperlexia and related disorders, such as Semantic-Pragmatic disorder. Materials, conferences, and useful sites are found here, along with personal stories. Hyperlexia is a communication or language disorder where children have precocious reading abilities accompanied by significant problems in verbal, learning and social skills.

Communication Disorders
http://www.healthtouch.com/level1/leaflets/118857/119760.htm

Informative online leaflets on aspects of speech and on communication disorders.

Net Connections for Communication Disorders and Sciences
http://www.mankato.msus.edu/dept/comdis/kuster2/welcome.html

An Internet guide for those with speech and language disorders.

Stuttering Frequently Asked Questions
http://www.casafuturatech.com/FAQ/faq.html

This text file is a shorter version of the book, *Stuttering, Science, Therapy and Practice* which is also available on the Internet. Answers to questions on childhood and adult stuttering, the science of stuttering, and resources for those who stutter.

Stuttering Homepage
http://www.mankato.msus.edu/dept/comdis/kuster/stutter.html

Information about stuttering and other fluency disorders such as cluttering. Provides links to support groups, research and publications, case studies, news, personal accounts, therapy and discussion forums. Lists famous people who stutter.

Developmental Disorders
See also: Mental Retardation, later in this chapter.

Developmental Disabilities Resource Center
http://www.caccb.org/ddrc/

The site for this Colorado-based center offers regional and general information on developmental disability resources. Includes "what is a developmental disability," frequently asked questions, glossary, agencies and job postings.

Developmental Disability Links
http://discovertechnology.com/Links/MRFInfo.htm

Includes mental retardation, brain injury, epilepsy, autism, fragile X syndrome, pervasive development disorder and Down syndrome links.

National Association of Developmental Disabilities Councils Home Page

http://www.igc.apc.org/NADDC/

NADDC promotes a national policy which enables individuals with developmental and other disabilities to be included in the community and to have the opportunity to make choices regarding the quality of their lives.

Treatment of Destructive Behaviors in Persons with Developmental Disabilities

http://text.nlm.nih.gov/nih/cdc/www/75.html

This is the text of a statement from the National Institutes of Health 1989 Consensus Development Conference.

Waisman Center's List of Web Sites

http://waisman.wisc.edu/www/mrsites.html

Lists dozens of websites about cognitive and developmental disabilities.

Down Syndrome

Diagnosis Down Syndrome

http://home1.gte.net/mcelwee/

This website informs you of the life realities that a person with Down syndrome can look forward to today. It provides statements from DS parents, as well as links, advice and support.

Down Syndrome: A Parent's Resource

http://www3.sympatico.ca/terry.edwards/Shelby.html

Information for parents of a child who has recently been diagnosed with Down syndrome. Includes a straightforward explanation of DS (or Trisomy 21), a description of common physical and other features of a DS baby, medical concerns, and a gallery of links and pictures of other family's children and sites.

Down Syndrome Health Issues

http://www.ds-health.com/

Down syndrome articles and medical essays on common health concerns of DS patients, research and resources. Site is maintained by a pediatrician who is also the parent of a child with DS.

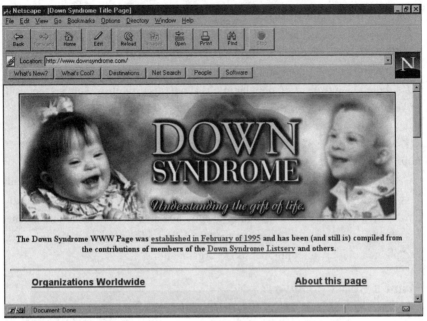

Down Syndrome WWW Page. *http://www.downsyndrome/com/*

Down Syndrome Listserv

http://www.nas.com/downsyn/dslistserv.html

Information on how to subscribe to this listserv group and to search archives.

Down Syndrome WWW Page

http://www.downsyndrome/com/

Articles, frequently asked questions, health care guidelines, organizations, resources, parent support groups, conferences, toy catalogs, and personal "Brag Pages" created about children with Down syndrome by their parents. Links.

DownsCity

http://www.downcity.com/

Cyber space and support for the Down syndrome community.

Recommended Down Syndrome Sites on the Internet

http://www.ds-health.com/ds_sites.htm

The list includes national and international organizations, comprehensive websites, medical resources, online magazines, DS clinics and foundations, education resources, family sites and more.

The Trisomy 21 Foundation
http://www.geocities.com/HotSprings/9438/t21hmpg.htm

The Foundation supports results-oriented research of practical and applicable benefit to infants, children and adults with Down syndrome. Site provides some facts about DS and clears up popular myths about this disability, which is the result of an additional chromosome 21.

UPSIDE!
http://www.telebyte.com/upside/upside.html

Self-described as an informal society of individuals, parents, and friends involved in the world of Down syndrome. Includes child-of-the-month, newsletters, short articles, upcoming events, and lots of web links and Usenet newsgroup addresses, listservers, as well as e-mail addresses, mailing addresses, and phone numbers for a number of DS organizations.

What's Up with Downs?
http://members.ttlc.net/~kehler/What'sUp.html

Includes information on TNI, or Targeted Nutritional Intervention, an alternative therapy that uses vitamins, minerals, amino acids and enzymes to address the metabolic disturbances associated with Down syndrome.

World Wide Information Pages about Down Syndrome
http://alf.zfn.uni-bremen.de/~downsyn/down10e.html

Down syndrome organizations from Europe, Asia, Australia, North America and South America.

Dyslexia

Dyslexia Archive
http://www.hensa.ac.uk/dyslexia.html

Contains information about dyslexia, including education, groups, events, articles and software. Also offers human-interest information, such as a list of famous people with dyslexia and personal stories.

Dyslexia 2000 Network

http://www.futurenet.co.uk/charity/ado/index.html

Information and advice on software, hardware and other tools for adult dyslexics. Link to the Adult Dyslexia Organization, which was founded by dyslexics to support others with dyslexia. Dyslexia checklist and further resources.

International Dyslexia Association

http://www.interdys.org/

This organization supports research and educational efforts for intervening with and teaching dyslexics. The site provides information on dyslexia in adults and children, and legal, legislative, scientific and technical updates.

Teens vs. Dyslexia

http://www.ldteens.org/

Site by teens with dyslexia, for teens with dyslexia. Includes study help, information on an annual teen conference, pages for teens to express their feelings, "parent stuff" and links.

Educational Issues

DO-IT

http://weber.u.washington.edu/~doit/

DO-IT (Disabilities, Opportunities, Internetworking, and Technology) seeks to increase the participation of those with disabilities in science, engineering and mathematics. The program supports high school students with disabilities who are interested in these fields and want to attend college through mentoring and summer-study programs, as well as by loaning computers and adaptive technologies for use in their homes. Newsletter, publications, video, and newsgroup information are provided as well.

Different Roads to Learning

http://www.difflearn.com/

Online catalog of learning materials and playthings for children with developmental delays and disabilities. Includes educational flash cards, manipulative toys and learning games. Describes each item and the skills it helps the child develop.

Marc Sheehan's Special Education Page

http://www.halcyon.com/marcs/sped.html

A huge list of special education links, both general and focussing on specific disabilities.

Special Education Resources on the Internet

http://www.hood.edu/seri/serihome.htm

Large collection of Internet-accessible resources for those involved in special education. This includes everything from physical disability and speech impairment, to learning disability, mental retardation and autism.

Employment Issues

See also: Legal Issues, later in this chapter.

Disabled Businesspersons Association

http://www.web-link.com/dba/dba.htm

The DBA is a nonprofit, public charity and educational organization that helps disabled entrepreneurs and professionals maximize their potential in the business world, and encourages the participation and enhances the performance of the disabled in the workplace.

Job Accommodation Network

http://janweb.icdi.wvu.edu/

An international, toll-free consulting service that provides information about job accommodations and the employability of people with disabilities. Information on the Americans with Disabilities Act is also provided.

Fragile X Syndrome

Fragile X Listserv

http://www.fraxa.org/listserv.html

An information exchange and online support group. To subscribe, send mail to *LISTSERV@LISTSERV.CC.EMORY.EDU* with the following command in the body of your e-mail message: *SUBSCRIBE FRAGILEX-L.*

Fragile X Syndrome

http://www.nih.gov/nichd/publications/news/fragilextoc.htm

Discusses the testing, diagnosis and treatment of fragile X. Also describes the mental, physical and behavioral characteristics, medical problems and learning difficulties frequently associated with this disease.

Fragile X Syndrome: Recognition in Young Children

http://home.coqui.net/myrna/fragile.htm

Explains the physical and developmental characteristics of fragile X syndrome in young and school-aged children.

FRAXA Research Foundation

http://www.FRAXA.org/

Supports research in treating fragile X syndrome, which is the number one inherited cause of mental retardation. Describes symptoms, causes, diagnosis and treatment, and provides links to other websites, MEDLINE, associations and references. Newsletter available.

General Resources

Ability OnLine Support Network

http://www.ablelink.org/

A penpal e-mail system that connects young people who have disabilities or chronic illness with disabled and non-disabled peers and mentors. In addition, the site offers information for patients, their families and friends about medical treatments, educational strategies and employment opportunities.

Disability Information

http://galaxy.einet.net/GJ/disabilities.html

A condensed collection of websites offering information on resources for the disabled. It contains many academic links and links to organizations based outside of North America.

Disabled Peoples' International

http://www.dpi.org/

A grass-roots network that includes individuals from over 110 countries, devoted to promoting the human rights of people with disabilities.

DRM WebWatcher

http://www.geocities.com/CapitolHill/1703/DRMwww.html

The Disabilities Resources Monthly guide provides an alphabetical list of online resources with links to specific disabilities, as well as to organizations whose scope is cross-disability. Includes resources to a number of disorders and diseases not typically grouped in the disabled category, such as arthritis and chronic fatigue syndrome.

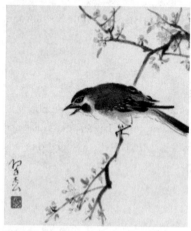

Information Resources for People with Disabilities. http://www.sd.soft. iwate-pu.ac.jp/sensui/index-e.html

Information Resources for People with Disabilities

http://www.sd.soft.iwate-pu.ac.jp/sensui/index-e.html

A long list of international weblinks, split into helpful sections including music, art and broadcasting; education; law; leisure and sports; products; publications; social support groups; technology, toys and travel; and work resources.

Internet Resources for Special Children

http://www.irsc.org/

Large amount of information and web links for parents, educators, medical professionals and other people who interact with disabled children. Topics include specific disability information, support groups for parents and family members, special education and legal resources.

Internet Resources on Disabilities

http://www.sped.ukans.edu/disabilities/

This University of Kansas site contains links to Internet resources concerning people with disabilities, including academic and social programs, online texts and other references sources. Information on technology for people with disabilities, and links to disability-related gophers.

Invisible Disability Index
http://www1.shore.net/~dmoisan/disability/index.html

An alphabetical list of many invisible disabilities (i.e., disabilities that are not readily apparent to others) with resources on the Internet. Included are ADD, Asperger's syndrome, brain injury, chemical sensitivity, chronic fatigue syndrome, chronic pain, deafness and hearing impairments, depression, diabetes, epilepsy, fetal alcohol syndrome, fibromyalgia, migraine, narcolepsy, reflex sympathetic dystrophy syndrome, repetitive stress and vision disorders.

Lubin's disABILITY Information and Resources
http://www.eskimo.com/~jlubin/disabled.html

This site offers a collection of net and non-net resources for people with disabilities and those who work with them. It is maintained by Jim Lubin, a respirator-dependent quadriplegic who types 17 words per minute using a sip-and-puff switch.

New England INDEX
http://NE-INDEX.Shriver.Org/

Serving mostly the New England area, this INDEX (INformation on Disabilities EXchange) invites users to call their specialists who can search a database for up-to-date information. Provides links to resources on the Internet, contains fact sheets and the "Exceptional Physician" newsletter.

New Mobility Interactive Café
http://www.newmobility.com/

This website for the disabled community provides news, resources and culture. It includes the magazine, *New Mobility*, a message board, chat area and a jobline.

Hearing Impairment
See also: Ear, Nose & Throat/Otolaryngology.

The American Speech-Language Association
http://www.asha.org/

This site is a resource for ASHA members, who are audiologists, speech-language pathologists, and speech, language, and hearing scientists. It also provides the general public information about communication disorders and careers.

AUDIES Net
http://www.tsi.it/contrib/audies/deafnet.html

Although this site is in Italian, most of the sites linked to are written in English. Medical and technology links are listed, along with dozens of research projects, academic sites and institutes around the world.

Beyond-Hearing Mailing List
http://www.webcom.com/~houtx/r-b-h.htm

To subscribe, send e-mail to: *majordomo@acpub.duke.edu* and leave the subject area blank. Type the following in the message: "subscribe beyond-hearing."

Common Diseases of the External and Middle Ear
http://www.bcm.tmc.edu/oto/studs/midear.html

Outline used for a course at Baylor University. It is not easy-reading.

Deaf/Hard of Hearing
http://www.familyvillage.wisc.edu/lib_deaf.htm

This site provides descriptions, names, mailing addresses, phone numbers and e-mail addresses for many organizations serving the deaf and hard-of-hearing community. It also directs browsers to e-mail lists, online magazines and other sites for the hearing impaired.

The Deaf Resource Library
http://www.deaflibrary.org/

World-wide resources to educate people about the culture of the deaf and hard of hearing. There is a huge number of resources.

DeafNation.com
http://www.deafnation.com./index.html

News, product information, jobs and the opportunity for online chatting are offered at this site.

Deaf Magazine
http://WWW.Deaf-Magazine.Org/

News and communication with other deaf computer users. To subscribe, send e-mail to: *listserv@listserv.deaf-magazine.org* and leave subject area blank, but in body, type: "subcribe deaf *firstname lastname*."

Deaf Queer Resource Center

http://www.deafqueer.org/

This site is interested in promoting deaf lesbian, gay, bisexual and transgender visibility on the web. Library and information resources are provided, along with a bulletin board which includes announcements, a calendar, penpal matches, discussion groups, and the Point of View Café.

Deaf World Web

http://deafworldweb.org/

Provides information and social/cultural resources for the hearing-impaired. Includes news, chat and discussion groups, as well as the searchable *Deaf Encyclopedia*.

Early Identification of Hearing Impairment in Infants and Young Children

http://text.nlm.nih.gov/nih/cdc/www/92txt.html

Full text of a statement from the National Institutes of Health Consensus Development Conference, which states that approximately 1 of every 1,000 infants is born deaf. Present and future screening plans are discussed.

FAQ about People with Hearing Loss

http://www.betterhearing.org/faq.htm

Includes incidence, symptoms, common myths and other questions and answers about hearing loss.

Gallaudet University

http://www.gallaudet.edu/

Admission and program information about the only four-year university for deaf and hard-of-hearing students. Graduate programs are also available. Gallaudet University is located in Washington, D.C. and supports the National Information Center on Deafness.

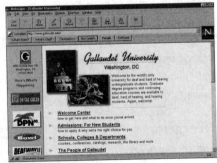

Gallaudet University.
http://www.gallaudet.edu/

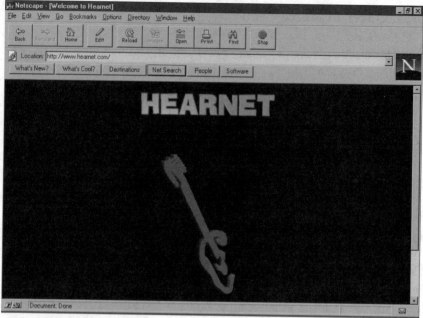

Hearnet. http://www.hearnet.com.

Hearing Help Online

http://www.betterhearing.org/

The Better Hearing Insitute homepage provides comprehensive information on hearing loss, tinnitus, and hearing aids, as well as a directory of hearing care providers.

Hearing Loss Resources

http://www.webcom.com/~houtx/

For those suffering from or interested in hearing loss. Primarily, this site is the vehicle of the SayWhatClub, an online group of late-deafened and hard-of-hearing individuals who support each other via e-mail. Includes essays and links to other hearing loss resources.

Hearnet

http://www.hearnet.com/

Information is provided to prevent hearing loss and tinnitus, especially among music industry professionals and music fans. Site includes "article of the month" and archives, frequently asked questions, tinnitus information, and more. It also sells products, sponsors a chatline, and makes referrals to hearing specialists.

National Institute on Deafness and Other Communication Diseases

http://www.nih.gov/nidcd/

This NIH branch supports and conducts research on the normal and disordered processes of hearing, balance, smell, taste, voice, speech and language. This site describes current research and offers NIDCD publications.

NIDCD Information Clearinghouse

http://www.nih.gov/nidcd/textonly/health/pubs_misc/eagle.htm

This database provides titles, abstracts and availability information on articles related to deafness and other communication disorders. It includes a lot of material that is not classified elsewhere.

Speech on the Web

http://fonsg3.let.uva.nl/Other_pages.html

Links to sites related to phonetics and speech sciences.

Speechreading (Lipreading)

http://mambo.ucsc.edu/psl/lipr.html

This site contains essays and resources about speech-reading. It begins with a 1648 essay entitled, "Philocophus: Or, the Deafe and Dumbe Mans Friend," an essay on lip-reading. Includes NATO studies and many more related websites.

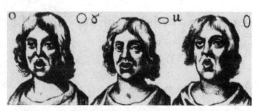

Speechreading (Lipreading).
http://mambo.ucsc.edu/psl/lipr.html

Travel Tips for Hearing Impaired People

http://www.netdoor.com/entinfo/herimaao.html

Advice on making travel arrangements. Provides useful phone numbers to services adapted for the deaf and hearing impaired.

Legal Issues

ADA Information Center

http://www.ada-infonet.org/ (Rocky Mountain Region)
http://www.adainfo.org/ (Mid-Atlantic States)

Informational documents, training materials, referrals and technical assistance about the Americans with Disabilities Act (ADA). Although these sites are hosted by regional organizations, most of the information pertains to everyone in the U.S.

ADA Information Center On-Line

http://adabbs.hr.state.ks.us/dc/

This site from Kansas State University provides government, general and news information and resources on the Americans with Disabilities Act.

Americans with Disabilities Act Document Center

http://janweb.icdi.wvu.edu/kinder/

ADA statute, regulations, guidelines, federally reviewed technologist sheets and other assistance documents.

Americans with Disabilities Act Information on the Web

http://www.usdoj.gov/crt/ada/

Links to ADA sites online.

Council for Disability Rights

http://www.disabilityrights.org/

News affecting the disability community and practical information on rights of the disabled. The best part is you don't have to be a lawyer to understand it.

Department of Justice ADA Home Page

http://www.usdoj.gov/crt/ada/adahom1.htm

The U.S. Department of Justice provides information about the toll-free ADA phone line, ADA enforcement programs, status reports, regulations, and grants.

The Disability Rights Activist

http://www.teleport.com/~abarhydt/

This site collects much of the information needed to work for the rights of the disabled. It includes action alerts, links to organizations and agencies, disability rights publications and indexes, and it provides accessibility guidelines.

Do I Have a Case?

http://www.swiftsite.com/adaman/

This website was made to help people decide whether to spend the time and the money to seek local legal counsel in order to initiate litigation when they believe they have been the victim of discrimination due to a disability.

Liberty Resources, Inc.: In the News

http://www.libertyresources.org/news/

News items of legal interest to the disability community.

Social Security Online

http://www.ssa.gov/SSA_Home.html

Information and publications on Social Security entitlement programs.

Mental Retardation

See also: Developmental Disabilities, earlier in this chapter.

American Association on Mental Retardation

http://www.aamr.org/

The mission of the AAMR is to advance the knowledge and skills of those who work in the field of mental retardation by helping the exchange of information and ideas. The site contains membership information, abstracts, convention inform-ation, training and career opportunities, and a list of disability resources.

Arc of the United States Home Page

http://TheArc.org/welcome.html

The Arc is the nation's largest voluntary organization serving children and adults with mental retardation and their families. There are over 1,000 affiliated chapters of the Arc, and this site describes the organization's mission and activities, which include research, advocacy, education and training for the mentally handicapped. Fact sheets provide information on services, groups, Social Security benefits, the ADA and community living. Some pages are available in Spanish. Links to online chapter sites.

Cognitive and Developmental Disabilities Resources

http://www.waisman.wisc.edu/mrsites.html

Includes links to many organizations and facilities that serve or research mental retardation.

Hydrocephalus Association Homepage

http://neurosurgery.mgh.harvard.edu/ha/

This site describes programs dealing with hydrocephalus, an abnormal accumulation of fluid in the brain. Includes articles and frequently asked questions.

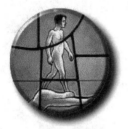

Institutes for the Achievement of Human Potential. *http://www.iahp.org/*

Institutes for the Achievement of Human Potential

http://www.iahp.org/

The goal of this organization is to raise the ability of all children, regardless of their present capabilities. It offers different programs and seeks to develop children who are brain-injured as well as those who are healthy.

Introduction to Mental Retardation

http://thearc.org/faqs/mrqa.html

Very good information in the form of basic questions and answers.

Mental Retardation and Developmental Disabilities

http://members.aol.com/MRandDD/index.htm

Includes an article entitled: "Introduction to American History of Mental Retardation," movies of interest, commentary, many links (with descriptions), and a message board.

President's Committee on Mental Retardation

http://www.acf.dhhs.gov/programs/pcmr/

Includes publications, and state and national resources.

Paralysis/Spinal Cord Injuries

American Spinal Injury Association
http://www.asia-spinalinjury.org/

Research, publication, news and information on ASIA. Seeks to foster treatment efforts to manage, prevent and cure spinal cord damage.

Christopher Reeve Paralysis Foundation
http://www.apacure.com/

In partnership with the American Paralaysis Association (APA), this Foundation supports research efforts to cure spinal cord research which focuses on treatments to limit the loss of function from spinal cord injuries as well as therapies to regenerate lost nerve cells and repair the damaged cord. You can find information about the research that is supported, as well as discussion and news.

Cure Paralysis Now
http://cureparalysis.org/

Site is devoted to the advancement of a cure for spinal cord paralysis. Includes frequently asked questions, news, chat rooms, research and many related links.

News from the Edge
http://www.from-the-edge.net/

One man's story of his new life after a spinal cord injury, as told through a series of letters to his friends and family.

Paralyzed.Com
http://www.paralyzed.com/

Free information about paralysis, spinal cord injuries, physical disabilities, resources for the disabled, accessibility issues, wheelchair resources, personal stories, mobility issues, people who are ventilator dependent, and more.

Spinal Cord Injury Information Network
http://www.spinalcord.uab.edu/

A comprehensive and organized source of spinal cord injury information and resources from centers, organizations, researchers and others. Includes links and frequently asked questions. Great information; straightforward and supported with references.

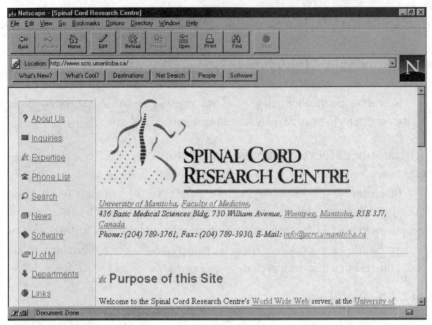

Spinal Cord Research Centre. http://www.scrc.umanitoba.ca/

Spinal Cord Research Centre
http://www.scrc.umanitoba.ca/

Describes the Centre's activities and research efforts to cure spinal cord injuries.

Spine and Peripheral Nerve Surgery
http://neurosurgery.mgh.harvard.edu/spine-hp.htm

The Neurological Service at Massachusetts General Hospital and Harvard Medical School provides information on spine evaluation and treatment, surgery, tumors, referrals, and links to related sites.

Polio

Polio Information Center Online
http://cumicro2.cpmc.columbia.edu/PICO/PICO.html

Includes information on the polio virus, vaccination, history, and links to other polio sites.

Polio Survivors' Page

http://www.eskimo.com/~dempt/polio.html

This page provides links to polio and post-polio resources, and includes announcements, articles and research. A great deal of material may be found on Post Polio Syndrome (PPS), a muscle fatigue syndrome that occurs in patients who have suffered from polio years before.

Post Polio Syndrome and Links to Same

http://home.earthlink.net/~polioinfo/

Those who survive polio may find that there are physiologic changes in their nervous system which result in a characteristic set of symptoms known as Post Polio Syndrome. Complications such as arthritis, scoliosis, and entrapment syndromes also frequently accompany paralytic conditions. This site includes fact sheets, information on government help, medication and the Social Security appeals process, as well as links to a number of personal homepages.

Post-Polio Syndrome Central

http://angus.interspeed.net/ppsc/

Many links with descriptions. Includes e-mail news and discussion groups.

Virtual Museum of the Iron Lung

http://members.xoom.com/lungmuseum/

History, personal stories, research, resources and photographs. The iron lung is a mechanical respirator that is often used to help sufferers from polio to breath. There is also a long list of links to other polio sites on the Internet.

Publications

ABILITY Magazine

http://www.abilitymagazine.com/

Contains interviews with well-known people involved with disability causes. Articles cover legal issues, new technology, travel and leisure, employment opportunities, national and local resources and human interest stories. Requires subscription, but excerpts from current and back issues are available for no charge.

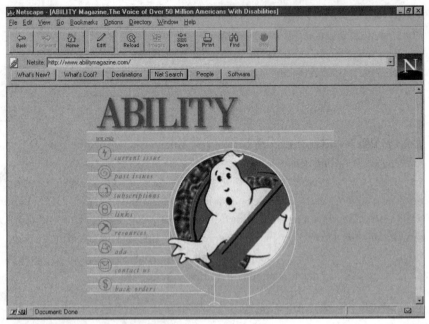

ABILITY Magazine. http://www.abilitymagazine.com/

Disabilities/Health Related Newsletters

http://www.dinf.org/disability_resources/newslett.htm

Long list of alphabetized links to online magazines and newsletters.

Mainstream Online

http://www.mainstream-mag.com/

Self-described as "the leading news, advocacy, and lifestyle zine for people with disabilities." This site covers many facets of disability culture, including disability rights, news and current affairs, products, technology, personal profiles, education, employment, relationships, housing, transportation, and recreation.

New Mobility Magazine

http://www.newmobility.com/magazine/

Recent issue and article archives are available for this lifestyle magazine for the disabled. It includes personal interviews, columns, book reviews, articles on alternative medicine, cures, drugs, mobility, arts, sports, sex, travel, etc. Subscription information and links to related sites are also provided.

Reach Out Magazine

http://www.reachoutmag.com/

Free web magazine and meeting place for people with disabilities all over the world. Requires only registration.

Special Child Magazine

http://www.specialchild.com/index.html

For parents and caregivers of kids with special needs. Covers success stories, horror stories, family issues, education and other topics.

Sibling Support

Sibling Support Project

http://www.chmc.org/departmt/sibsupp/

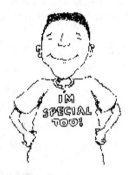

National program dedicated to the brothers and sisters of people with special health and developmental needs. Site offers support and information to both child and adult siblings. Workshops, newsletters and listservers discuss the concerns and needs of these individuals. Directory offers listing of sibling programs and books about disabilities and illness for young readers.

Sibling Support Project.
http://www.chmc.org/
departmt/sibsupp/

Social Issues

PeopleNet DisAbility DateNet Home Page

http://chelsea.ios.com/~mauro/

This page was created by a writer who has been disabled since the age of five. It contains articles, stories, poems and resources concerning love, dating, sex, intimacy and contraception as experienced by disabled individuals.

Rick and Joni's Home Page

http://www.access.digex.net/~vandyke/

Information about the Disabled-Able Travel Service, amputee resources with information about prosthetics, and links to social clubs and disability chatlines.

Romance and Resources for the Disabled

http://disableddating.com/

Celebrity corner, shopping and meeting places, and teen chat.

Spina Bifida

See also: Brain & Brain Disorders.

Children with Spina Bifida

http://www.waisman.wisc.edu/~rowley/sb-kids/index.html

This site serves as a resource page for parents of children with spina bifida, which is also called myelomeningocele. Includes mailing list information, words of encouragement, information resources, articles, research, photos and personal web page links, as well as links to related sites.

Information on Spina Bifida and Hydrocephalus

http://www.spinabifida.org/general.htm

These pages were written for teachers of children with spina bifida, but the information is useful to parents and others. It describes the problems and challenges kids with spina bifida and hydrocephalus face, from latex allergy, to handwriting, to socializing with other children.

John's Spina Bifida Page

http://www.sapyta.com/jsbp.html

What spina bifida is, chat areas, mailing lists, wheelchair manufacturers online, personal pages and online publications.

Spina Bifida Association of America

http://www.sbaa.org/

The mission of this organization is to promote the prevention of spina bifida and to assist those who have it. Services include a referral program, bimonthly newsletter, meetings, scholarship fund and publications.

Spina Bifida Information

http://nyneurosurgery.org/child/myelomeningocele/spina/bifida.htm

Introduction, prenatal detection, obstetrical considerations, outcome, treatment options, complications and more related to spina bifida.

Spina Bifida Occulta

http://www.icondata.com/health/pedbase/files/SPINABIF.HTM

Clinical information on this spinal defect.

Understanding Spina Bifida

http://seals.com/publish/understanding/usb.html

Spina bifida occurs when the spinal cord does not form properly during fetal development.

Sports

Special Olympics International

http://www.specialolympics.org/

Special Olympics is a nonprofit, international program of sports training and competition for individuals with mental retardation. More than one million athletes in nearly 150 countries participate in 22 sports. This site describes the games, provides information on volunteering, coaching and competing, and offers information and links to U.S. chapters, and world-wide regional programs.

National Sports Center for the Disabled

http://www.nscd.org/

Outdoor recreation for children and adults with disabilities.

Rick Hansen Institute

http://www.rickhansen.org/

Wheelchair athlete and author Rick Hansen co-founded this institute that aims to remove barriers limiting people with disabilities from reaching their full potential. The Institute also strives to help find a cure for paralysis.

Visual Impairment

See also: Eye/Optometry & Ophthalmology.

American Council of the Blind

http://www.acb.org/

Provides general information about the ACB and recent issues of their monthly publication, *The Braille Forum*. Also offers updates from Washington, D.C. and ACB affiliates, as well as resources about blindness, braille, product catalogs and financial help.

American Foundation for the Blind

http://www.igc.apc.org/afb/

Offers information on blindness, low vision and related issues, as well as access to AFB newsletters, the *Journal of Visual Impairment and Blindness*, and the AFB catalog of books. AFB activities fall within the non-medical aspects of blindness and vision impairment.

Associated Services for the Blind Information Page

http://www.libertynet.org/~asbinfo/

Speech-friendly option available at this site, which describes ASB activities and mission. Also offers recorded periodicals, including over 25 magazines on subjects ranging from archeology to home cooking and computers to science.

Archives of the Visually Impaired Computer Users' Group List

http://maelstrom.stjohns.edu/archives/vicug-l.html

Search past issues by month, author, or topic. Archives cover from February, 1997 to the present.

Blind Net

http://www.blind.net/blindind.htm

Factual information about blindness, general information, and links to organizations of and for the blind. The motto is: "blind people need equality, not random acts of senseless kindness."

Blind Related Links

http://www.seidata.com/~marriage/rblind.html

Offers many links to resources of interest to the blind, including adaptive technology, training, publications, employment, medical and government sites.

Blindness Resource Center

http://nyise.org/blind.htm

Collection of websites related to assisting the blind and visually impaired. Provides a brief description of most of the sites, which include organizations, software and technology, schools and research sites, information on braille, translators, deaf-blindness, eye diseases, libraries and vendors.

BLIST: The Comprehensive Index of Blindness-Related Emailing Lists

http://www.hicom.net/~oedipus/blist.html

Information on over 65 e-mail groups online.

Dotmaker's Home Page

http://www.azstarnet.com/~dotmakr/index.html

Resources and information links for the blind, visually impaired, and deaf and blind. Offers sites of interest to braille users, including the computerized braille tutor, and a long list of homepages maintained by blind computer-users.

Guide Dog Laws

http://www.seeingeye.org/laws.html

Type in the state or province (for Canada) abbreviation to receive a description of the regional laws relating to guide dogs.

Louis Braille

http://www.duxburysystems.com/braille.html

Autobiographical information.

National Federation of the Blind

http://www.nfb.org/default.htm

This group was founded to help the blind help themselves and is the largest organization serving the blind in the U.S., according to this site. The NFB's activities and events are described, and information about *The Braille Monitor* magazine may be found. In addition, it features information for children describing what it is like to be blind, as well as links to braille resources, research, technological, legal and legislative information.

National Library Service for the Blind and Physically Handicapped

http://lcweb.loc.gov/nls/nls.html

A free library of braille and recorded materials that is circulated through cooperating libraries. Search the online catalog at this site to see what is available. Book reviews, legal information, and a list of network libraries for blind and physically handicapped individuals may be found here.

Outpost

http://home.earthlink.net/~mail4tdb/

A "speech-friendly" site created for the blind computer user as well as for those who seek information in accessible format. Contains links and material about adaptive technology companies, demos, guide dogs, automated online banking, shopping and products for the blind.

Recordings for the Blind and Dyslexic

http://www.rfbd.org/

National headquarters of this nonprofit organization that serves people who cannot read standard print because of a visual, perceptual or other physical disability. Site describes RFB&D's library, provides links and a catolog of services.

Resources for Parents and Teachers of Blind Kids

http://www.az.com/~dday/blindkids.html

Useful links, especially for parents who are interested in home-schooling their child.

Royal National Institute for the Blind, UK

http://www.rnib.org.uk/

This site was designed not only to serve and provide information for blind and partially-sighted computer users, but also to demonstrate how an Internet site can be designed to be usable by the visually impaired. The RNIB events, publications and products are described, and fact sheets on the eye and visual impairments are provided, along with an international guide to agencies and other links. There is a demonstration of a braille translation software program, entitled "Braille It!"

Scotter's Low Vision Land

http://www.community.net/~byndsght/

Also known as "Beyond Sight: Low Vision Resources." Scotter has assembled a list of resources for the blind and visually impaired, and offers computer assistance to any fellow vision-impaired individual. Internet resources listed include newsgroups, listservers, bulletin boards, online books and other sites. A brief summary of each site is provided.

The Seeing Eye Information Center

http://www.seeingeye.org/info.html

Based in Morristown, New Jersey, this center teaches guide dogs for the blind. Site offers a lot of information on how to apply for a guide dog, a guide dog history reading room, canine guidelines, and much more.

Vision Impairment

http://www.tmx.com.au/guidedogs/vision/

Learn what some people with vision impairments do see by reading their first-hand accounts. Site also explains the major causes of vision impairment.

DRUGS / PHARMACOLOGY

> *Covered in this chapter*: Antibiotics; Aspirin; Children; Consumer Sites; Drug Databases; Elderly; General Resources; Mental Health; Organizations; Publications; Prozac; Ritalin; Toxicology.
>
> *Related chapters*: Alternative Medicine; Pain Management.

Antibiotics

Antibiotic Resistance

http://www.cdc.gov/ncidod/dbmd/antibioticresistance/Default.htm

Fact sheet from the Centers for Disease Control and Prevention, and links to professional and patient information.

Antibiotics: Facts You Should Know

http://www.district-1.org/july98/p070798.html

Information for patients about antibiotics, including side effects, resistance, dosage and disposal.

The Challenge of Antibiotic Resistance

http://www.sciam.com/1998/0398issue/0398levy.html

Feature article from *Scientific American.*

Penicillin and Other Antibiotics

http://helios.bto.ed.ac.uk/bto/course-info/third-yr/micro3m/penicill.htm

Illustrated text describes the penicillin and its activity, as well as other clinically important antibiotics.

What the Heck is an Antibiotic?

http://falcon.cc.ukans.edu/~jbrown/antibiotic.html

Feature article from "Bugs in the News," a regular online scientific column written for the curious lay public.

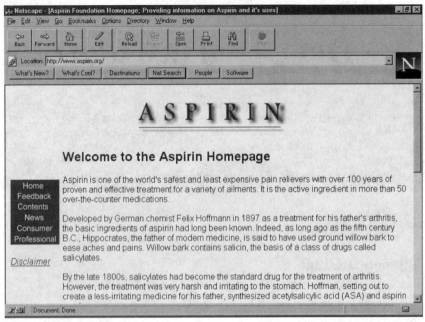

The Aspirin Foundation. http://www.aspirin.org/

Aspirin

The Aspirin Foundation of America
http://www.aspirin.org/

A central source of information on aspirin and aspirin products. It provides information for consumers and professionals, and news updates.

Aspirin: The Daily Apple
http://thedailyapple.com/level3/ds3/ddasphm.htm

The subtitle to this article is, "Familiarity breeds contempt, but for Aspirin it shouldn't." This article describes some of the benefits aspirin has shown in treating heart disease, cancer and Alzheimer's, and provides contraindications.

Aspirin Trivia Game
http://www.bayerus.com/aspirin/game/

Quiz to test your knowledge of aspirin.

Children

Antibiotics for Kids: Overprescribed?

http://www.onhealth.com/ch1/in-depth/item/item,2287_1_1.asp

More than two-thirds of babies receive antibiotics in their first six months. Description and physician's perspective are offered here.

Kids Aren't Just Small Adults: Medicines, Children and the Care Every Child Deserves

http://babybag.com/articles/fdaotc.htm

Safety tips.

KidsMeds

http://www.kidsmeds.com/

Pediatric drug information and consultation to parents. It is comprised of a group of pharmacists who are trained in pediatric pharmacy. The site offers information sheets and articles, a list of poison control centers, and an e-mail service whereby within 24 hours you will receive a free, e-mailed response to questions you have concerning pediatric medications.

OTC Dosing Guide

http://www.drpaula.com/topics/otcdosages.html

Shows parents what dose is advisable for their child, based on weight.

Questions to Ask about Psychiatric Medications for Children and Adolescents

http://www.aacap.org/factsFam/medquest.htm

Suggestions from the American Academy of Child and Adolescent Psychiatry.

Consumer Sites

Ask a Pharmacist Medication Counseling

http://www.geocities.com/HotSprings/8953/

If you e-mail a question, a pharmacist will provide you a referenced answer. There is a voluntary fee of $5.00. Link to online chat as well.

Consumer Information

http://www.ndmainfo.org/consumerInfo/consumerInfoFrame.html

Consumer information on the safe and appropriate use of over-the-counter medications. From the Consumer Healthcare Products Association.

Drugstore.com

http://www.drugstore.com/

You can shop at this online drugstore and get your prescription filled.

How to Read the Prescription

http://www.ns.net/users/ryan/rxabrv.html

List of common medical abbreviations which you may encounter on a doctor's prescription.

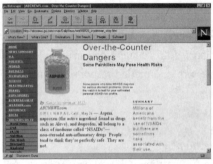

Over the Counter Dangers.
http://abcnews.go.com/onair/DailyNews/
wnt990526_snyderman_story.html

Over-the Counter Dangers

http://abcnews.go.com/onair/Daily News/wnt990526_snyderman_story. html

This article discusses some of the potential dangers of non-steroidal anti-inflammatory drugs, or NSAIDS.

PlanetRx

http://www.planetrx.com/

Online pharmacy and drugstore.

Prescription Drugs Reference Page

http://home.cyberave.com/~hsquare/drugmain.htm

The *PDR Family Guide To Prescription Drugs* provides information on the major FDA approved prescription drug products. This site offers disease overviews, drug profiles, and a number of appendices that include recommended vaccinations and poison control centers. Local health care resources are also available (e.g., help in locating a nearby physician, specialist, or hospital).

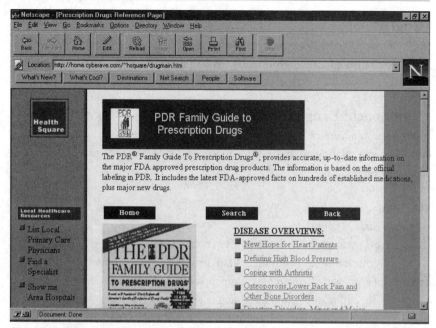

Prescription Drugs Reference Page. *http://home.cyberave.com/~hsquare/drugmain.htm*

Drug Databases

Clinical Pharmacology Online

http://www.cponline.gsm.com/

Excerpts from full drug monographs are available or, with subscribership, the entire monographs, which include dosage, contraindications, interactions, adverse reactions, costs, product ID, and classifications.

Drug Formulary

http://www.intmed.mcw.edu/drug.html

As well as providing basic formulary information, also includes analgesic drug guidelines, an antibiotic guide and further web resources.

Drug Information and Databases

http://www.coreynahman.com/druginfopage.html

There are a number of databases listed here, some of which are disease-specific (e.g., the AIDS/HIV Drug Database and the Diabetes Drug Database). They are rated by the webmaster and some descriptive text is offered.

DrugDB

http://pharminfo.com/drugdb/db_mnu.html

A database of drug information with links to articles and specific drug resources; browsable by generic and trade names.

Healthtouch: Drug Information Search

http://www.healthtouch.com/level1/p_dri.htm

This site claims to have information on over 10,000 prescription and over-the-counter drugs.

Rx List

http://www.rxlist.com/

A free, searchable, database of more than 4,000 prescription and over-the-counter drug products. Also provides some patient information, monographs on herbal treatments, homeopathic and Chinese herbal medicines, drug specific online discussions, RxLaughs and more.

Rx Med Prescribing Information

http://www.rxmed.com/prescribe.html

For physicians.

Elderly

Drugs and the Older Adult

http://www.crha-health.ab.ca/hlthconn/items/drugsoa.htm

Discusses why older adults may encounter more complications from taking medications, and suggests six questions anyone prescribed a medication should ask his or her doctor.

Medication Center for Seniors

http://www.studycenter.org/senmeds.html

This Center advocates informed, safe use of necessary medicines (prescribed, over-the-counter, or other remedies) with the goal of maintaining or enhancing personal wellness. Information sheets and other materials must be ordered, and there is a fee.

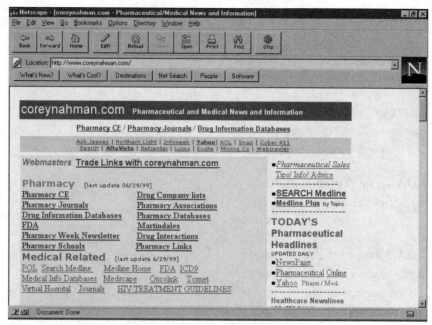

Coreynahman.com: Pharmaceutical and Medical News and Information.
http://www.coreynahman.com/

Medications and Older Adults

http://www.fda.gov/fdac/features/1997/697_old.html

Feature article from the Food and Drug Administration also offers advice on cutting costs and questions to ask the doctor.

Prescription Safety for Seniors

http://www.safewithin.com/seniorsafe/sen.prescrip.cgi

List of safety tips for seniors prescribed a drug.

General Resources

Coreynahman.com: Pharmaceutical and Medical News and Information

http://www.coreynahman.com/

Valuable information and news of new drugs, free online journals, continuing education, MEDLINE search, drug and medical databases, links, information and resources for AIDS, diabetes, cancer, heart disease, ENT and more. Updated daily.

Doctors' Guide to New Drugs or Indications

http://www.pslgroup.com/NEWDRUGS.HTM

This site contains a long list of news items covering recently-approved drugs, and new indications for drugs that were previously available.

Edmund's Home Page/Pharmacy Sites

http://www.li.net/~edhayes/rx.html

Lists dozens of pharmacy sites and offers a directory of U.S. pharmacy schools.

FDA Drug Approvals List

http://www.fda.gov/cder/da/da.htm

Updated weekly. Read disclaimer at beginning.

FDA News and Publications

http://www.fda.gov/opacom/hpnews.html

Press releases, papers and current publications of the U.S. Food and Drug Administration.

Hardin Meta Directory: Pharmacy and Pharmacology

http://www.arcade.uiowa.edu/hardin-www/md-pharm.html

Links to lists of Internet sites.

Internet Self-Assessment in Pharmacology

http://www.horsetooth.com/ISAP/

For health professionals, this self-study guide includes lecture outlines and pharmacological information on approximately 300 drugs, as well as exam questions and answers with explanations and clinical cases. Access to this service is free to all interested health care providers and educational users.

Links of Interest in Pharmacology

http://www.museum.state.il.us/isas/health/farmacol.html

Includes journals, associations and organizations and toxicology sites from around the world.

PDRnet.com

http://www.pdrnet.com/

Access to the PDR database, which includes a complete entry of each drug in the following: *Physicians' Desk Reference, PDR for Ophthalmology,* and *PDR for Nonprescription Drugs,* as well as MEDLINE, AIDSLINE, AIDSDRUGS, AIDSTRIALS and DIRLINE literature searches. This service is free to all MDs and DOs in full-time patient care.

Pharmacology Central

http://www.pharmcentral.com/

View the three-dimensional chemical structure of various classes of drugs.

PharmInfoNet

http://pharminfo.com/

The Pharmaceutical Information Network contains a drug database, frequently asked questions (FAQs) and publications. Links to diseases and discussion groups, as well as to related Internet sites. Excellent resource.

PharmWeb

http://www.pharmweb.net/

International pharmaceutical links and services. Lots of information.

Mosby's GenRx

http://www.mosby.com/Mosby/PhyGenRx/

Prescribing information, drug interactions, and patient information in the form of a book, a CD, an Internet tool or an intranet application. Description of products and purchasing form.

U.S. Pharmacopoeia Drug Information

http://www.usp.org/

Educational leaflets on prescription and non-prescription medications and their uses. USP is a private, nonprofit organization that seeks to disseminate unbiased information about drugs.

Virtual Library Pharmacy

http://www.pharmacy.org/

Includes associations, schools, jobs, pharmaceutical companies, journals and books, databases, government sites, databases, listservers and newsgroups on pharmacy-related topics.

"Virtual" Pharmacy Center

http://www-sci.lib.uci.edu:80/~martindale/Pharmacy.html

Guide to pharmacy, pharmacology, clinical pharmacology and toxicology resources on the web. Human and animal drug databases, drug dose calculators, drug information and research, dictionaries, online journals, and much more.

World Wide Drugs

http://community.net/~neils/new.html

More links to drug sites on the web. Includes homeopathic and alternative medicine remedies.

Mental Health

Internet Mental Health: Medications

http://www.mentalhealth.com/p30.html

Monographs containing information on dozens of drugs, from Adapin (Doxepin), an antidepressant; to Zyprexa (Olanzapine), an antipsychotic. Information includes pharmacology, indications and contraindications, warnings, adverse effects, dosage and research. There are also links to medication and medication research, magazine articles and booklets.

Medications for Mental Illness

http://www.athealth.com/NIH_medication.html

Online booklet shows how and why medications may be used as a part of the treatment for mental health problems. It has special sections on antipsychotic, antimanic, antidepressant, and antianxiety medications, as well as special considerations for children, pregnant women and seniors. There is also an index of medications.

Psychopharmacology Tips

http://uhs.bsd.uchicago.edu/dr-bob/tips/tips.html

You can search psychopharmacology tips, in which practitioners submit their questions and experience regarding medications and disorders; read Rx Qx (prescription questions); or join in psycho-babble, a chat room.

Organizations

American Academy of Pharmaceutical Physicians

http://www.aapp.org/

Offers information on this group and how to join it, as well as news, a member's forum, journals, research tools and a career counseling section.

American Society of Health-System Pharmacists

http://www.ashp.org/

This is a society whose members are pharmacists who work in hospitals, health maintenance organizations, long-term care facilities, home care agencies, and other components of health care systems. It provides accreditation and educational programs, as well as a number of publications.

Publications

Drug Topics

http://www.drugtopics.com/

A twice-monthly news magazine for pharmacists and the pharmaceutical community. Includes continuing education articles, news flashes, new products and cover stories. Free to qualified recipients.

Pharmacological Reviews

http://pharmrev.aspetjournals.org/

Access table of contents and abstracts for free, or view full text with subscription. Offers current issue online, or search through article archives.

Pharmacy Week
http://www.pharmacyweek.com/
Pharmacy salary and employment information. Includes resumés and a list of past articles.

U.S. Pharmacist
http://www.uspharmacist.com/
View the current issue of this magazine. Includes feature articles and departments, editorials, news, links and an index to earlier issues.

Prozac

Fluoxetine Drug Monograph
http://www.mentalhealth.com/drug/p30-p05.html
Information on Prozac (fluoxetine) which is classified as an antidepressant, antiobsessional and antibulimic.

Is Prozac for You?
http://www.adlist.com/psychiatry/prozac.html
Whether use of the antidepressant fluoxetine HCl (Prozac) is advisable.

Prozac and Other Prozac-Like Drugs
http://breggin.com/prozac.html
This site discusses what it believes are the dangers of using fluoxetine.

Ritalin

Factline on the Non-Medical Use of Ritalin
http://www.drugs.indiana.edu/pubs/factline/ritalin.html
Prescriptions for Ritalin have increased more than 600% in the last five years, and it is believed that this drug is often used inappropriately or recreationally. This site describes the "non-medical" abuse of this drug and its potentially dangerous health consequences.

Toxicology

Alan Barbour's Forensic Toxicology Page
http://userzweb.lightspeed.net/~abarbour/
Great collection of forensic toxicology links.

Links of Interest in Toxicology
http://www.museum.state.il.us/isas/health/toxicol.html
Includes links to numerous toxicology societies and organizations, toxicology journals and toxicology research sites.

Society of Environmental Toxicology and Chemistry
http://www.setac.org/
Nonprofit professional organization.

Toxicology and Pharmacology
http://www.santel.lu/SANTEL/toxico/toxico.html
Toxicology and pharmacology links, including newsgroups, journals, organizations, academic programs, drug and substance abuse.

Toxicology Web Sites
http://www.lib.ttu.edu/biology/tox-web.htm
This list comes from the University of Texas Tech.

EAR, NOSE & THROAT / OTOLARYNGOLOGY

Acoustic Neuroma

Acoustic Neuroma Association Home Page
http://ANAusa.org/

A patient-organized support and information group for people who have tumors affecting the cranial nerves, such as acoustic neuroma. Frequently asked questions, detection and treatment information are provided.

Acoustic Neuroma Resources
http://www.shorelinks.com/anr/neuroma.html

Collection of information sources, personal stories, support groups, newsgroups and bulletin boards dealing with acoustic neuroma. Also branches out into resources on vestibular disorders, brain tumors and neurooncology. Links with descriptions.

Information on Acoustic Neuroma
http://itsa.ucsf.edu/~rkj/IndexAN.html

Epidemiology, pathology, growth characteristics, clinical manifestations, medical tests, surgery, radiation therapy and research, as well as illustrations of acoustic neuroma.

Bell's Palsy

Bell's Palsy Exercises
http://www.mindspring.com/~mattcn/medical/bpexercises.htm
Suggestions from people who have suffered from this condition.

Bell's Palsy Intro Page
http://www.bellspalsy.com/
Bell's palsy is a condition that results in partial paralysis of the face. The primary cause is suspected to be a virus. This site briefly describes the symptoms, treatment and recovery processes, and will provide referrals to facilities that deal with this disorder.

The Bell's Palsy Network
http://www.bellspalsy.net/
This site includes frequently asked questions, online chat forum, links and references.

Bell's Palsy Resource Center
http://www.findinfo.com/bellspalsy.htm
Information and many links to general information about Bell's palsy. Also offers links to chat rooms and bulletin boards, personal stories, treatments, and foundations.

Ear Anatomy and Health

The Cochlea
http://www.bp.sissa.it/cochlea/
A graphic tour of the inner ear. Find online zipped video applications, and links to related sites.

Cochlear Implants in Adults and Children
http://text.nlm.nih.gov/nih/cdc/www/100.html
Text of the National Institutes of Health Consensus Development Conference statement. Addresses the issue of cochlear implants thoroughly and straight-forwardly.

Diseases of the Ear

http://www.hsc.wvu.edu/som/otolaryngology/ears.htm

Dizziness, cochlear implants, Ménière's disease, hearing loss, otitis media and Bell's palsy are briefly described.

Ear Diseases

http://galaxy.einet.net/galaxy/Medicine/Diseases-and-Disorders/Otorhinolaryngologic-Diseases/Ear-Diseases.html

Articles and organizations.

The Ear Foundation

http://www.theearfound.com/

There are a suggestions for those with hearing or ear disorders, including how to get a quiet table at a restaurant, travel tips for ears while flying, online support groups, downloadable articles, and more.

Ear Surgery Information Center

http://www.earsurgery.org/

More than just ear surgery information, this site also describes how the ear functions, its anatomy, different ear diseases and injuries to the ear. Also includes glossary and research information.

Ideology Forum: Video Otoscopy

http://www.li.net/~sullivan/ears.htm

Clinical video otoscopy images for audiologists who may employ video otoscopy (VO) in their practices. There is a lot of information here in the form of case presentations, frequently asked questions and images. For health professionals.

Noise and Hearing Loss

http://nlm.nih.gov/nih/cdc/www/76txt.html

Statement from the National Institutes of Health Consensus Development Congress regarding contribution to, susceptibility for, protection and prevention of hearing loss.

Shea Center for Ears Hearing and Balance, Inc.

http://www.ears.com/

Access to a news forum and resources devoted to the diagnosis and management of diseases of the ears, hearing and balance.

Virtual Tour of the Ear
http://inst.augie.edu/~hanavan/ear/hearmech.htm

Information on the hearing mechanisms, including the outer, middle and inner ears, auditory nerve and central auditory processing disorders. Links to audiology and audiological resources are also offered.

Ear Infections

Acute Otitis Media (Earache)
http://kidshealth.org/parent/common/otitis_media.html

Signs and symptoms, description, duration, contagiousness, prevention, professional and home treatment for this inflammation of the eardrum.

Ear Infections
http://scendtek.com/darren/earhome.html

Answers to some frequently asked questions.

Ear Infections: Facts and Stats
http://www.earinfections.com/html/infections/facts.html

After the common cold, middle ear infection is the most common illness in children. Site covers treatment options, symptoms and prevention, and answers frequently asked questions.

Ménière's Disease

Ménière's Disease
http://www.psych.ucsb.edu/~smits/meniere.htm

Ménière's is characterized by ear pressure, discomfort, and fullness; fluctuating hearing loss; fluctuating ringing in the ears; and episodic vertigo.

Ménière's Disease
http://members.idnsi.com/sgm/meniere.htm

Information including symptoms, treatments and different diagnoses.

Symptoms and Incidence of Ménière's Disease

http://oto.wustl.edu/men/mn1.htm

Provides a detailed description of the symptoms and incidence of this disease, with case studies.

Nose, Smell & Taste

Sinus Disease

http://www.ent-consult.com/sinus_disease_pro.html

Description of sinus disease and environmental factors.

Smell and Taste

http://www.nih.gov/nidcd/health/st.htm

About smell and taste and disorders that involve these senses. Also provides a list of organizations that are national in scope and that focus on hearing, balance, smell, taste, voice, speech, and language. From the National Institute on Deafness and Other Communication Disorders, a branch of the National Institutes of Health.

Smell and Taste Disorders

http://www.entnet.org/smelltaste.html

Explains how smell and taste work, in layperson's language. Also describes some things that can go wrong.

Smell Database

http://mc2.cchem.berkeley.edu/Smells/index.html

Interesting site provides the chemical and common name of dozens of smells, describes what it smells like, and gives the melting and boiling point, color, state and molecular model. For instance, 2-Propene-1-sulfinothioic acid S-2-propenyl ester, common name Allicin, is the substance that gives garlic its distinctive odor.

Foreign Body in a Nose

http://www.clark.net/pub/electra/cse0309.html

What to do and what not to do if a child has a foreign object stuck in his nose.

Nosebleeds (Epistaxis)

Care and Prevention of Nosebleeds
http://www.netdoor.com/entinfo/epistaao.html
Shows what to do to stop a nosebleed and prevent it from re-bleeding.

Management of Epistaxis
http://www.physsportsmed.com/issues/aug_96/davidson.htm
Explains bloody noses and when they may be cause for alarm.

Organizations

American Academy of Otolaryngology, Head and Neck Surgery
http://www.entnet.org/
The world's largest organization of physicians dedicated to ear, nose and throat problems. Offers information for members as well as for patients (e.g., fact sheets on hearing loss, sinusitis, Bell's palsy, smell and taste loss, and more). Other information includes clinical indicators, links to their official journal, research efforts, a virtual museum, and web links.

Professional Organizations and Institutes
http://www.bcm.tmc.edu/oto/othersf.html
Alphabetized, long list of links to otolaryngology organizations in the U.S. and internationally; list of support organizations and of related medical organizations.

Otolaryngology/Otorhinolaryngology & ENT Resources

Dr. Grossan, the On-line ENT Consultant
http://www.ent-consult.com/
Lots of information on sinus and nose problems, ear problems, sore throats and other temperomandibular joint/ENT conditions. Special section on diving.

Ear, Nose and Throat Disorders
http://hml.org/CHIS/topics/ent.html
Informational sites and support group links.

General Otorhinolaryngology Patient/Family Resources
http://www.slis.ua.edu/cdlp/WebCoreAll/patientinfo/otorhinolaryngology/general.htm
Provides links to a few ENT sites.

Hardin MD: Otolaryngology and Hearing Disorders
http://www.lib.uiowa.edu/hardin/md/oto.html
Collection of websites with large, medium and small lists of links to otolaryngology resources.

Otolaryngology Resources on the Internet
http://www.bcm.tmc.edu/oto/others.html
Provides links to discussion groups, academic programs, publications and research about otolaryngology and related areas of study.

Otorhinolaryngologic Diseases
http://www.mic.ki.se/Diseases/c9.html
This long list of links is part of the Karolinska Institute's resource directory. It includes ear diseases, laryngeal diseases, pharyngeal diseases and nose diseases.

Sore/Strep Throat

Childhood Infections: Strep Throat
http://www.kidshealth.org/parent/common/strep_throat.html
Advice for parents.

Sore Throat Solutions
http://www.health-line.com/articles/hl9605dt.htm
Health-line remedies.

Strep Throat Fact Sheet
http://www.kparikh.com/janim/strept.htm
Basic information.

Temperomandibular Joint Disorders

Temperomandibular Disorders
http://www.nidr.nih.gov/news/pubs/tmd/main.htm
Pamphlet from the National Oral Health Information Clearinghouse.

Temperomandibular Joint Disorder; Books, Links and People
http://www.tmjd.linkable.org/
Also contains disability links.

Temperomandibular Joint Syndrome
http://www.thriveonline.com/health/Library/illsymp/illness506.html
TMJ syndrome results from pain and inflammation in the temporomandibular joint, which is the joint on either side of the jaw that opens and closes the mouth, and adjoining muscles. Site provides good description, signs and symptoms, and general advice on how to treat TMJ problems.

Tinnitus

American Tinnitus Association
http://www.teleport.com/~ata/
Information about this nonprofit organization which helps fund tinnitus research and supports educational efforts and prevention efforts to protect ears and hearing. Information about tinnitus, including self-help advice, brochures and a quarterly newsletter from the ATA.

Information about Tinnitus
http://users.bart.nl/~tomdeman/tinnitus.htm
For those with tinnitus or those who have a loved one with the disorder.

Tinnitus
http://www.asha.org/consumers/brochures/tinnitus.htm
An online brochure that answers many patient questions regarding tinnitus. Tinnitus can be a high-pitched ringing in one or both ears, or it may be a buzzing, whistling, popping, hissing or roaring noise. Tinnitus may be constant or may come and go.

Tinnitus Information Network
http://members.aol.com/MyTinnitus/index.html

Definitions, causes, treatment and treatment centers, chat rooms and miscellaneous information.

Tonsils

Tonsillitis
http://www.lvm-systems.com/lvminter/SELFCARE/Tonsil.htm

Symptoms and questions to ask. Flowchart for self-care procedures.

Tonsils and Tonsillectomies
http://kidshealth.org/parent/healthy/tonsil.html

Explanation of the procedure. Knowing the facts can help ease one's fear.

The Tube and Tonsil Homepage
http://www.ent.holowww.com/welcome.html

Information about common ear, nose and throat problems. Includes earaches, ear infections, perforations of the ear, adenoid problems, tonsillectomy and more.

Vestibular Disorders

Coping with Dizziness: Resources for Vestibular Disorders
http://www.conciliocreative.com/dizzy/

A good place to start for information on comes to locating information on the Internet about dizziness, vertigo, balance problems, and other vestibular disorders. Includes organizations, support groups, personal stories, articles, newsgroups, mail lists, treatment, testing, and multimedia sites, among other resources.

In Balance: Vestibular Disorders Support Group
http://www.best.com/~lyceum/inbalance/

Support and help for individuals suffering from vestibular disorders such as dizziness, balance problems, hearing loss, ringing and/or pain in the ears.

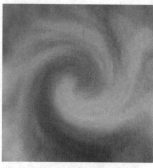

Vertigo, Dizziness, Vestibular Disorders

http://www.seanet.com/~tzhre/vertigo.htm

Links for those who suffer from these conditions.

Vestibular Disorders Association (VEDA)

http://www.teleport.com/~veda/

Vertigo, Dizziness, Vestibular Disorders. http://www. seanet.com/~tzhre/vertigo.htm

VEDA provides information and support to people suffering from inner ear/balance disorders. Site offers a lot of material, including an overview of the various vestibular disorders which covers symptoms, statistics, causes, diagnosis and treatment. It also describes specific manifestations such as labyrinthitis, neuronitis and Ménière's disease. Links to support groups, local and online, and to books, conferences and workshops are also provided.

EATING DISORDERS

Anorexia

Anorexia
http://www.neca.com/~cwildes/

A touching account of a woman with the disease; information and support.

Anorexia and Bulimia
http://www.rcpsych.ac.uk/public/help/anor/anor_frame.htm

Online pamphlet discusses these eating disorders.

Anorexia Nervosa
http://wellweb.com/INDEX/QANOREX.HTM

Describes this disorder and provides a summary of bodily effects as well as current research.

Anorexia Nervosa General Information
http://mentalhelp.net/factsfam/anorexia.htm

Discusses symptoms, causes, treatment and research.

The Skinny: A Webzine for Anorexia and Bulimia
http://www.angelfire.com/ca/TheSkinny/index.html

This online 'zine provides articles on eating disorders, health, book reviews, poetry, lowfat recipes, an advice column, links and more.

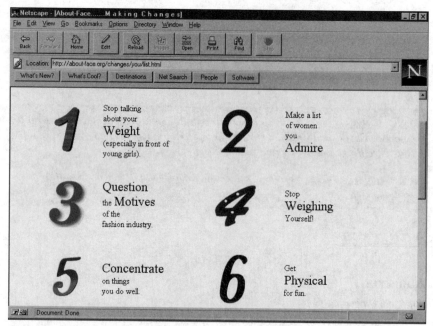

*Suggestions of what you can do to make changes (Note: list continues). At: **About Face.***
http://about-face.org/changes/you/list.html

Body Image

About-Face!

http://about-face.org/

This creative site includes facts about body image, as well as ways to combat negative and distorted images of women. They say it best: "By deconstructing media images, we teach critical thinking skills and we invite your opinions in an ongoing discussion about societal assumptions, the world we live in and our cultural priorities and values."

Body Icon

http://nm-server.jrn.columbia.edu/projects/masters/bodyimage/

"The media promote a biologically unattainable ideal. The diet industry promises to deliver it. Food has become a tempting taboo. Plastic surgery has upped the ante of perfection." A master's project by students at Columbia University Graduate School of Journalism, this attractive site discusses cultural (and market) forces that affect individuals' perception of their body.

Body Image: Health Versus Obsession

http://www.monash.edu.au/health/ pamphlets/BodyImage/index.htm

Find out your body image perception and learn about the body image problem. Separate tests/assessments for males and females.

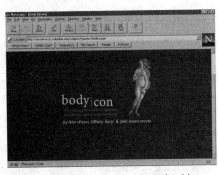

Body Icon. *http://nm-server.jrn.columbia. edu/projects/masters/bodyimage/*

Body Image: Parent and Teacher Guide

http://www.chatelaine.com/read/health/ptguide.html

Questions about body image to discuss with girls.

Body Image Project

http://www.justthink.org/BIP/

Uses multimedia, curricula and workshops to help young girls and women challenge negative messages media feeds them about body image. Includes webzine and forum.

BodyPositive

http://www.BodyPositive.com/

Defines healthy weight as the weight you are when you are living a reasonable life. Includes newsletter and online forums, discusses inner parenting, children and weight, how to change your inner dialog, and more.

Bulimia

Ability's Bulimia Page

http://www.ability.org/bulimia.html

A number of links to sites providing information on bulimia, including diagnostic criteria, symptoms, help and frequently asked questions.

Bulimia

http://www.laureate.com/nedo/nedobulimia.asp

Important facts, warning signs, medical consequences, treatment options, and a personal recovery story.

Coping with Bulimia

http://www.shpm.com/articles/eating/other/bulimia2.html

This article appeared in *Self-Help & Psychology* magazine. It provides key points on what bulimia is, how it begins, and advice for those seeking help for themselves or for someone they know who suffers from bulimia nervosa.

Fact Sheet: Bulimia Nervosa

http://www.noah.cuny.edu/illness/mentalhealth/cornell/conditions/bulimia.html

Provides definition, description of symptoms, cause, course, treatment and self-management of this eating disorder.

Complications

Dangers and Complications of Eating Disorders

http://www.concernedcounseling.com/eatingdisorders/eatingdisorders complications.htm

Many damaging medical and psychological complications can result from eating disorders.

Dental Ramifications of Bulimia

http://members.aol.com/dentistry/bulimia.html

Bulimia can have harmful effects on the teeth.

Health Implications of Obesity

http://text.nlm.nih.gov/nih/cdc/www/49txt.html

This National Institutes of Health Consensus Development Conference Statement adressing obesity, how it affects health, how it affects longevity, the appropriate uses of height-weight tables, which medical conditions weight loss is recommended for, and what areas future research should focus on.

Myer's Objective Information on Obesity, Weight Control, Eating Disorders, and Related Health Conditions

http://www.weight.com/

The goal of this site is to provide unbiased medical information on obesity and related issues. Definition of obesity, complications, diets and obesity, sexual abuse and obesity, treatments, fad diets, and much more.

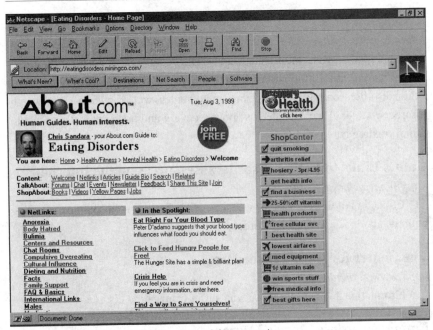

Eating Disorders. *http://eatingdisorders.miningco.com/*

Symptoms and Complications of Bulimia Nervosa
http://www.healthguide.com/english/brain/eating/bulimia.htm

Description of some of the behaviors and characteristics common to individuals who suffer from bulimia.

General Resources

About.com: Eating Disorders
http://eatingdisorders.miningco.com/

Anorexia, body hatred, bulimia, centers, family support, compulsive eating, obesity, risk factors, self-help, and much more.

All About Eating Disorders
http://eatingdisorders.mentalhelp.net/

Symptoms, treatment, online resources, organizations, support and research.

ANRED
http://www.anred.com/index.html

Anorexia Nervosa and Related Eating Disorders, Inc., is a nonprofit organization that provides information about anorexia nervosa, bulimia nervosa, binge eating disorder, compulsive exercising, and other less well-known food and weight disorders. Material includes details about recovery and prevention. There is a lot of information here.

Cath's Links to Eating Disorders Resources on the Internet
http://home.nvg.org/~cath/ed/

Collection of links to various websites and information on compulsive eating, bulimia, anorexia and related disorders.

The Center for Eating Disorders
http://www.eatingdisorder.org/

Information and help for those who suffer from eating disorders.

Eating Disorders Mirror Mirror
http://www.mirror-mirror.org/eatdis.htm

Great information and support.

Eating Disorders Online
http://caringonline.com/

Links included at this site are divided into three major categories: news and resources, topics (e.g., athletics, biology, body image and diet), and personal thoughts (poetry, stories, quotes, discussion). It has has a great deal to offer.

The Eating Disorders Site
http://closetoyou.org/eatingdisorders/

Information, support, and resources such as ED self-tests, vitamin deficiencies, body-mass index calculator, normal eating, and more.

The Harvard Eating Disorders Center
http://www.hedc.org/

Dedicated to research and education on eating disorders. This site offers information, help for family and friends, information for those who think they may have a problem with their eating habits, and further resources.

Less Well Known Eating Disorders
http://www.anred.com/lesser.html

Anorexia, bulimia, compulsive and binge eating are not the only kinds of eating disorders, but they are the most common. Additional disorders identified here include bigarexia, pica, night-eating syndrome and several others.

Lucy Serpell's Eating Disorders Resources
http://www.iop.bpmf.ac.uk/home/depts/psychiat/edu/eat.htm

General information, academic resources, associations, physical problems and more. Links were chosen for their high quality content.

Something Fishy Website on Eating Disorders
http://www.something-fishy.org/

This is a great source for information and support on anorexia nervosa, bulimia nervosa, compulsive overeating and other eating disorders. Signs and symptoms, dangers, cultural issues, medications and other resources are offered, along with articles on stress management and recovery.

Family and Friends

Confronting a Person with Anorexia or Bulimia
http://www.healthtouch.com/level1/leaflets/anad/anad013.htm

Suggestions on approaching someone who you believe has an eating disorder.

Eating Disorders Theme Page
http://www.cln.org/themes/eating.html

Although the site was designed to provide information for students and teachers on eating disorders, anyone with concerns about these problems will find it helpful.

Eating Disorders Warning Signs
http://www.kidsource.com/nedo/warning.html

Includes physical problems associated with eating disorders as well as suggestions on how to help someone with anorexia or bulimia.

Positive Voices
http://www.ednewsletter.com/
This newsletter is devoted to helping families cope when a loved one is suffering from an eating disorder. You can receive the first issue free and check out recent topics covered in the newsletter at this site. Subscription information is also provided.

Symptoms of Eating Disorders
http://icarus.med.utoronto.ca/fndweek1/symptoms.htm
Many links with descriptions.

Understanding Eating Disturbances or Disorders
http://www.healthtouch.com/level1/leaflets/anad/anad013.htm
This guide was written for families or friends of someone with an eating problem.

Healthy Eating
See also: Diet & Nutrition.

Eat Well, Live Well
http://www.healthyeating.org/
Discusses healthy eating habits.

Healthy Weight Network/Healthy Weight Journal
http://www.healthyweightnetwork.com/
The mission of this site and the newsletter it produces is to promote healthy eating habits and attitudes. They state: "Recognizing that weight is an easily exploitable health and social concern, we are further committed to exposing deception, reshaping detrimental social attitudes, and promoting good health at any size." This site provides articles to this end, exposes weight loss fraud and diet quackery, and discusses normal eating.

Males

Male Body Image

http://www.infoplease.com/spot/mbi1.html

"For men, more than ever, looks count." Six-part article covers the male body image concerns and trends. Addresses eating disorders and obsessive exercising behaviors. Originally appeared in *The Boston Phoenix.*

Males

http://caringonline.com/eatdis/topics/males.htm

These links to articles about men with anorexia, bulimia or other eating disorders again shows that eating disorders are not "female diseases."

Males and Eating Disorders

http://www.primenet.com/~danslos/males/home.html

Although one out of every ten people with an eating disorder is male, most resources you find are directed toward helping women who suffer from these illnesses. However, this site provides information and links to sites that deal with men and eating disorders, eating disorders in general, and provides stories of men who have suffered.

Obesity and Compulsive/Binge Eating

Affirmations for People Suffering from Compulsive Eaing

http://www.fatfairygodmother.com/affirmations.htm

Ten affirmations to hang on your fridge.

Alternatives to Binging-Purging

http://www.mirror-mirror.org/altbin.htm

List of activities you can do to prevent you from binging and feeling badly about it afterward.

Centers for Overcoming Overeating

http://www.overcomingovereating.com/centers.html

List of centers around the country.

Compulsive Eaters Anonymous-HOW

http://www.ceahow.com/

A 12-step organization for controlling compulsive eating patterns through fellowship and support.

Overeaters Anonymous

http://www.overeatersanonymous.org/

Overeaters Anonymous describes itself as a fellowship of individuals who are recovering from compulsive overeating. There are approximately 9000 meetings in 60 countries around the world. This site shows you how to find one convenient for you. In addition, you can also participate in an online meeting. Site describes OA philosophy, including the 12 steps and the 12 traditions.

Overeaters Anonymous Homepage

http://www.oa.org/

Another OA site describing this 12-step program.

Overeaters Recovery Group

http://recovery.HIWAAY.net//

Lists many different e-mail groups, as well as Overeaters Anonymous weekly meetings on the Internet.

When Food Becomes an Obsession

http://www.reach4life.com/news28.html

Approximately 1 to 2 million Americans suffer from binge eating disorder, a disease that, according to this site, "is about more than willpower."

Organizations

Academy for Eating Disorders

http://www.acadeatdis.org/

Organization for professionals devoted to treating eating disorders.

American Anorexia/Bulimia Association, Inc.

http://www.aabainc.org/

General information on eating disorders as well as information geared for those who suffer from the problem, those who know someone who is suffering from the problem, and health care professionals. This organization is dedicated to the prevention and treatment of eating disorders. It supports research as well as promotes social attitudes that enhance a healthy body image.

Eating Disorders Organizations

http://www.something-fishy.org/ed-4.htm

List of organizations online and offline, including contact information and descriptions.

Recovery

Eating Disorders: Body Image Betrayal

http://www.geocities.com/HotSprings/5704/edlist.htm

Helpful material for those struggling with an eating disorder. Includes a long list of alternatives to eating disorder behavior and a checklist for identifying one's feelings, as well as many other resources.

Eating Disorders Recovery Online

http://www.edrecovery.com/

Site offers programs as well as individual consultations for those who suffer from eating disorders. In addition, it describes the latest information on eating disorders, including what they are, who has them, some of the causes, warning signs, what to do if you or someone you know shows signs of having an eating disorder, and a set of guidelines for family members.

Getting Help

http://www.mirror-mirror.org/gethelp.htm

There *is* help available, and people with eating disorders will need help to overcome their problem. Treatment should probably include individual, family and group therapy, support groups, medical and nutritional counseling, and in some cases medications or hospitalization. Site helps to take you from the point of realizing you have a problem, to the point of being able to get help.

Medications for Eating Disorders

http://www.something-fishy.org/meds.htm

Here is a list of medications sometimes used for treating eating disorders. Provides indications, considerations, side effects, and drug interactions.

Optimal Eating Articles

http://healthyeating.com/articles.html

These articles from different sources discuss recovery from eating disorders.

Serotonin and Eating Disorders

http://pharminfo.com/pubs/msb/seroton.html

Article from Pharminfo presents information on treating eating disorders pharmaceutically.

Treatment and Recovery

http://www.anred.com/tx.html

Explains that recovery from an eating disorder is possible, and describes what it involves.

EMERGENCY MEDICINE & CRITICAL CARE

Critical Care

CCM-L

http://www.sfhs.edu/ccm-l/

Site provides subscription information for the International Critical Care Internet Discussion Group. Includes discussion of specific questions that are subtmitted, a forum, and a journal club. Topics addressed include daily activities in a critical care arena, determination of resuscitation status, management of scarce resources, and implications of the latter. Archives of discussions and other interesting sites are also found. List is easy to subscribe (or unsubscribe) to.

Critical Care Connection

http://www.springnet.com/criticalcare/top.htm

Links to over 50 critical care resources organized into the following areas: drugs, general critical care, professional issues, cardiac monitoring, cardiovascular disorders, pulmonary artery pressure, pulmonary, and point-of-care testing.

Critical Care Forum

http://ccforum.com/

Registration is the only requirement for participation. Facilities include an official journal for the forum, paper and web reports, reviews, dispatches, links and conference information.

Critical Care Humor Page
http://ccm-l.med.edu/jokes/
Lots of laughs, but little decorum...

Critical Care Web
http://w3.one.net/~gloriamc/critcare.html
Long list of links to critical care, anesthesiology, cardiology, emergency and trauma, neurology, pediatric critical care, pulmonary/respiratory care and transplantation sites on the web. Many of the links have to do with critical care nursing issues.

Emergency Medicine Links
http://www.lib.uiowa.edu/hardin/md/emerg.html
Hardin MD provides links to meta-lists divided into large, medium and small.

MedWebPlus Critical Care
http://www.medwebplus.com/subject/Critical_Care.html
Links to critical care resources, broken down by subject.

Pediatric Critical Care Medicine
http://www.invivo.net/bg/reaped2.html
Long list, showing pediatric emergencies (e.g., involving acute epiglottis, croup, asthma) and more general pediatric critical care websites.

PedsCCM: Pediatric Critical Care
http://PedsCCM.wustl.edu/
Information tool for professionals who care for critically ill and injured infants and children. Clinical resources, research, organizations and meetings, parent resources and more.

Society of Critical Care Medicine
http://www.sccm.org/
Critical care and society news, journals, education, consumer pages and links.

WWW Sites of Interest to Intensive/Critical Care
http://anzics.herston.uq.edu.au/ICUWebs.HTM
There are several sites of interest here.

"We Can't Kill Your Mother" & Other Stories of Intensive Care

http://www.mtsinai.org/pulmonary/books/icu/contents.html

This book presents interesting medical and ethical challenges encountered in the ICU. It was written by Lawrence Martin, M.D., and relates his real experiences.

Disaster Relief

American Red Cross

http://www.redcross.org/

Contains news, donation information, international and domestic disaster updates, emergency guides, Red Cross history and services, local chapter contacts, volunteer opportunities and a virtual museum.

Church World Service Emergency Response

http://www.ncccusa.org/CWS/emre/

This international relief and development organization of the National Council of Churches works through partnership with faith-based organizations in disaster-affected communities by providing seed money, materials, counsel and technical assistance, educational materials and communication efforts.

International Medical Corp

http://www.imc-la.com/

A nonprofit humanitarian relief organization whose mission is to save lives and relieve suffering through health interventions and medical training that build local capacity and self-reliance in war-torn and impoverished regions of the world.

Internet Disaster Information Network

http://www.disaster.net/

Provides the Internet community with news on ongoing and historical disaster situations around the world.

ReliefWeb

http://wwwnotes.reliefweb.int/

Global information project to provide news of and assistance for those suffering in cases of complex emergencies and natural disasters. It is a project of the United Nations Office for the Coordination of Humanitarian Affairs.

WHO Division of Emergency and Humanitarian Action
http://www.who.int/eha/

This agency is responsible for coordinating the international response to emergencies and natural disasters in the health field, in close partnership with other member agencies of the United Nations Inter-Agency Standing Committee (IASC), and within the framework set out by the United Nations Department of Humanitarian Affairs (DHA). Information on areas in need, discussion zone, violence and injury prevention, research and resources.

World Association for Disaster and Emergency Medicine
http://www.pitt.edu/HOME/GHNet/wadem/wadem.html

Provides knowledge, techniques, education and policy information, and publications. Encourages the dissemination of information about disaster and emergency medicine.

Emergency Home Safety

Common Simple Emergencies
http://www.clark.net/pub/electra/cse0.html

This site promotes a book by the same name, and also includes many case presentations online. It offers what to do, what not to do, discussion and references for many conditions, from penis-caught-in-a-zipper to pharyngitis (sore throat).

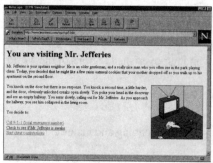

CPR Simulation Scenarios
http://www.lessstress.com/simintro.htm

Virtual simulation for administering CPR to someone in trouble. Choose from bystander CPR simulator for adult, child and infant. CPR information, and other simulators also available.

CPR Simulation Scenarios:
http://www.lessstress.com/cpr/cpr1.htm

Home Safety Tips

http://www.farmersinsurance.com/fi3260.html

Includes suggestions on home fire protection, childproofing your home, backyard safety, first aid tips, bicycle safety, hurricane safety and more.

Learn CPR

http://www.learncpr.org/index.html

Illustrated guides detailing CPR methods. Also has games, links, frequently asked questions, and information on how to help choking victims.

Emergency Preparedness

Disaster Resources

http://www.ag.uiuc.edu/~disaster/disaster.html

Side provides consumer information on how to prepare for a disaster, what to do after a disaster, how to get help after a disaster, how to help disaster victims, and other disaster resources.

Earthquake Information

http://quake.wr.usgs.gov/

Maps and lists of recent earthquakes, how to prepare for an earthquake, frequently asked questions, research and other resources. From the United States Geological Survey.

Emergency Preparedness Information Exchange

http://hoshi.cic.sfu.ca/epix/

Emergency/disaster management topics information and guidelines. Includes personal preparedness, organizations, government plans and more.

FEMA for Kids

http://www.fema.gov/kids/

The Federal Emergency Management Agency teaches kids about disasters, and what they can do to help their family in a disaster.

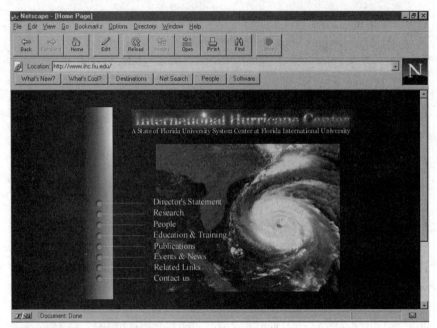

International Hurricane Center. http://www.ihc.fiu.edu/

International Hurricane Center

http://www.ihc.fiu.edu/

Conducts research to predict storm impact and trains individuals and communities about hurricane preparedness.

General Resources

Department of Public Safety Online: Medic Alert Program

http://www.ou.edu/oupd/medalert.htm

The Medic Alert emblem is worn around the neck or wrist, and contains important information about the wearer's medical problem(s), name, and contact number to reach medical file information. On-call 24 hours a day.

Emergency Medical Humor

http://home.cwnet.com/catspaw/emshumor.htm

For the emergency room crowd.

Emergency Medicine and Primary Care Home Page

http://www.embbs.com/

Educational resources for emergency and primary care physicians and allied health care providers. Collections of relevant clinical photographs, radiographs, and EKGs; lectures, job opportunities and timely clinical information. Also includes patient care simulations and links to additional related websites.

Emergency Medicine Internetwork Gateway

http://oac.hsc.uth.tmc.edu/uth_orgs/emer_med/

Information about the University of Texas program, as well as interesting emergency medicine cases, resources and links.

Emergency Medicine Lectures

http://www.vh.org/Providers/Lectures/EmergencyMed/EmergencyTitle.html

Lectures on what to do in cases of psychiatric emergencies, hypertensive emergencies, and acute respiratory failure.

Emergency Sciences WWW Site List

http://www.district.north-van.bc.ca/eswsl/www-911.htm

A list of known fire, rescue, EMS and emergency service sites that can be found on the Internet. At the time of this viewing, 2223 websites were included.

ER Watch

http://www.erwatch.com/

Searchable database of emergency room cases from 100 U.S. hospitals.

Global Emergency Medicine Archives

http://gema.library.ucsf.edu:8081/

A unique online journal serving the emergency medicine Internet community.

Intensive Care and Emergency Medicine Archives

http://www.sciencekomm.at/journals/medicine/inten.html

Dozens of journals related to critical care.

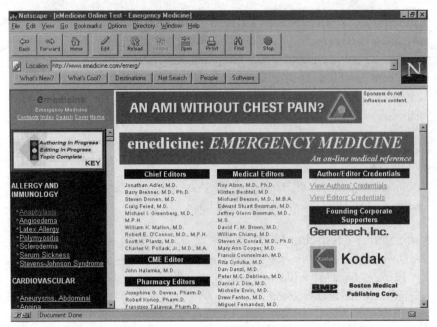

Online Emergency Medicine Reference. *http://www.emedicine.com/emerg/*

Online Emergency Medicine Reference

http://www.emedicine.com/emerg/

Full text of book covering emergency medicine from allergy and immunology, to trauma and orthopedics. Includes authors' and editors' credentials, a thorough contents, index and search.

Paramedic's CyberBase

http://paramedic.i.am/

Describes what a paramedic does.

Virtual ER

http://www.virtualer.com/

Includes tutorials, clinical and radiological images, a medical library, an emergency medicine professional network, residence and fellowship information, and links.

Yahoo's Emergency Services

http://www.yahoo.com/Health/Emergency_Services/

Yahoo provides links to many emergency services sites, including ambulance services, natural disaster medical systems, organizations, and more.

Injury Control

Injury Control Resource Information Network

http://www.injurycontrol.com/icrin/

Internet-accessible resources related to the field of injury control and prevention. Injury specific resources include fire safety, burns, poisonings, firearms, violence, and occupational safety. Recent research and links to governmental, professional and commercial sites are provided, as well as many posting and discussion areas.

Injury Prevention Resources on the Net

http://www.albany.edu/sph/injur_8a.html

Thoughtful descriptions accompany these links to sites involving injury prevention, public safety and public health.

National Center for Injury Prevention and Control

http://www.cdc.gov/ncipc/ncipchm.htm

This organization works to reduce morbidity, disability, mortality, and costs associated with injuries. It provides facts, data and other resources on various forms of injury, from gang violence to bicycle safety. NCIPC works closely with other federal agencies; national, state, and local organizations; state and local health departments; and research institutions. Links to numerous sites.

National SAFEKIDS Campaign

http://www.safekids.org/

To prevent unintentional injury to children, this organization educates adults and children, provides safety devices to families in need, and advocates for laws to empower families and communities to protect children ages 14 years and under. Site provides fact sheets, frequently asked questions, and a family safety checklist. Information on state and local coalitions.

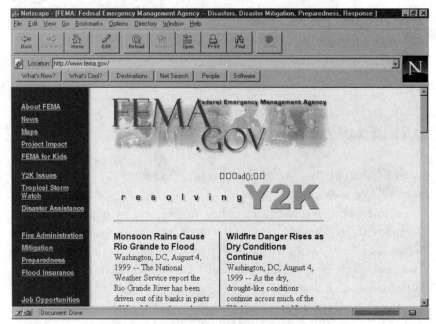

Federal Emergency Management Agency. http://www.fema.gov/

Ten Leading Causes of Death, United States, 1993-1995

http://www.cdc.gov/ncipc/osp/leadcaus/ustable.htm

Table highlights leading causes of death, broken down by age group.

Organizations

American Trauma Society

http://www.amtrauma.org/index.htm

This voluntary nonprofit organization is dedicated to the prevention of trauma and the improvement of trauma care.

Federal Emergency Management Agency

http://www.fema.gov/

FEMA provides emergency relief to areas declared National Disasters. The site offers news about floods, tornadoes, and other disasters, and about efforts to aid victims of these events. It sponsors programs in emergency preparedness and training, and provides assistance to help people get back on their feet.

International Committee of the Red Cross

http://www.icrc.org/

International agency that helps victims of war and internal violence. Site has news, description of operations by country, discussion of special issues and topics, and international humanitarian law.

Trauma

American Association for the Surgery of Trauma Webnet

http://www.aast.org/

Self-described as providing "scientific information regarding the care of the trauma patient." Includes prevention, prehospital care, resuscitation, operative care, critical care, rehabilitation and trauma system design. Hyperlinks to other trauma resources and discussion groups on the Internet.

Trauma and Injury Prevention WWW Servers

http://rmstewart.uthscsa.edu/traumasites.html

Links to trauma and injury prevention websites, accompanied by a brief description. Includes professional organizations, research and academic centers.

TraumAID Project

http://www.cis.upenn.edu/~traumaid/

TraumAID is a program developed to assist physicians with the diagnosis and treatment of critical care and trauma patients. After the patient has been stabilized, the physician supplies some information and TraumAID proposes goals that need to be addressed as well as produces a plan that will maximize the chance of meeting these goals.

Trauma.Org: Care of the Injured

http://www.trauma.org/

The main feature of this site is the Traumabank, which contains images, articles, case presentations and links divided by specific trauma area specialties, from neurotrauma, to trauma anesthesiology. Connections to Trauma Chat and archives are also offered.

UTHSCSA Trauma Home Page

http://rmstewart.uthscsa.edu/

The University of Texas Health Science Center at San Antonio focuses on issues dealing with injury, injury prevention and surgical critical care. Information for health care professionals, patients and the public is provided. Specifically, find advice on pediatric emergency treatment, safety and injury prevention are offered, as well as links to web pages on critical care and emergency prevention.

Wilderness Medicine

AEE Wilderness Safety and Emergency Care Home Page

http://www.princeton.edu/~rcurtis/wildsafe.html

Safety management resources, wilderness first aid resources and first aid training.

High Altitude Pathology Institute

http://www.geocities.com/CapeCanaveral/6280/

High altitude pulmonary edema, chronic mountain sickness and other illnesses related to altitude are addressed.

Medical Herpetology

http://www.xmission.com/~gastown/herpmed/med.htm

Lists medical herpetology (the study of reptiles and amphibians), emerging diseases, and wilderness medicine websites.

Mountain Rescue Association

http://www.mra.org/

This is a volunteer organization dedicated to saving lives through rescue and mountain safety education. Site describes training programs, general and membership information.

OA First Aid & Safety Home Page

http://www.princeton.edu/~oa/safety/index.shtml

Outdoor action resources include guides to planning a safe trip, first aid in the wilderness and under specific circumstances (i.e., in cases of high altitude sickness etc.), information on water purification, wind chill chart and many more tools to promote outdoor safety.

Outdoor Action Program

http://www.princeton.edu/~oa/oa.html

Wilderness first aid and safety for outdoor recreations, from rock climbing, biking and camping, to caving.

Snakebyte Emergency First-Aid Information

http://www.xmission.com/~gastown/herpmed/snbite.htm

What to do (and what not to do) if bitten by a venomous snake.

Wilderness Emergency Medical Services Institute

http://www.wemsi.on.ca/

The Institute provides education, promotes research, and offers direct assistance in emergency medical services. Site provides curriculum, as well as technical information (such as a personal wilderness medical kit list), information on legislative issues, and more.

The Wilderness Medicine Institute

http://wmi.nols.edu/

Offers courses, articles and books.

ENDOCRINOLOGY

Acromegaly

Acromegaly
http://www.niddk.nih.gov/health/endo/pubs/acro/acro.htm

Information on this disorder that results when the pituitary gland produces an excess of growth hormone. Includes incidence, causes, treatment and resources.

Addison's Disease

Addison's Disease
http://www.niddk.nih.gov/health/endo/pubs/addison/addison.htm

Addison's Disease is a rare endocrine disorder involving the adrenal gland, and it is characterized by weight loss, muscle weakness, fatigue and darkening of the skin. Site describes AD symptoms, diagnosis and treatment, and offers suggested reading.

Addison's Disease: The Facts You'll Need to Know
http://www.medhelp.org/www/nadf3.htm

Basic information on Addison's. Includes description, symptoms, causes, treatment and related diseases.

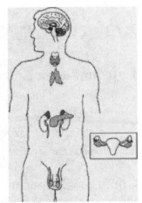

Addison's Disease.
*http://www.niddk.nih.gov/
health/endo/pubs/addison/
addison.htm*

National Adrenal Disease Foundation
http://www.medhelp.org/nadf/
Addison's, Cushing's and congenital adrenal hyperplasia are some of the diseases of the adrenal gland on which you can find information.

Cushing's Syndrome

Cushing's Support and Research Foundation
http://world.std.com/~csrf/
Information on Cushing's disease and Cushing's syndrome for patients, professionals, and the general public.

Cushing's Syndrome
http://www.niddk.nih.gov/health/endo/pubs/cushings/cushings.htm
Online brochure discusses this rare hormonal disorder.

Cushing's Syndrome Bulletin Board
http://www.support-group.com/cgi-bin/sg/get_links?cushings
Support group. Post a message or browse. Includes frequently asked questions and related links.

Endocrine Function & Disorders

Case Studies in Endocrine Disorders
http://www.mcl.tulane.edu/classware/pathology/medical_pathology/endocrine_cases/casesTop.html
Seven different cases covering evaluation of pituitary, thyroid, parathyroid, adrenal, and reproductive endocrinology topics.

Common Endocrine Diseases
http://members.xoom.com/endocrine/faqframe.htm
General information on thyroid diseases, adrenal disease and pituitary diseases.

The Hormones of the Human

http://www.ultranet.com/~jkimball/BiologyPages/H/Hormones.html

Examines the properties of endocrine chemical signaling.

Endocrine Diseases

http://www.mic.ki.se/Diseases/c19.html

The Swedish Karolinska Institute has assembled an extensive list of links to Internet sites focusing on endocrinology in general, as well as to sites addressing specific diseases afflicting the organs of the endocrine system: e.g., diabetes mellitus, Addison's disease, Cushing's syndrome, breast diseases, pituitary diseases, parathyroid diseases, thyroid diseases, Kallmann Syndrome and endocrine gland neoplasms.

Endocrinology and Hepatology Journals

http://www.sciencekomm.at/journals/medicine/endoc.html

List and links to endocrinology journals on the Internet.

Endocrine Web

http://www.endocrineweb.com/index.html

Patient information on thyroid, parathyroid, adrenal, and pancreas disorders, including diabetes and osteoporosis information. There is a very large amount of information on endocrine disease, conditions, hormone problems, and treatment options including all types of thyroid, parathyroid, and adrenal surgery. There are also chat rooms, support groups, a user forum and a doctor search.

Endocrinology Databases

http://museum.state.il.us/isas/data2.html

The Illinois State Academy of Science maintains this site which provides tables showing the standard ranges of concentration of pituitary, steroid, thyroid and other hormones as well as levels of the insulin-like growth factors in humans (by age) and in other animals.

Endocrinology Home Page

http://www.endocrinology.com/

Information on diabetes, thyroid and parathyroid disorders, adrenal disorders, pituitary disorders, osteoporosis, weight management and sexual dysfunction. A directory of endocrinologists and of endocrinology organizations is also available.

Links of Interest to Endocrinologists

http://www.geocities.com/HotSprings/1833/endolinks.htm

This site contains numerous references to endocrinology associations and journals, and points to sites providing patient information on endocrinology, as well as to guidelines and medical resources for physicians.

MedWebPlus' Endocrinology

http://www.medwebplus.com/subject/Endocrinology.html

Another choice starting-place for researching endocrinology topics. This site provides links to endocrine-related sites that include case studies, consumer health information, pediatric endocrinology and toxicology.

Publications Online: Endocrine and Metabolic Diseases

http://www.niddk.nih.gov/health/endo/endo.htm

NIDDK information for patients and the general public on acromegaly, Addison's disease, Cushing's syndrome, familial multiple endocrinoneoplasia, hyperparathyroidism and prolactinoma. A description of each disease, its cause, prevalence, symptoms, treatment and suggested readings are provided. Also offers a directory of organizations addressing endocrine and metabolic diseases.

Organizations

American Association of Clinical Endocrinologists

http://www.aace.com/

Offers professional information for AACE members and non-members about practice guidelines, continuing education opportunities, jobs, legislative updates, discussion groups and CPT coding issues as related to endocrinology. In addition, site offers access to the online edition of *The First Messenger*, a bi-monthly newsletter, and other Association publications.

Endocrine Society

http://www.endo-society.org/

This organization is devoted to the research, study and clinical practice of endocrinology. This site is well-organized and well-written, and it offers professionals and patients information on endocrine-related topics. In addition, *Endocrine News* is free to approved applicants, and it contains editorials, articles, and technical news.

The Society for Endocrinology

http://www.endocrinology.org/

The major endocrine society outside of North America. This organization seeks to advance endocrinology and public education in endocrinology. The site offers access to electronic journals (if you are a member), free full-text articles, conference and membership information.

Pancreas

See also: Diabetes.

Endocrine Diseases of the Pancreas

http://www.endocrineweb.com/pancreas.html

Discusses the endocrine functions of the pancreas, pancreatic endocrinic hormones and their function.

Parathyroid Disorders

Parathyroid Disease

http://www.endocrine-surgery.com/parathyroid.html

The parathyroid glands regulate calcium levels in the body. Site explains the function of these glands, and disorders that can occur.

Your Parathyroid

http://www.parathyroid.com/

Discusses parathyroid diseases and their treatments. Information for patients.

Pathology

Endocrine Pathology Index

http://www-medlib.med.utah.edu/WebPath/ENDOHTML/ENDOIDX.html

Images of the thyroid, pituitary, parathyroid, adrenal glands, and the islets of Langerhans. Includes both normal and diseased samples.

Pituitary Disorders

See also: Acromegaly and Cushing's Syndrome, earlier in this chapter.

The Pituitary Center at Vanderbilt University Medical Center

http://www.pituitarycenter.com/

Learn more about pituitary disease and this Center's clinical services.

Pituitary Cancer

http://oncolink.upenn.edu/disease/pituitary/

Symptom management; physician and patient information.

Hypopituitarism

http://www.healthanswers.com/adam/top/view.asp?filename=000343.htm

Basic information on this hormonal disorder of the pituitary gland.

PTNA Home Page

http://www.pituitary.com/

The Pituitary Tumor Network Association site includes ask the experts, bulletin board, a physician's section, and information and symptoms describing acromegaly, Cushing's syndrome, hormonal imbalances, and many other disorders.

Reproductive Endocrinology

See also: Sexual & Reproductive Health.

Links of Interest in Reproductive Endocrinology

http://www.museum.state.il.us/isas/oblink2.html

Includes fertility clinics around the country.

Midlife Passages

http://www.midlife-passages.com/

Endocrinology, and male and female menopause.

Reproductive Endocrinology

http://www.collmed.psu.edu/obgyn/repend.htm

Describes treatment options for couples desiring pregnancy, disorders of the female reproductive system, and post menopausal care.

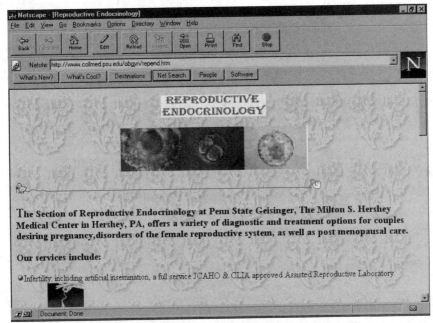

Reproductive Endocrinology. http://www.collmed.psu.edu/obgyn/repend.htm

Reproductive Endocrinology and Infertility

http://www.stanford.edu/dept/GYNOB/rei/

Site is maintained by the Division of Stanford Health Services, which helps those with fertility and reproductive problems, and addresses infertility as related to the endocrine system.

Thyroid Disorders

American Foundation of Thyroid Patients

http://www.thyroidfoundation.org/

This organization was formed by thyroid patients to provide information and support for other patients. Site offers Foundation information and material on thyroid disease symptoms, as well as links. Members receive a quarterly newsletter and free physician referral.

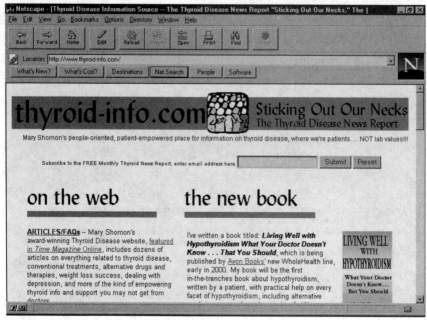

Sticking Out Our Necks. *http://www.thyroid-info.com*

Diagnosing Thyroid Disorders

http://www.hsc.missouri.edu/medicine/thyroid/thyindex.html

Describes the different thyroid disorders and various thyroid function tests. Presents case studies in the form of a "thyroid quiz," and offers links to other thyroid and endocrine sites.

Health Guides on Thyroid Disease

http://home.ican.net/~thyroid/English/Guides.html

The Thyroid Foundation of Canada offers educational guides for patients and the public that provide general information on thyroid disease and on specific manifestations of thyroid disease (Grave's, hypothyroidism, thyroiditis, etc.), thyroid disease in childhood, late in life, or during pregnancy; thyroid surgery and thyroid cancer.

Hyperthyroidism

http://www.thyrolink.com/baskin/ch4.htm

Explains the symptoms and causes.

Hypothyroidism

http://www.endocrineweb.com/hypo1.html

When the body lacks sufficient thyroid hormone, hypothyroidism results. Site describes symptoms, potential dangers, diagnosis and treatment. Links to further thyroid information as well.

Sticking Out Our Necks: The Thyroid Disease News Report

http://www.thyroid-info.com/

Online, biweekly patient-oriented newsletter compiles news from around the world related to thyroid disease causes, treatments, drugs and research, highlights new weblinks of interest, and features stories that focus on living well thyroid disease. Past articles have focused on losing weight, alternative thyroid drugs and natural medicine, dealing with depression, hair loss, support groups and more.

Thyroid Disease

http://thyroid.about.com/mlibrary.htm

Great index of resources on thyroid disease from About.com.

Thyroid Foundation of Canada

http://home.ican.net/~thyroid/Canada.html

Information in French and English for thyroid patients and their families. Includes educational materials, pamphlets, contacts, meetings, lectures and events, as well as links to an international directory of organizations devoted to the thyroid. A quarterly publication entitled "Thyrobulletin Newsletter" is free with membership.

Thyroid Home Page

http://www.thyroid.com/

As well as information specific to the Santa Monica Diagnostic Center, this site offers patient information on thyroid function and anatomy, hypothyroidism and hyperthyroidism. Describes the diseases and their symptoms, treatment, etc. Patient and physician links to articles, books, associations and online services are also provided. "Thyroid fun stuff" includes famous people with thyroid disorders and thyroid jokes.

Thyroid Neck Check

http://www.aace.com/pub/spec/tam99/card99.html

All you need is a glass of water and a mirror to check out your thyroid gland.

ENVIRONMENTAL HEALTH

Children's Health

Children's Environmental Health Network
http://www.cehn.org/cehn/index.html

Provides information and resources to help protect children and fetuses from environmental health hazards.

Children's Health Environmental Coalition
http://www.checnet.org/

Grassroots organization that seeks to protect children from hazards in the environment that may lead to cancer or other illness. Risk assessment, parents' forum, science facts and ways to take action, including how to make your household safer and legislative actions.

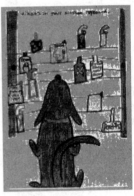

Children's Health Environmental Coalition.
http://www.checnet.org/

Mothers and Others Online
http://www.mothers.org/

Educates consumers about product and lifestyle choices that are safe and ecologically suitable.

Tips to Protect Children from Environmental Threats
http://www.epa.gov/children/tips.htm

Brought to you by the EPA. Simple suggestions about limiting your child's exposure to smoke, lead poisoning, pesticides, sun and radon exposure.

Genetic Engineering

Genetic Engineering and Its Dangers
http://online.sfsu.edu/~rone/gedanger.htm

Essays about genetic engineering, genetically engineered food, biowarfare, and genetically engineered humans.

Genetic Engineering of Crops
http://www.zoo.toronto.edu/zooweb/s199s04/cropge.html

According to this site, crops already tested include corn, barley, broccoli, carrot, chicory, cranberry, eggplant, gladiolus, grape, pea, pepper, raspberry, strawberry, sugarcane, sweet potato, watermelon, wheat and many others.

Hazardous Substances/Toxicology
See also: Emergency Medicine & Critical Care; Public Health.

Agency for Toxic Substances and Disease Registry
http://www.atsdr.cdc.gov/

This Agency provides public health assessments of waste sites, health consultations concerning specific hazardous substances, health surveillance and registries, response to emergency releases of hazardous substances, applied research in support of public health assessments, information development and dissemination, and education and training concerning hazardous substances. The site contains national alerts and public health advisories, the HazDat Database, and information on the assessments described above. Also find ToxFAQ, summaries about hazardous substances, a chart of minimum risk levels (MRLs), a list of the top 20 hazardous substances, glossary, and toxicology profiles. Pages addressing children's health, and pages written especially for children, parents and teachers.

Chem-Tox.Com
http://www.chem-tox.com/

Links to research finding health disorders resulting from exposure to common chemicals and pesticides. Illnesses identified include brain cancer, neuroblastoma, neurological disorders, immune system dysfunction, asthma, allergies, infertility, miscarriage, and child behavior disorders including learning disabilities, mental retardation, hyperactivity and ADD (attention deficit disorder).

ExToxNET: The Extension TOXicology NETwork

http://ace.orst.edu/info/extoxnet/

Provides a variety of information about exposure to toxicants, and environmental chemistry information about pesticides. Includes fact sheets, news, technical information, newsletter, and additional resources. Frequently asked questions have been prepared on a number of topics, such as diet and cancer, food safety issues, household hazardous waste, indoor air pollution, pesticides, safe drinking water, and soil (gardening and chemicals).

Federal Laws, Regulations & Policies

http://www.iet.msu.edu/regchrt/regchrt.htm

Explains the laws that govern hazardous chemicals in language the lay public can understand.

Hazardous Substances and Public Health

http://www.atsdr.cdc.gov/HEC/hsphhome.html

Quarterly newsletter published by the Agency for Toxic Substances and Disease Registry.

HazDat: Hazardous Substance Release/ Health Effects Database

http://www.atsdr.cdc.gov/hazdat.html

Provides information on hazardous substances released on from Superfund sites or due to emergency events. Maintained by the Agency for Toxic Substances and Disease Registry (ATSDR). The database includes site characteristics, contaminants found, contaminant media and maximum concentration levels, impact on population, community health concerns, ATSDR recommendations, exposure routes, physical hazards at the site/event, and other data.

Natural Hazards Center

http://www.Colorado.EDU/hazards/

The Center is a clearinghouse for information on natural hazards and human adjustments to hazards and disasters. It produces periodicals and publications, provides lists and indices of disaster information, and provides a library database on hazardous substances.

Pesticide Information Profiles

http://ace.ace.orst.edu/info/extoxnet/pips/ghindex.html

Provides information on the health and environmental effects of pesticides. Information included: trade and other names, regulatory status, chemical class, description, formulation, toxicological effects, ecological effects, environmental fate, physical properties, exposure guidelines and manufacturer.

Multiple Chemical Sensitivity

Environmental Illness Links

http://www-hsl.mcmaster.ca/tomflem/envir.html

Long list from the Health Care Information Resources.

Multiple Chemical Sensitivity

http://www.supernet.net/~jackibar/mcs.html

Suggestions on living a non-toxic lifestyle.

Multiple Chemical Sensitivity

http://www.seanet.com/~tzhre/mcs.htm

Links to related sites.

Resources for the Chemically Sensitive or Environmentally Ill

http://www.snowcrest.net/lassen/ mcsei.html

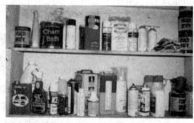

Multiple Chemical Sensitivity.
http://www.seanet.com/~tzhre/mcs.htm

Directory for individuals wishing to avoid excessive use of synthetic and chemical products. Includes organizations, magazines, newsgroups and services.

Understanding Multiple Chemical Sensitivity

http://mentalhelp.net/archives/editor7.htm

Editorial that questions direct linkage of chemicals with physical symptoms, and suggests that the problems may require some mental scrutiny, as well.

Organizations

American Environmental Health Foundation

http://www.aehf.com/

AEHF is a nonprofit organization that seeks to further the practice of environmental medicine. Site offers educational materials on air quality, food contaminants and more, as well as a product catalog.

Environmental Health Project

http://www.crosslink.net/~ehp/

EHP assists development organizations to address environment related health problems. It focuses on the prevention of acute respiratory infections, diarrheal diseases, and malaria; and it provides technical assistance in the areas of water supply, sanitation, wastewater, solid waste, and air pollution. Sponsored by the U.S. Agency for International Development, its projects are world-wide.

National Center for Environmental Health

http://www.cdc.gov/nceh/ncehhome.htm

Information on the Center, its programs and publications. Includes fact sheets and online brochures. The organization seeks to apply research, educate, recommend standards, and train state and local health agencies.

U.S. Environmental Protection Agency

http://www.epa.gov/

This EPA's mission is "to protect human health and to safeguard the natural environment." This site describes the many EPA programs and Agency operation, provides access to environmental news, laws and regulations, databases on environmental facts and publications; and to other information relevant to the scientific community business and industry. In addition, there are pages for teachers, students, kids and concerned citizens.

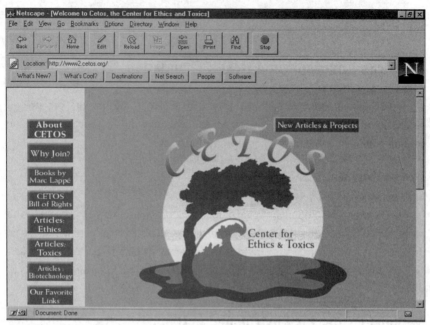

Center for Ethics and Toxics. http://www2.cetos.org/

Public Environmental Education

Center for Ethics and Toxics
http://www2.cetos.org/

This nonprofit, environmental organization is committed to preventing unconsenting exposure to hazardous chemicals, devices, or drugs and to formulating toxic substance policies based on sound ethical analysis. It seeks to do this with research, public education, and watchdog efforts. Site provides articles on ethics, biotechnology, and toxics, pesticide reports, and material describing the Center's philosophy.

Emergency Response Notification Center of the EPA
http://www.epa.gov/ERNS/

Find out the details about the top 10 oil and hazardous substance spills this past month, past year, and overall. Database, fact sheets, headlines.

Envirofacts

http://www.epa.gov/enviro/index_lojs.html

Access the Environmental Protection Agency databases on air, chemicals, hazardous waste, risk management, Superfund, toxic release, drinking water and more from this site.

Environmental Health and Safety Resources

http://www.uwm.edu:80/People/rjg/ehslinks/ehslinks.html

Set of links on environmental-occupational health, safety, and risk management topics gathered by the University of Wisconsin-Milwaukee.

Environmental Health Clearinghouse

http://www.infoventures.com/e-hlth/answers.html

Questions and answers about problems related to environmental exposure. Major subjects are home, air, water, food, disease and radiation.

Environmental Health Patient Education

http://www.vtmednet.org/diner/env.htm

Information on mercury, lead, radon, pesticides, air quality and other contaminants, for the general public.

Health and Fitness: Environmental Health

http://www.fanafana.com/Consumers/Health-and-Fitness/Environmental-Health/

Links to articles and sites discussing the health risks of air pollution, lead poisoning, radiation exposure and other issues.

Institute for Environmental Toxicology

http://www.iet.msu.edu/

Promotes public awareness of environmental issues. Includes newsletter and documents about environmental toxicology and specific chemicals.

National Environmental Protection Publications

http://www.epa.gov/ncepihom/nepishom/

Full-text access to over 7,000 EPA documents.

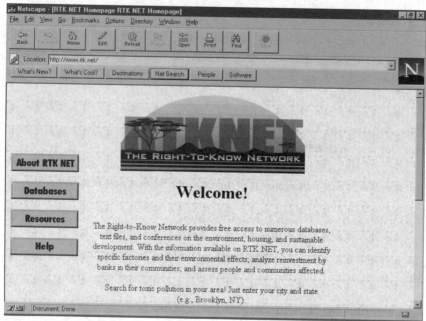

The Right-to-Know Network. *http://www.rtk.net/*

National Institute of Environmental Health Sciences
http://www.niehs.nih.gov/

Research on environment-related diseases, as well as press releases, journal links, information clearinghouse, and background on scientific programs. Community outreach efforts and kids' pages are also offered.

Nelson Institute on Environmental Medicine
http://charlotte.med.nyu.edu/

Center for research on the health effects of environmental pollution. Part of the New York University School of Medicine. Site describes the facility and staff, as well as the community outreach, research and training programs it supports.

Right-To-Know Network (RTK Net)
http://www.rtk.net/

Free access to government databases relating to environment, housing and sustainable development issues. You can use this resource to "identify specific factories and their environmental effects; analyze reinvestment by banks in their communities; and assess people and communities affected." Input your city name, and you can learn of toxic polluters in your neighborhood.

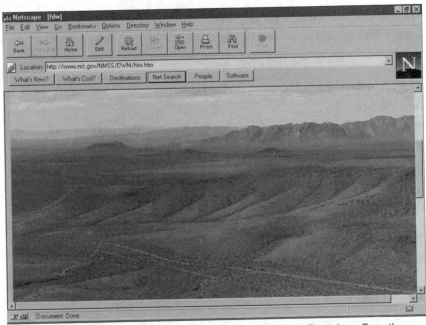

Yucca Mountain, NV, proposed site of High Level Nuclear Waste Repository. From the
U.S. Nuclear Regulatory Commission Website. *http://www.nrc.gov/NMSS/DWM/hlw.htm*

Radiation

Ask a CHP
http://www.iem-inc.com/askset.html
Ask a certified health physicist (CHP) questions you have on radiation and radioactivity, or learn about radioactivity basics.

History of Radiation Protection
http://www.sph.umich.edu/group/eih/UMSCHPS/hist.htm
Essays and other items addressing the history of radiation protection, radiation and health physics.

Radiation and Health Physics Home Page
http://www.umich.edu/~radinfo/
Written for the general public, students and the health physics community. Provides a great introduction to radiation, as well as professional and educational resources, organizations, research and "hot topics."

Radiation Information Network
http://www.physics.isu.edu/radinf/index.html

Links to sites about radiation and radiation safety.

U.S. Nuclear Regulatory Commission
http://www.nrc.gov/

News and information on nuclear reactors, nuclear materials, radioactive waste, radiation protection and emergency response. Also offers a reference library.

Radon

EPA's Position on Radon
http://www.epa.gov/iaq/radon/

Radon is a known lung carcinogen. Site shows you how to test the levels of radon in your house, and how to reduce your risk of exposure.

Understanding Radon
http://www.discoverit.com/at/phi/article.html

This inert radioactive gas is considered to be a serious health problem. Article written for the general public describes the risk and what you can do about it.

EYES / OPTOMETRY & OPHTHALMOLOGY

Anatomy

Anatomy
http://www.eyenet.org/public/anatomy/anatomy.html
> Identifies basic parts of the eye.

Anatomy, Physiology & Pathology of the Human Eye
http://users.aol.com/mont714/tutorial/the_eye/framxmpl.html
> Great tutorial and overview of the eye.

Anton's Ophthalmic Scrap Book
http://www.geocities.com/Eureka/Park/2021/index.html
> Eye drawings and photographs.

Cow's Eye Dissection
http://netra.exploratorium.edu/learning_studio/cow_eye/
> Good method for kids and students to learn about the anatomy of the eye.

Eye Websites
http://members.tripod.com/auyeung/color/eye.htm
> Links to many sites that discuss the eye and how it functions.

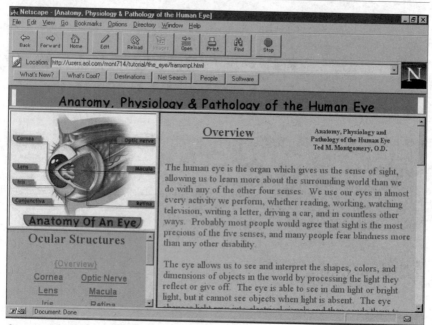

Anatomy, Physiology& Pathology of the Human Eye. http://users.aol.com/mont714/
tutorial/the_eye/framxmpl.html

Cataracts

See also: Surgery - Cataract Surgery.

American Society of Cataract and Refractive Surgery

http://www.ascrs.org/

This is the homepage for member ophthalmologists specializing in cataract and refractive surgery. It offers Society news as well as eye care information, *Eye World Magazine Online*, legislative and government updates, and a marketplace section which provides information on industry news, stocks, and a listing of eye care vendors. Links to other professional societies.

Cataract Fact Sheet

http://www.eri.harvard.edu/Documentation/cataracts.html

What is a cataract, and what happens during cataract surgery?

Cataract Information for Patients

http://www.nei.nih.gov/publications/cataracts.htm

Online pamphlet from the National Eye Institute.

Cataracts

http://bewell.com/hic/cataracts/

Basic information and answers to common questions about cataracts.

Clinical Trials

See also: Clinical Trials chapter.

Clinical Trials

http://www.nei.nih.gov/neitrials/index.htm

Database of clinical trials supported by the National Eye Institute.Tells how doctors may participate in a trial and how to refer a patient to a trial.

Conjunctivitis

Conjunctivitis

http://kidshealth.org/parent/common/conjunctivitis.html

Pink eye (conjunctivitis)s a very contagious infection inside the eyelid. This site provides basic information for parents. Description, prevention, incubation, duration, and when to call in a professional.

Conjunctivitis (Pink Eye) Patient Information

http://lib-sh.lsumc.edu/fammed/pted/pinkeye.html

Brief description of signs, symptoms and treatment.

Medical Self-Care: Conjunctivitis

http://www.healthy.net/library/books/healthyself/pinkeye.htm

Self-care tips and flow-chart of questions to ask.

Contact Lenses & Glasses

20/20 Magazine

http://www.2020mag.com/default.htm

Attractive optical industry magazine covers the newest technology, fashion, and latest trends in product innovations.

Contact Lens Council Questions and Answers
http://www.iglobal.com/CLC/clc-02.htm

Explains the different types of contact lenses, care and maintenance, and general wear. Contact lens history, statistics, and a small glossary of terms are also provided.

Glasses
http://www.beakman.com/glasses/eyeglasses.html

Describes how eyeglasses work to correct vision.

Lens Options
http://sola.com/consumer/lenses/index.html

Describes different kinds of glasses, lens materials, and other options.

Corneal Transplant

Corneal Transplant: Overview
http://www.adam.com/ency/article/003008.htm

Very basic information.

Corneal Transplant
http://www.nova-vista.com/cts/ctsintro.htm

Introduction, history, donor tissue, indications for surgery, preparing for surgery, surgery, post-surgery, risks and frequent questions.

Eye Banks
http://dir.yahoo.com/Health/Medicine/Ophthalmology/Eye_Banks/

Links to eye banks around the United States.

Dry Eye Syndrome

Dry Eye Syndrome
http://www.ccberry.com/eyes/dryeye.htm

One out of five Americans suffers from this condition, which is due to poor quality or insufficient tear production. Links, and good information for patients.

Eye Care and Eye Disorders

Eye Care FAQS

http://www.eyenet.org/public/faqs/faqs.html

Frequently asked questions and answers covering eye conditions of the elderly, eye conditions of the young, and other eye care issues.

Eye Care: Related Links

http://www.nerdworld.com/nw1041.html

Nerd World Media's long list of sites related to eye care, including acupressure, contact lenses, eye strain, questions and answers about glaucoma, eye diseases, eye surgery and eye-robics. Includes links with descriptions.

Eye Information

http://www.noah.cuny.edu/eye/eye.html

Many links. Information on common eye health topics, anatomy, function, diseases and eye care. Good starting place.

Eye Page

http://haas.berkeley.edu/~dowis/eye/eye.html

Forum for professionals to discuss issues relating to the eye care industry with each other, as well as a tool to to enable communication between eye professionals and the public on eye care and treatment.

Eyenet

http://www.eyenet.org/

Information from the American Academy of Ophthalmology. Includes member information, online education center, find an ophthalmologist, patient information, products and publications.

EyeWorks

http://www.cvworld.com/forsight/eyeworks/index

Explains how the eye works, what to expect from your vision as you age, what it means to have 20/20 vision, tips for healthy eyes, and information on common eye conditions, from astigmatism to styes.

National Eye Institute
http://www.nei.nih.gov/

Information for researchers, health care professionals, the general public and patients, educators and the media on the research and activities being carried out or supported by the NEI. Includes publication list of brochures for patients, fact sheets, and other resources.

National Eye Research Foundation Public Information
http://www.nerf.org/okdr.html

Includes information on orthokeratology, a non-surgical method of reshaping of the cornea and correcting vision.

Glaucoma

Glaucoma FAQ
http://www.iglou.com/KEC_eyedocs/glaucoma.htm

What glaucoma is, what causes it, types of glaucoma and symptoms, detection and treatment. Links to related sites are provided.

Glaucoma Mailing List
http://www.geocities.com/HotSprings/Resort/3929/index.html

Eye care links, frequently asked questions, personal stories from glaucoma patients, and information on joining the glaucoma mailing list.

The Glaucoma Network
http://www.glaucoma.net/

Offers glaucoma questions and answers, medications and side effects, and patient compliance, as well as information on the services of the Glaucoma Associates of New York.

Consumers Guide to Glaucoma
http://www.eyecare.org/consumer/disease/gl.html

Basic information on glaucoma, the third leading cause of blindness in the United States.

The Glaucoma Foundation

http://www.glaucoma-foundation.org/info/

Dedicated to public education and research. Site includes information about glaucoma, patient's guide, doctor's corner, mailing list, newsroom and *Eye to Eye*, a quarterly newsletter.

Glaucoma Research Foundation

http://www.glaucoma.org/

Information on glaucoma, the Foundation and its activities. Features selected articles from eye care journals that are summarized in layperson's language, as well as a glaucoma discussion group.

Macular Degeneration

Age-Related Macular Degeneration

http://www.nei.nih.gov/publications/armd-p.htm

Information for patients from the National Eye Institute. Large typeface.

American Macular Degeneration Foundation

http://www.macular.org/

As yet, there is no cure for macular degeneration, the leading cause of blindness for those age 55 and over. Information on this disease, help and advice, newsletter, bulletin board and a state-by-state directory of eye care facilities can be found at this site.

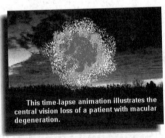

This time-lapse animation illustrates the central vision loss of a patient with macular degeneration.

From: The American Macular Degeneration Foundation.
http://www.macular.org/

Macular Degeneration

http://209.64.11.10/Disease%20Center/diseases/amd.asp

Article from the Health Connection describes this disease and its prevalence.

Optical Illusions and Perception

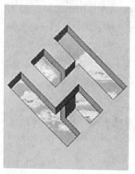

Al Seckel's Home Page
of Perception, Illusions...
http://www.klab.caltech.edu/
~seckel/index.html

Al Seckel's Home Page of Perception, Illusions, and Their Neuronal Correlates

http://www.klab.caltech.edu/~seckel/index.html

This site claims to house hundreds of illusions. There are different levels of explanation, from easily-understood to rigorous proofs.

B-Eye

http://cvs.anu.edu.au/andy/beye/beyehome.html

See the world through the eyes of a honeybee.

Optical Illusions

http://www.sciencecentre.sk.ca/science/optical.htm

Great site for children to view basic optical illusions.

The Joy of Visual Perception: A Web Book

http://www.yorku.ca/eye/

Interesting and you can learn a lot. Table of contents includes optical illusions, color, distance perception, motion perception and much more. Lots of links.

Organizations

The American Optometric Association

http://www.aoanet.org/

Information for consumers from this association of more than 32,000 eye care professionals. Includes common vision conditions, eye diseases, children's vision, contact lenses, sports, eye care tips, first aid and corneal modifications. Media center includes press releases and news briefs.

Eye Vision Organizations

http://bioport.com/organize/eyes.htm

Links to U.S. and Canada organizations.

The Low Vision Research Group

http://vision.psych.umn.edu/www/lovnet/lovnet.html

This organization's purpose is to foster communication among those who investigate low vision, and to advance research in that field. The site provides information on new research, frequently asked questions, support and discussion groups and other resources of interest to the low vision community.

Vision Council of America

http://www.visionsite.org/

Dedicated to teaching consumers about quality eye care and eyewear, the Vision Council offers consumers articles and hints on eye care. "Frame Game" is a interactive method of checking out what frames will look good on you, based on your face shape.

Refractive Surgery

I Know Why Refractive Surgeons Wear Glasses

http://members.aol.com/eyeknowwhy/index.htm

This site challenges some of the claims of refractive surgery, and contains links to many eye and vision care sites.

International Society of Refractive Surgery

http://www.isrs.com/

Patient information, how to locate a doctor, and members-only areas.

Laser Eye Surgery: The Refractive Surgery Patient Information Center

http://www.eyeinfo.com/

General information on what refractive surgery is, how to choose a surgeon, different kinds of surgical treatments, anatomy and optics, complications, and "random thoughts." Bulletin board and links to other refractive surgery sites are also offered.

NoGlasses.com: Laser Vision Correction
http://www.noglasses.com/

Laser vision correction can fix nearsightedness, farsightedness, and astigmatism. Description of procedures, who qualifies, side effects, and more.

Radial Keratotomy Homepage
http://www-or.stanford.edu/~mob/RK/

Presents answers to frequently asked questions, and less frequently asked questions. Personal experiences are also expressed. Links to surgeons and surgery centers, as well a to other RK websites.

The Vision Correction Website
http://www.lasersite.com/index.htm

Anatomy of the eye, information about PRK (Photorefractive Keratectomy) and LASIK ("LAser in SItu Keratomileusis") laser surgeries, as well as about radial keratotomy.

Retinitis Pigmentosa

A Guide to Retinitis Pigmentosa
http://www.brps.demon.co.uk/Graphics/G_Guide.html

Describes living with retinitis pigmentosa, a hereditary degeneration of the retina which can lead to night blindness and gradual vision degradation. Also includes medical aspects of this disease.

Retinal Implant Project
http://rleweb.mit.edu/retina/

This site describes the goal and theory behind a research project which seeks to develop a silicon-chip eye implant that can restore vision for patients suffering from retinitis pigmentosa and macular degeneration.

John Wenberg's Retinitis Pigmentosa Page
http://www.jwen.com/rp/rp.html

RP links, articles, mailing lists, research and more.

Vision Tests

Colour Vision Test

http://www.umist.ac.uk/UMIST_OVS/UES/
COLOUR0.HTM

Includes test and explanation of different types of color-blindness.

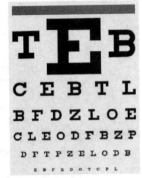

Macular Degeneration Eye Test

http://www.eyesight.org/eyetest2.html

Simple test for this disease.

Test Your Vision

http://www.2eyeballs.com/eyetest/eyetest.html

This site also provides general eye information.

Test Your Vision.
*http://www.2eyeballs.com/
eyetest/eyetest.html*

Vision Test

http://www.smbs.buffalo.edu/oph/ped/disclaim.htm

Online vision acuity test.

FAMILY MEDICINE

Clinical Resources

Clinical Practice Guidelines
http://text.nlm.nih.gov/ftrs/pick?collect=ahcpr&dbName=0&cc=1&t= R934300997

The National Institutes of Health Agency for Health Care Policy and Research offers 19 different downloadable clinical practice guidelines on various health issues (e.g., acute care, Alzheimer's disease, smoking). The site also includes access to reference guides for clinicians, and consumers' guides, in both English and Spanish.

Diagnostic Procedures Handbook
http://www.healthgate.com/dph/html/index.shtml

Enter the name of the procedure or browse through alphabetical list to find synonyms, where it is used, procedures it commonly includes, indications, contraindications, patient preparation, aftercare, special instructions, complications, equipment, technique, data acquired, normal findings, limitations, and references.

Intern-in-the-Middle-of-the-Night
http://lib-sh.lsumc.edu/fammed/intern/intern.html

Created to keep interns company during their long nights on call, this site is "a hypertext collection of short 'how to' handouts that are ideal to put into a 'peripheral brain.'" Topics in cardiology to urology, as well as general medicine.

MD Consult

http://www.mdconsult.com/

"The ultimate clinical library" for physicians. It includes access to articles from 48 journals, 35 reference books, over 600 clinical practice guidelines, patient education handouts, drug information and updates, CME programs, and other tools for physicians. It all works together in one continuously updated tool designed to help you answer clinical questions and stay current in medicine. Fee, but 10-day free trial period to test it out.

National Guideline Clearinghouse

http://www.guidelines.gov/index.asp

This public resource provides a comprehensive database of evidence-based clinical practice guidelines and related documents produced by the Agency for Health Care Policy and Research (AHCPR), in partnership with the American Medical Association (AMA) and the American Association of Health Plan (AAHP). Search by key word, or browse through disease/condition, treatment/intervention, or organization.

Physical Exam Study Guides

http://www.medinfo.ufl.edu/year1/bcs/clist/

Vital signs and system exam check lists.

University of Iowa Family Practice Handbook

http://www.vh.org/Providers/ClinRef/FPHandbook/FPContents.html

Electronic clinical reference source that places an emphasis on the diagnosis and treatment of common medical illnesses. Chapters study different medical specialties, with a special section on AIDS.

Discussion Groups

Internet Resources for Family Doctors: Mailing Lists

http://www.ncl.ac.uk/~nphcare/WONCA/resource/othlist

Describes many mail lists family physicians are invited to join.

STFM Online

http://www.stfm.org/listserv/lists.html

List of e-mail discussion groups dealing with family medicine.

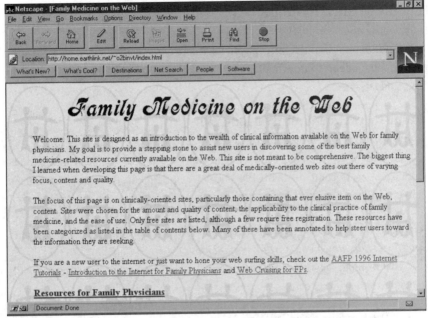

Family Medicine on the Web. *http://home.earthlink.net/~o2binvt/index.htm*

Links

A Family Physician's Web Starter
http://dragon.labmed.umn.edu/~john/bookmark.html
> Includes clinical links and non-clinical links collected by one family physician.

Family Medicine at About.com
http://familymedicine.miningco.com/
> About.com provides a great set of links and features topic-specific articles and sites. Chat groups, forums and marketplace.

Family Medicine on the Web
http://home.earthlink.net/~o2binvt/index.html
> Resources for family physicians. Includes clinical resources, lists and directories, professional journals, professional societies, patient education, and government health agencies.

Family Medicine Online
http://www.aafp.org/family/

Information about family physicians and the medical specialty of family practice. Includes resources for health care professionals and policymakers, patients and students.

Family Practice, Family Medicine
http://www.uib.no/isf/guide/family.htm

List of links from the Primary Care Internet Guide. Includes newsgroups, organizations, documents, textbooks and continuing medical education resources, university departments and residency programs, from all around the world.

Hardin MD Family Medicine & Primary Care
http://www.lib.uiowa.edu/hardin/md/fam.html

List of links to large and medium-length sites that list sites relating to family medicine and primary care.

Internet for the Family Physician
http://users.eponet.it/glacchia/familymd.htm

Links to primary care resources, online journals, drug resources, literature search, organizations, continuing medical education, patient education, guidelines, and more.

Links of Interest in Family Medicine
http://www.museum.state.il.us/isas/health/fammed.html

Links to societies and associations, journals and more.

MedicineNet
http://www.medicinenet.com/Script/Main/hp.asp

"Doctor-produced" medical information. Covers diseases, procedures, treatments, first aid, medical dictionary and more.

MedWebPlus Family Practice
http://www.medwebplus.com/subject/Family_Practice.html

Over 125 categorized links to sites on the Internet.

Sites of Interest to Family Physicians
http://www.uwo.ca/fammed/clfm/sites.html

From the Canadian Library of Family Medicine, this site provides organizations, clinical information, medical education, continuing education, journals, guidelines and other Internet resources for family practitioners.

VOLC-R Family Medicine Related Internet Sources
http://griffin.vcu.edu/~dimlist/

Links to medical and primary care resources for patients and health care professionals. Includes continuing medical education, journals, medical informatics, specialty medicine, drug information, educational sites, governmnet sites, sites of interest to physicians, medical students and residents, mail lists, managed care resources, and more.

Organizations

American Academy of Family Physicians
http://www.aafp.org/

This professional organization serves more than 88,000 family physicians, family practice residents, and medical students in the United States. Site offers a great deal of information for members and patients alike. Includes continuing medical education, practice management, socioeconomic concerns, career opportunities, statistics, publications and more.

American Board of Family Practice
http://www.abfp.org/

Certifies and recertifies family practice doctors to assure consumers that they have completed and maintained the necessary training/experience to provide quality care to the individual and the family. Site describes the certification process, provides future exam dates, review courses, and more.

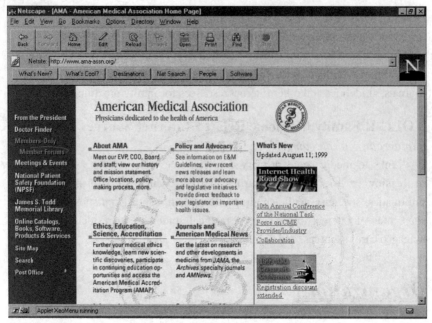

American Medical Association Home Page. http://www.ama-assn.org/

The American Medical Association

http://www.ama-assn.org/

The AMA represents physician interests in improving health care and medical education. The homepage describes the organization, and provides access to JAMA, the journal of the American Medical Association, as well as to other AMA publications and services. The AMA offers medical education advancement programs, advances policy and advocacy efforts of behalf of its members, and presents consumer health information as well as membership privileges.

Health on the Net Foundation

http://www.hon.ch/

HON's mission is to help individuals, medical professionals and health care providers to realize the potential benefits of the Internet. This site offers individuals suffering from a specific illness or disability access to relevant information and links to support communities. HON features a full listing of health information and support community sources, together with testimonials.

World Organisation of Family Doctors

http://www.wonca.org/

Information on the activities of WONCA, an international organization whose mission is to foster high standards of care in family medicine. It does this by providing support, a forum for the exchange of ideas, a newsletter and publications; and by representing WONCA members and interacting with organizations around the world.

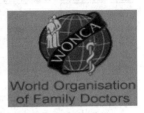

http://www.wonca.org

Patient Education/Fact Sheets

Annotated List of Patient Educational Materials

http://www.vh.org/Patients/PatientsAnnotatedList.html

From anesthesia to surgery, a great deal of information for patients.

CareSheets

http://www.infolane.com/pamp/

New patient education sheets every month. Order form available at website.

Patient Education

http://www.vtmednet.org/diner/home.htm

Covers topics such as alcohol abuse, allergies, asthma, cancer, cardiovascular health, diabetes and much more.

Patient Education Menu

http://lib-sh.lsumc.edu:80/fammed/pted/pted.html

Health problems, health maintenance, and information on drugs.

Professional Resources

Doctor's Guide to the Internet (Professional Edition)
http://www.pslgroup.com/docguide.htm
According to its mission statement, the purpose of this site is to save doctors "countless hours of fruitless browsing while providing them with a comfortable and friendly environment from which to derive the most value from the Internet." It includes patient information and resources, medical news and alerts, new drugs, medical conferences, and financial, business, travel and leisure sections.

InfoMedical.Com Medical Resource Directory and Search Engine
http://www.infomedical.com/nindex.htm
Search engine for the medical business. Categories include: company types, manufacturers, distributors, products, organizations and services.

Physician's Guide to the Internet
http://www.webcom.com/pgi/
Physician lifestyle section, clinical practice, postgraduate education, "funstuff" and medical news and links.

Rural Family Medicine
http://www.ruralfamilymedicine.org/
Resources for rural physicians and educators. Provides information about rural America, rural health issues, health resources and clinical topics dealing with agromedicine.

Publications

American Family Physician
http://www.aafp.org/afp/
Offical journal for the American Academy of Family Physicians.

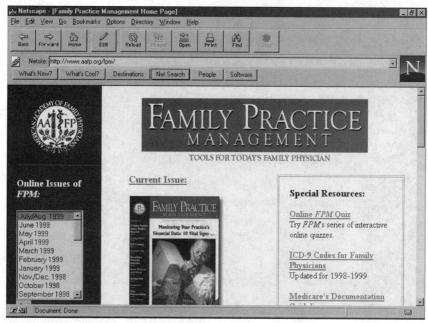

Family Practice Management. http://www.aafp.org/fpm/

Family Practice Management

http://www.aafp.org/fpm/

Article from the monthly issue, archives and tools for family practitioners are provided. This journal seeks to advance the goals of family practitioners in today's health care environment, i.e., functioning in a world where managed care and other pressures may make it hard to stay in control of one's career and one's desire to serve.

Health Gazette

http://www.freenet.scri.fsu.edu/HealthGazette/gazette.html

New articles on family health topics appear quarterly, or look at previous editions. The treatment of acne, domestic violence, St. John's wort, and melatonin were some subjects covered in earlier gazettes. Written by a family physician.

The Journal of Family Practice

http://www.jfampract.com/

Research, clinical reviews, and commentary for family practice physicians.

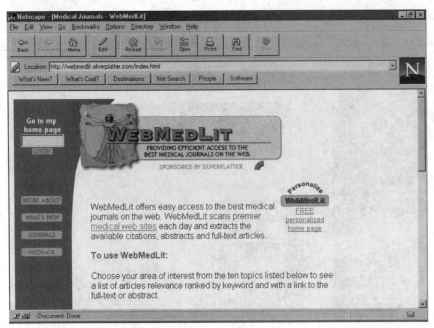

WebMedLit. http://webmedlit.silverplatter.com/index.html

Internet Medical Journal

http://www.medjournal.com/

Online journal of family practice and general medicine.

WebMedLit

http://webmedlit.silverplatter.com/index.html

This tool scans over a dozen premier medical journal's websites each day and extracts the available citations, abstracts and full-text articles. Choose from among ten major areas of interest, or create your own search criteria.

FITNESS

Aerobics & Jazzercise

Aerobic Activities
http://www.fitnesslink.com/exercise/aerobic.htm

Ten different exercises that can provide an effective aerobic workout, with links to Internet sites.

Aerobics and Fitness Association of America Telefitness Center
http://www.afaa.com/

The Aerobics and Fitness Association of America certifies aerobics instructors, personal trainers, step instructors, weight training instructors, and kickboxing instructors. Site offers member benefits, education opportunities, *American Fitness Magazine*, and feature health articles.

Bonnie's Jazzercise Page
http://users.ccnet.com/~bonnie/

Answers common questions about jazzercise, tips for starting, and links.

Jazzercise
http://www.jazzercise.com/

Includes jazzercise news and articles, as well as specifics about the jazzercise industry and how to become an instructor.

Lisa's Jazzercise Mega-Site
http://www.physical.com/

Meet and chat with other jazzercise fans, learn new music to try, search for a class near you, read fitness facts, and link to other sites.

Rebel Ropers
http://freestyle-jumproping.com/
Free-style jump-roping as a fun cardiovascular exercise. Includes explanation, tips and promotional material. Links.

Tae-Bo
http://www.bodytrends.com/taeanim.htm
Information on this new, trendy fitness workout.

Turnstep.com
http://www.turnstep.com
Browse through frequently asked questions about aerobics, the aerobics dictionary, and adaptive aerobics. Includes access to over 5,000 aerobics patterns submitted from people all over the world, and links to aerobics music.

What Is Aerobic Exercise and Why Should I Do It?
http://k2.kirtland.cc.mi.us/~balbachl/aeroprin.htm
Definition of aerobic exercise and a description of some of its benefits.

Bicycling

Bicycle Discussion Lists on Internet
http://eksl-www.cs.umass.edu/~westy/cycling/cycling-on-internet.html
Includes sections of mailing lists and section of Usenet newsgroups.

Bicycles FAQ
http://www.cis.ohio-state.edu/hypertext/faq/usenet/bicycles-faq/top.html
Answers to frequently asked questions, primarily about mountain biking.

Bicycling
http://bicycling.about.com/
Net links with description, feature stories, live chat and bicycling newsletter.

BICYCLING Magazine
http://www.bicyclingmagazine.com/
The world's largest cycling publication. Includes chat rooms, bike-finder, training center, message boards, repairs and riding techniques.

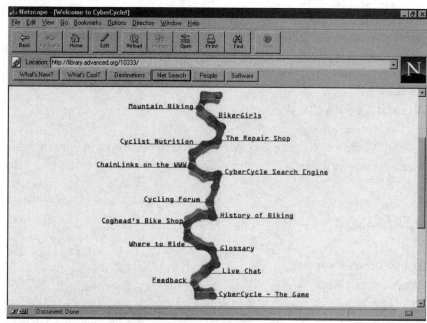

CyberCycle. http://library.advanced.org/10333/

Bike Culture Encycleopedia and Bycycle
http://bikeculture.com/home/

    These publications for bike afficianodos are available online.

Cyber Cyclery
http://cycling.org/

    Hundreds of electronic mail lists, links to over 3000 related sites, cyber mart, forums, cycling world happenings and bike groups.

CyberCycle
http://library.advanced.org/10333/

    Lots of information on biking for pleasure or sport. Includes cyclist nutrition, glossary, and a history of biking, as well as bicycle repair, advice on where to ride, web links and chat room.

Roger Marquis' Cycling Page
http://www.roble.com/marquis/

    Tips about bike racing, as well as noteworthy coaching and cycling links.

Trento Bike Pages

http://www-math.science.unitn.it/Bike/

These pages contain information on and images of mountain biking in Europe and the Mediterranean.

WOMBATS on the Web

http://www.wombats.org/

The WOmen's Mountain Bike And Tea Society, a network of women "who share a passion for pedaling in the dirt."

Exercise

About.com: Exercise

http://exercise.about.com/

A huge number of links to sites on different kinds of exercising, exercising for beginners, exercising at work, pregnancy and exercising, and much more. "Spotlight" features exercise articles.

American Council of Exercise Online

http://www.acefitness.org/

Fact sheets on nutrition and exercise, hotline and online publication.

Cybercise

http://www.cybercise.com/

Includes the cybercise forum on fitness-related issues; cybercise sound room (with music to exercise by); fitness supplies and fitness events around the world. Nutrition information provided as well.

Exercise Demonstrations

http://exercise.about.com/blexercisedemos.htm?pid=2756&cob=home

Click on a muscle group and view a video clip demonstration and written instructions for exercises that target that area.

Fitness Fundamentals
http://www.hoptechno.com/book11.htm

Online pamphlet provides you with the basic information you need to begin and maintain a personal physical fitness program. The guidelines are intended for the average healthy adult and tell you what your fitness goals should be, as well as how often, how long and how hard you must exercise to achieve them.

Perpetual Motion World Wide Web Sites
http://www.teleport.com/~pmotion/

News, commentary, and links to other fitness-related sites; archive and subscription information on "Don't Stop Moving," their newsletter.

Stretching and Flexibility
http://www.cs.huji.ac.il/papers/rma/stretching_toc.html

The subtitle to this site is "everything you never wanted to know," but it is valuable information. Discusses types of stretching and how to stretch. The document is viewable in pieces online, or you can download it in full as a *.pdf or zipped postscript file.

Fitness Links & Tips

Elaine's Physical Fitness and Health Links
http://www.elainecase.com/ecfit.html

Long list of alphabetized links to fitness and health sites on the Internet.

Fitness
http://segment.ucsf.edu/brent/fitness/fitness.htm

Links to fitness, weight lifting and body building sites.

Fitness Files
http://rcc.webpoint.com/fitness/index.htm

Fitness fundamentals, how to start a fitness program and find an activity that is right for you, how to avoid injuries, and practice first aid and proper eating habits.

get active!

FitnessFiles.
http://rcc.webpoint.
com/fitness/index.htm

Fitness Jumpsite
http://primusweb.com/fitnesspartner/
Site contains advice about fitness, exercise, dieting and health. Articles are straightforward and positive, and suggestions are realistic and encouraging. Links.

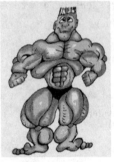

FitnessLink
http://www.fitnesslink.com/
Offers articles and tips on fitness; lists books, magazines, newsgroups, mailing lists and related Internet links. Fitness news is updated daily.

Fitness Matters
http://lifematters.com/fitnesn.html
Fitness, nutrition and weight management. Includes book reviews, news and feature articles.

FitnessLink. http://www.fitnesslink.com/

Fitness Online
http://www.fitnessonline.com/index.asp
Information, tools, news and products for consumers interested in achieving their fitness goals, be it weight loss, muscle gain, increased energy or good health.

Health and Fitness World Guide Forum
http://www.worldguide.com/Fitness/hf.html
Subjects covered here include anatomy, strength training, cardiovascular exercise, eating well, and sports medicine.

Internet's Fitness Resource
http://www.netsweat.com/
Information on exercise and fitness. Lots of links.

New Balance Cyberpark
http://newbalance.com/
This beautiful site focuses on running, walking, health and fitness.

Shape Up America
http://shapeup.org/
Provides information on safe weight management and physical fitness. Determine your body-mass index, develop a meal plan suitable for your health, take a health and fitness quiz and download information. Pages for fitness professionals.

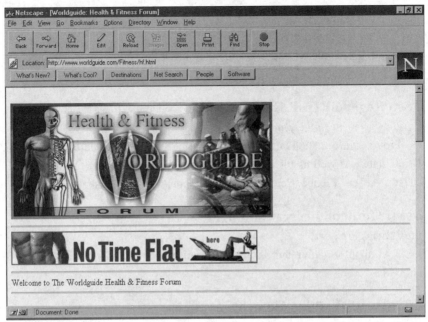

Health and Fitness World Guide Forum. *http://www.worldguide.com/Fitness/hf.html*

Stepping Stones: Practical Tools for Achieving Your Goals

http://www.flpinstitute.com/steppingstones/

Monthly newsletter providing advice and support on how to change your lifestyle to reach your fitness, health and emotional goals.

World Fitness

http://www.worldfitness.org/

Advice, commentary and information on getting fit. Includes ask the expert, and information for instructors and personal trainers.

Hiking & Walking

DayHiker

http://www.dayhiker.com/

Extreme day hike information. FYI, extreme day hikes are defined as "day hikes which are rigorous, exciting, unique, with interesting sights and terrain." Includes hiking tips and a hike directory.

Dirty Sole Society
http://www.barefooters.org/

A site for people who love going barefoot all the time, or who are barefoot hikers, dancers, etc.

Gorp Regional Trail Guides
http://www.gorp.com/gorp/activity/hiking/hik_guid.htm

Provides information on hiking trails, hiking stories and resources for each of the 50 states, as well as for Europe, Australia, the South Pacific, New Zealand, Canada, Africa, Mexico, Central America, South America, and the Caribbean.

Great Outdoor Recreation Pages
http://www.gorp.com/

Lots of information and discussion about outdoor activities and wilderness attractions.

Hiking and Walking Homepage
http://www.teleport.com/~walking/hiking.html

Offers information on hiking and walking clubs, places to go hiking, appropriate gear, philosophy and trail guides.

National Historic Trails
http://www.gorp.com/gorp/resource/us_trail/historic.htm

Descriptions of famous routes to travel by foot, bike or car. For example, it describes the Lewis and Clark National Historic Trail, the Pony Express National Historic Trail, and the Trail of Tears National Historic Trail, among others.

National Recreation Trails
http://www.gorp.com/gorp/activity/hiking/natrectr.htm

These trails range from one to 40 miles long.

National Scenic Trails
http://www.gorp.com/gorp/resource/us_trail/nattrail.htm

Descriptions of great long-distance footpaths such as the Appalachian Trail, the Pacific Crest, and the Continental Divide.

Ruth's Power Walking Page

http://members.aol.com/PowerWalkr/index.html

Web page provides information and inspiration on the fitness aspects of walking. It includes frequently asked questions, articles and links, as well as information on marathons and other walking activities.

Volksmarch and Walking Index

http://www.ava.org/

Volksmarch is a non-competitive, 6-mile walk, around which numerous volkssport clubs are based. Site provides information on how to join, upcoming events and walks, articles, and e-mail groups.

Walking

http://walking.miningco.com/

Netlinks for everyone from beginners, to marathon walkers, to trekkers. Includes email groups, clubs, products and magazines, not to mention directory of walks internationally and in North America. "Spotlight" draws your attention to feature articles.

Walklist

http://www.ava.org/walklist.htm

To join this discussion group, send an e-mail to: *lyris@telelists.com* and in the message, write either "subscribe walklist *your_emailaddress*" or "join walklist *your_emailaddress.*"

Martial Arts

Martial Arts

http://martialarts.about.com/

Guide to Internet resources on the martial arts.

The Martial Arts Dojo Directory & Search Engine

http://www.martial-artists.com/

Find a *dojo* or martial art school for a specific style, or browse through their alphabetical list.

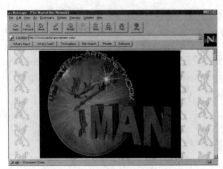

The Martial Arts Network.
http://www.martial-arts-network.com

The Martial Arts Network

http://www.martial-arts-network.com/

Electronic forum dedicated to promoting the future of martial arts. Offers news, awards, magazines, information, t.v. guide and chat rooms.

Martial Arts Resources Page

http://www.middlebury.edu/~jswan/martial.arts/ma.html

Articles by martial arts experts as well as links to general martial arts sites; pages on judo, karate, *tai chi chuan* and less well-known martial art forms. Also connects to mail lists, stuff to buy, newsletters, magazines, and other martial-arts related resources.

Organizations

American Council of Exercise

http://www.acefitness.org/

Organization certifies exercise instructors and equipment.

Department of Kinesiology and Health Science W3

http://www.tahperd.sfasu.edu/sfakin.html

At the Stephen F. Austin State University. Department description and curriculum.

Department of Kinesiology, Kansas State University

http://www.ksu.edu/kines/

Programs, courses, faculty and research information, and application for admission.

National Athletic Trainers' Association Education Council

http://www.cewl.com/

Links for athletic health care professionals. Clinical and continuing education, grants and accreditation.

Running

Cool Running
http://www.coolrunning.com/
News and races, race results, editorials, forums and mail.

Dead Runners Society
http://storm.cadcam.iupui.edu/drs/drs.html
Information on the listserv and numerous links to other related sites. Contrary to its name, this is a discussion group for runners who are very much alive. To subscribe, send e-mail to: *listserv@listserv.dartmouth.edu* with the message: "SUB DRS *yourname.*"

Peak Performance
http://www.siteworks.co.uk/pperf/index.html
This is a scientific newsletter devoted to improving stamina, strength and fitness. Sample articles and subscription information are provided.

Road Runners Club of America
http://rrca.org/
Information about this club and how to join, publications, programs, contacts and forums. Also offers running news updates and links. RRCA represents 630 member clubs with 180,000 members.

Runners World Online
http://www.runnersworld.com/
Daily news and articles. Departments include running for beginners, running injuries, women and running, nutrition, travel and training shoes.

Running Network
http://www.runningnetwork.com/index.html
Information clearinghouse on running. Lots of marathon and regional information as well as running publications.

Running Page
http://www.runningpage.com/
Information about upcoming races, running clubs, places to run, running related products, magazines, and other information.

Running Research News
http://www.rrnews.com/
Written by exercise physiologists. Information about subscribing.

Ultramarathon World
http://Fox.NSTN.Ca/~dblaikie/
For athletes who run distances even longer than the standard marathon of 52.195 kilometers, or 26.2 miles.

U.S.A. Track and Field Road Running Information Center
http://www.usaldr.org/
Running news, and information on races and championships, records and rankings.

Women's Running
http://www.womens-running.com/
Provides information, inspiration and support for women runners.

Sports

CBS SportsLine
http://www.sportsline.com/
News for the sports-addict.

Go, Girl!
http://www.gogirlmag.com/
Free, bimonthly magazine dedicated to getting women of all ages and fitness levels involved in sports.

House of Boxing
http://www.houseofboxing.com/
All about boxing, including ranking, scoring, news, schedules and profiles and boxing links.

Muscle & Fitness
http://www.muscle-fitness.com/musclefitness/index.asp?catid=185
Online version of this popular monthly muscle magazine.

Snowboarding FAQ
http://www.nyx.net/~mwallace/sb_faq.html
Includes information on equipment, technique and jargon.

Sportfit.com
http://www.sportfit.com/
Sports-specific fitness information, such as training tips, glossary, online training log, and more.

SportQuest
http://www.sportquest.com/
"The Virtual Resource Center for Sports Information." Pick a sport, or pick a fitness topic. Links and information on sports training.

The Sports IQ Center
http://members.tripod.com/sportiq/
Includes chatrooms, trivia tests, links, scores and games you can download.

SportsForWomen.com
http://www.justwomen.com/
Lots of news on women's sports, including the latest scores and feature articles. Also includes chat room.

WWW Women's Sports Page
http://fiat.gslis.utexas.edu/~lewisa/womsprt.html
General and sports-specific pages for women.

Yahoo Recreation: Sports
http://dir.yahoo.com/Recreation/Sports/
Everything from Archery to Wrestling (and ever hear of Korfball or Sandboarding?).

Sports Medicine

Double Dutch Physical Therapy Link Connection
http://www.hia.net/pdesmidt/physicaltherapy.htm
Includes physical therapy news, links, education, research and more.

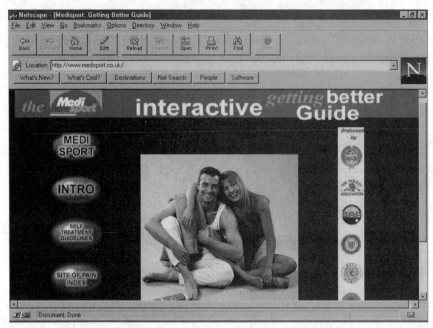

Medisport Interactive Getting Better Guide. *http://www.medisport.co.uk/*

Dr. Pribut's Running Injuries Page

http://www.clark.net/pub/pribut/spsport.html
Internet articles and links.

MedFacts' Sports Doc

http://www.medfacts.com/sprtsdoc.htm
Allows you to "play doctor." Twenty-four virtual patient examinations.

Medisport Interactive Getting Better Guide

http://www.medisport.co.uk/
Includes the "Site of Pain Index" self-treatment guidelines.

MSPWEB: Medicine in Sports Pages on the Web

http://www.mspweb.com/
Broken down into organizations, schools and universities; magazines and online journals; clinics and practices; and other points of interest.

Sports Medicine and Orthopedic Surgery

http://www.sports-medicine.com/
Submit a question relating to sports medicine to Dr. Stuart Zeman.

Tools

Activity Calorie Calculator
http://www.primusweb.com/fitnesspartner/jumpsite/calculat.htm
Input your weight and length of time exerted to find the number of calories burned for various kinds of activities.

Body Mass Index
http://www.shapeup.org/bmi/index.html
Explanation and calculation of your body mass index.

Calculate Your Body Fat Percentage, Circumference Method
http://www.he.net/~zone/prothd2.html
For both men and women.

HealthCalc Network
http://www.healthcalc.net/hcn/tools.htm
Find your target heart rate, calculate your energy expenditure and body mass index, take a walking test, or learn about nutrition and exercise.

Rob Wood's Home of Fitness Testing
http://fitness.testing.8m.com/
Tests your aerobic and anaerobic system, flexibility, body composition, agility, and other fitness indicators.

Weight Training

AtoZ Fitness and Bodybuilding Links
http://www.atozfitness.com/
Online fitness resource contains over 700 links. Bulletin board, mailing list, training and nutrition articles, as well as opportunities to save money on fitness services and products.

Bill Pearl's Bodybuilding and Fitness Web Circle
http://www.billpearl.com/billpearl.asp?key=list&site=frsa
Describes the different websites that are members of this circle.

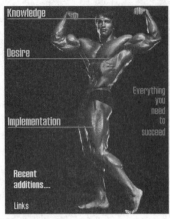

Muscle101.
http://www.muscle101.com/

Biofitness Health Club

http://www.biofitness.com/

Scientific plans for weight training and aerobic training.

A Bodybuilder's Complete Reference Guide (soon to be: Muscle101)

http://www.muscle101.com/

Knowledge, desire, and implementation are everything you need to succeed, according to this site. Use the information on this page to learn how to burn fat and build muscle.

Faith Sloan's Bodybuilding Site

http://www.frsa.com/bbpage.shtml

Includes female and male body building galleries, articles, discussion forum, business directory, competitions and results, links and statistics on Faith Sloan, a professional competitor and the creator of this site.

Greg's Weight Plan for Beginners

http://www.thriveonline.com/shape/weights/weights.step3.html

"Eight Essential Exercises for Weight Training Newbies."

Master Trainer

http://ageless-athletes.com/

Articles and training advice, personal coaching, frequently asked questions and links to other body building sites.

Weight Training

http://www.fitabc.com/wttrain/

Describes specific weight training exercises.

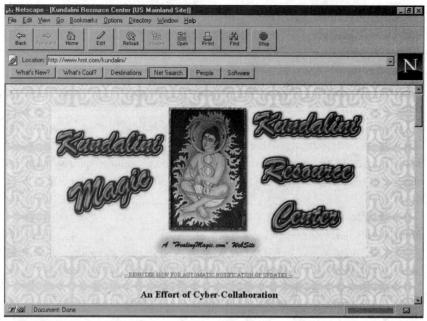

Kundalini Resource Center. http://www.hmt.com/kundalini/

Yoga

The Dhyanyoga Centers
http://www.dyc.org/

Learn about Kundalini Maha Yoga and the mental and physical benefits of meditation.

IndoLink Yoga
http://www.indolink.com/Health/yoga.html

Introduction to yoga, including yoga for stress management; yoga for fitness; digestion, breathing and yoga; specific poses that can help relieve stress; and other articles showing the benefits of this physical art form.

Kundalini Resource Center
http://www.hmt.com/kundalini/

Kundalini articles, events, frequently asked questions (FAQs) and mailing list.

Shoshoni: A Yoga Retreat Center

http://www.shoshoni.org/

A yoga and meditation retreat center in the Colorado Rockies.

Sivananda Yoga "Om" Page

http://www.sivananda.org/

Learn about the various techniques and teachings of Yoga and Vedanta, and about the different activities of the Sivananda Yoga Vedanta Centers. Provides yoga news, frequently asked questions, and a newsletter, as well as "spiritual utilities," shockwave chakras, information on yoga and prison programs, and more.

Yoga Class

http://www.yogaclass.com/welcome.html

Leads you to Yoga Central, which explains yoga basics and invites you to learn more. Provides links, e-mail list, recommended reading and other material. Very attractive site that includes video clips and descriptions of poses.

YogaNet

http://www.yogajournal.com/

This is the online resource for the bimonthly magazine, *Yoga Journal*. You can check out the table of contents of the recent issue, and learn how to subscribe, as well as purchase yoga products.

GRANTS & FUNDING FOR RESEARCH

AHCPR Funding Opportunities

http://www.ahcpr.gov/fund/

The Agency for Health Care Policy and Research supports research projects that examine the availability, quality, and costs of health care services; ways to improve the effectiveness and appro- priateness of clinical practice, including the prevention of disease; and other areas of health services research, such as services for persons with HIV infection. AHCPR also supports small grants, conference grants, and training through dissertation grants and National Re- search Service Awards to institutions and individuals. This site provides an overview of the funding process, policy notices and an application.

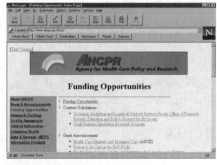

AHCPR Funding Opportunities.
http://www.ahcpr.gov/fund/

Biomedical Sciences Funding Information

http://www.arisnet.com/biomed.html

This site describes some governmental and non-governmental funding sources available for the field of biomedicine, and it includes contacts and deadlines for application. It lists federal and private sources of grants, fellowships, scholarships, contracts and awards to colleges and universities, research centers, and individuals that can be found in the *Biomedical Sciences Report*, which is available every six weeks from ARIS publications (link provided).

Centers for Disease Control and Prevention Funding Opportunities

http://www.cdc.gov/od/pgo/funding/funding.htm

Describes research funding programs available from the CDC.

Community of Science
http://www.cos.com/

COS is a network of scientists and research organizations whose mission is to help members find funding, collaborate with colleagues, and promote their research. Site offers *COS Funding Opportunities* (a database of grants on the web) and *COS Funding News* (which provides weekly highlights from *COS Funding Opportunities*). Members have direct access to complete information on more than 15,000 grants.

Database: NIH Guide to Grants and Contracts
http://grants.nih.gov/grants/guide/index.html

The *NIH-Guide* is distributed weekly via e-mail and contains detailed information on the programs supported by the National Institutes of Health. It is the official publication of NIH policies, procedures, and availability of funds. This site contains the current and back issues of the guide. The NIH considers applications for the support of basic or clinical biomedical, behavioral, and bioengineering research.

FEDIX
http://web.fie.com/fedix/

Federal Information Exchange Funding Opportunities. This is a database providing information on the funding opportunities available to the educational and research communities from a dozen federal agencies. Participating agencies include the National Institutes of Health, the Agency for International Development, the Department of Agriculture, the Department of Veterans Affairs and the Environmental Protection Agency, as well as many others.

Funding First
http://www.fundingfirst.org/

Works to strengthen the nation's committment to funding for medical research.

A Grant Getter's Guide to the Internet
http://web.calstatela.edu/academic/orsp/grantguide.html

The subtitle to this site is: "a brief summary of available grant information and where to find it." It includes a large number of links.

Grant Writing Tips List

http://www.njc.org/Library/resources/Grant_tips.html

Discusses the elements of a successful grant application, how to submit the grant and what to expect once you have submitted it.

GrantsNet

http://www.dhhs.gov/progorg/grantsnet/index.html

This is a tool for finding information about grants offered by the Department of Health and Human Services and other federal programs.

GrantsWeb

http://sra.rams.com/cws/sra/resource.htm

Lists many U.S., Canadian and international government and private grants funding resources, and offers policy information, circulars and legislation information. Includes some grant forms online and offers links to related sites.

Health and Medical Sciences Update

http://fundingopps2.cos.com/news/health/

Site offers a sampling of new and updated health and medical sciences award information available from the Community of Science Funding Opportunities.

Health Resources and Services Administration

http://www.hrsa.dhhs.gov/grants.htm

Describes grants available from HRSA's Bureau of Primary Health Care, the Bureau of Health Professions, the Bureau of Maternal and Child Health, and the HIV/AIDS Bureau.

Medical Research Council of Canada

http://www.hinetbc.org/information/2fmed.htm

Operating (research) grants, major equipment grants, research scholarships, fellowships, studentships, and workshop support are offered to qualified Canadian recipients working in the field of health sciences.

MOLIS Scholarship Search

http://www.fie.com/molis/scholar.htm

Search this database for information on scholarships available to minorities. Qualified applicants include high school seniors, college and graduate school students from the United States.

National Institute of Environmental Health Services
http://www.niehs.nih.gov/external/grant.htm
Describes extramural grant opportunities and allows you to request applications directly.

National Institute of Nursing Research
http://www.nih.gov/ninr/
Supports grants to universities and other research organizations and conducts research intramurally at laboratories in Bethesda, Maryland. Broad mandate in the management of patients during illness and recovery to the reduction of risks for disease and disability and the promotion of healthy lifestyles.

National Science Foundation Grants & Awards
http://www.nsf.gov/home/grants.htm
The National Science Foundation is an independent U.S. government agency responsible for promoting science and engineering. It invests over $3.3 billion per year in almost 20,000 research and education projects in science and engineering. This site describes funding opportunities, proposal criteria and preparation, and other information required to apply for financial support.

The NIH Center for Scientific Review
http://www.drg.nih.gov/
The Center for Scientific Review (CSR) is part of the National Institutes of Health and assists in the formulation of grant application review policies and procedures. It aids in assigning NIH grant applications to supporting institutes, and provides for scientific review of most NIH research grants.

NIH Grant Application Forms
http://chroma.med.miami.edu/forms/
Downloadable grant applications.

NIH Office of Extramural Research
http://www.nih.gov/grants/oer.htm
This page acts as a service for researchers, research administrators, research organizations and others interested in NIH grant programs. NIH funding opportunities, grants policy, awards data, and receipt dates are available at this site.

NLM Extramural Programs

http://www.nlm.nih.gov/ep/extramural.html

Describes the grants and other assistance mechanisms available from the National Library of Medicine. Research and resource grants, individual fellowships, institutional training grants, publication and conference grants are awarded to selected domestic public and private, nonprofit institutions involved in health science research, education or practice.

Robert Wood Johnson Home Page

http://www.rwjf.org/main.html

The Robert Wood Johnson Foundation is one of the largest philanthropic organization in the United States exclusively devoted to health and health care. Grants are awarded in support of three goal areas: assuring that all Americans have access to basic health care at reasonable cost; improving the way services are organized and provided to people with chronic health conditions; and reducing the personal, social and economic harm caused by substance abuse (tobacco, alcohol, and illicit drugs). This site describes the Foundation's principles and projects, and provides instructions for applying for a grant.

Research Sponsors

http://www.cs.virginia.edu/research/sponsors.html

Links to grant and funding agencies. Prepared by the University of Virginia.

University of Wisconsin Medical School Research Resources

http://www.biostat.wisc.edu/research/research.html

This site provides links to many medical research resources, as well as access to databases of interest to biomedical researchers.

HEALTH ADMINISTRATION

American College of Healthcare Executives

http://www.ache.org/

General information about this professional society for health care executives. Site provides access to ACHE publications, membership information, and a description of upcoming ACHE educational programs. The career resource center describes workshops, and offers a career guide and links to related sites.

American College of Medical Practice Executives

http://www.mgma.com/acmpe/index.html

This group supports and promotes the personal and professional growth of both physician and management health care leaders to work collaboratively to advance the profession of health care systems management. It offers certification and scholarships, programs and other services.

American Hospital Association

http://www.aha.org/

The goal of the AHA is "to make federal policy-making relevant to the real work of taking care of people and keeping them well." By advocating in the courts and in Congress, providing national leadership on legal issues that affect health care, and acting forcefully on quality and accreditation issues, the AHA brings the hospital and health system a voice to bear on decisions that affect its members.

Health Administration and Management Resources

http://www.execpc.com/~stjos/admin.html

Clinical outcomes, clinical practice guidelines, health economics and finance, health services administration, quality improvement, electronic journals and government resources.

Community Health Care Management
http://www.chcm-mag.com/

This magazine provides information and resources for executives and managers of community health centers across the country, and allows them the opportunity to interact. It reports on the non-clinical issues surrounding the day-to-day operations of clinics that strive to offer affordable, quality medical care to the underserved in their communities. Site provides access to current issue online, as well as to magazine archives.

DocBoard
http://www.docboard.org/

Administrators in Medicine/Association of State Medical Board Executive Directors allows you to look through its health professional licensing database.

Health Administration Discussion Lists
http://mel.lib.mi.us/health/health-hospital-lists.html

Presents over a dozen mail lists to join, from community health, to health care reform, to managed care.

Health Administration Responsibility Project
http://www.harp.org/

HARP is a resource for patients, doctors, and attorneys who wish to establish the liability of managed health care organizations and nursing facilities for "the consequences of their decisions." That is, it assists those who are concerned that the quality of patient care is at risk in today's managed care environment. HARP provides information on law, links to cases, and general advice on fighting a denial. There is also a listserver where questions and ideas can be posted and discussed.

Health Care Administration on the World Wide Web
http://www.tsufl.edu/library/8/special/health.htm

Includes links to some of the best starting points, government sites, academic/ research organizations, associations and journals that address health care administration.

Health Care HR
http://www.healthcarehr.com/

The health care administrator and recruiter's guide to the Internet. Links and monthly newsletter for health administrators.

Health Communication Resources

http://www.emerson.edu/acadepts/cs/healthcom/Resources/HOME.HTM

How to effectively communicate health-related information to the public. Includes public health goals; the role of communication in disease prevention and health promotion; communication models, theories and practice, and more.

Health Hippo

http://hippo.findlaw.com/

A collection of policy and regulatory materials related to health care. From advanced directives to vaccines, links are categorized by topic and by type of reference. Additional areas include: insurance, policy and administration, antitrust laws, fraud and abuse issues, medical devices, reproductive rights and tax exempt status.

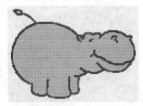

Health Hippo.
http://hippo.findlaw.com/

Healthcare Financial Management Association

http://www.hfma.org/

The HFMA is comprised of over 34,000 financial management professionals employed by hospitals, managed care organizations, medical group practices, and other health care organizations. It offers members educational programs, professional guidance, career development, and inter-field communication. This site describes the organization's activities and publications, posts job announcements and classified ads, and provides information on HFMA chapters and how to join.

HospitalLink

http://www.hospitallink.com/

Convenient connection to hospital websites and resources around the nation.

Knowledge Inc.

http://www.knowledgeinc.com/

Conferences, upcoming events and information about Knowledge Inc., which offers executives information on how to enhance knowledge, technology and performance. The company publishes a newsletter, available for a fee.

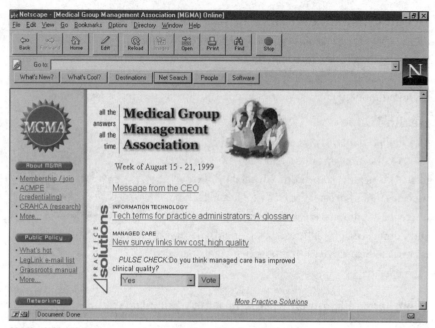

Medical Group Management Association. http://www.mgma.com/

Medical Group Management Association
http://www.mgma.com/

Supports medical group practice development and advancement nationwide. Includes a branch for health care executive's needs as well as a branch for their research and leadership missions.

Practice Choice
http://www.practicechoice.com/

Physician and health care professionals' job resources. Search for a position or post an announcement of an opening at your facility.

Toolbox for Health Administrators
http://www.pohly.com/admin.shtml

Contains articles, information and links to other websites pertinent to managers and administrators working in health care. You can find information about health economics, medical and insurance legislation, industry news, legal issues, regulatory, compliance, policy, business planning resources, human resources, careers, terminology and more.

HEALTH CARE CAREERS & EDUCATION

Careers in Health Care

Active Learning Centre Home Page
http://www.med.jhu.edu/medcenter/quiz/home.cgi

This site contains self-assessment tests/databases in different areas of knowledge, e.g., microbiology, pharmacology and vaccines.

Biological Sciences Career Exploration Links
http://www.uhs.berkeley.edu/CareerLibrary/links/header.cfm?Field=4

These links can help you explore your career interests. Includes occupational information about the nature of the work, working conditions, training and/or educational requirements, job outlook, and earnings; and lists of graduate, professional, and other educational programs. Also gives information of special interest to multicultural populations.

Careers in Health Care
http://www.science.lander.edu/jobs/Careers_in_Health_Care.html

A nice site linking to various resources on the web that offer information on health care careers.

Health Careers Index
http://www.mccg.org/healthcareers/

This guide assists high school students (and others) to explore the various health careers. It is divided into 15 career areas, which include 60 specific health occupations.

Health-Related Careers
http://mama.indstate.edu/dls/ug/preprof/careers.html

Descriptions of career opportunities in the health sciences, from Anesthesiologist Assistant to Veterinarian. Includes a description of the job, salary information, training necessary for this career, and national contact(s).

Medical and Health Career Descriptions
http://www.furman.edu/~snyder/careers/medical.html

Contains links to sites with medical and health-related career descriptions.

Continuing Education
See also individual specialties.

Center for Instructional Support
http://www.uchsc.edu/CIS/

This site provides resources to enhance the health professional's educational, research, leadership and management skills, and offers resources for career and personal development. Information on educational journals, conferences and workshops is offered, as well as fellowship and funding opportunities.

SearchCME
http://www.searchcme.com/

Continuing medical education (CME) information on more than 5,000 medical conferences indexed by medical specialty, geographic location and date.

WebDoctor Continuing Medical Education Resources
http://www.gretmar.com/webdoctor/cme.html

Index of continuing medical education resources, multi-media text books and patient simulations available on the Internet.

Dentistry

See also: Dentistry.

American Association of Dental Schools

http://www.aads.jhu.edu/

National organization for dental education lists U.S. and Canadian dental schools, hospital and other dental education programs, students and faculty. Links to sites of interest and information on conferences, dental news and updates are available from this site.

Dental Schools

http://www.aads.jhu.edu/links.html

Links to dental schools in the United States and Canada.

Dental Student Educational Resources

http://www.hsdm.med.harvard.edu/pages/dentstud.htm

Presents biomedical sites of interest to dental students, covering topics such as biochemistry, embryology, histology, immunology, microbiology, neuroscience, pathology, pharmacology and physiology.

Dentistry Careers

http://www.mccg.org/healthcareers/dentist.htm

This Internet resource guide for high school students describes what it is like to be a dentist, dental assistant and dental hygienist.

International Dental Schools Directory

http://www.dentalsite.com/dentists/intsch.html

Directory and links to dental schools around the world.

Professional Connection

http://www.oralb.com/pro/index.htm

Articles, journal abstracts and clinical abstracts for dental health professionals.

So, You Want to Be a Dentist?

http://www.vvm.com/~bond/home.htm

Kirk Bond, D.D.S. created this site to answer some basic questions that individuals who are considering entering the field of dentistry may have. It describes different kinds of dentists, provides dental images and interesting sites.

Web Sites for Dental Students

http://www.dentalsite.com/dentists/denstu.html

Links to dental student pages and resources, dental school sites, histology sites and publications.

Employment

America's Health Care Source

http://www.healthcaresource.com/

Site matches employers and job seekers, provides a list of educational seminars around the country, and links to professional, educational and licensure websites.

Future Med

http://ourworld.compuserve.com/homepages/futuremed/

Overseas employment opportunities for health care professionals.

Health Care Job Store

http://www.healthcarejobstore.com/

Find health care jobs, manage your career, sign up with a job search agent, view employer profiles, work on your resumé and more at this site for health care professionals. The list of related sites is dizzying.

Health Care Recruitment Online

http://www.healthcareers-online.com/Welcome.htm

Health care job database; information on relocating, and career management.

MedBulletin

http://www.medbulletin.com/

Free medical employment resource that posts physician job listings, health care job listings, and provides directories of employers, recruiters and residency programs.

Medical and Health Care Job Openings

http://www.nationjob.com/medical

Search through job listing by location, position type, salary or key word.

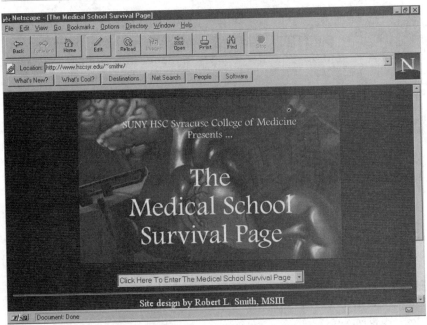

The Medical School Survival Page. http://www.hscsyr.edu/~smithr/

Health Care Education

Fellowship and Residency Database
http://www.ama-assn.org/freida/
Searchable database of graduate medical education and combined specialty programs.

The Medical Education Page
http://www.scomm.net/~greg/med-ed/
News, frequently asked questions, medical courses, medical schools, educational references and indices.

The Medical School Survival Page
http://www.hscsyr.edu/~smithr/
Everything the med school student needs from the Internet. Site provides resources for basic sciences, clinical clerkships, medical journals, medical references, diseases by specialty and much more.

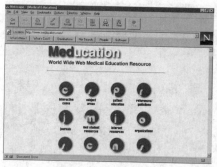

Meducation. http://www.meducation.com/

Meducation

http://www.meducation.com/

Meducation's main goal is to provide efficient, selected links to the vast amount of medical information available on the Internet. It offers a great deal of material, including medical student references and aids, interactive cases, journals, medical news and educational software.

Nursing

See also: chapter entitled Nursing.

Health Interactive Continuing Education for Nurses and Other Health Professionals

http://www.rnceus.com/

Courses in general, cardiac, diagnostics, geriatric, GI/GU, medical/surgical, and pediatric/perinatal nursing.

Cybernurse.com Careers

http://www.cybernurse.com/careers.html

General information for those interested in becoming nurses. Links to job sites.

NursingCenter.com

http://www.nursingcenter.com/

Offers continuing education, career development, journals and other resources for nurses and those studying to become nurses.

Nursing Jobs

http://www.wwnurse.com/nursingjobs/index.html

You can search for a nursing job or post a listing of an open position.

Healthcare Education and Resources for Nurses

http://www.swandesign.com/LRC.html

Provides links to nursing education and research resources online.

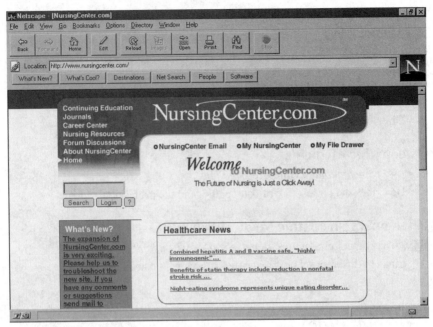

NursingCenter.com. *http://www.nursingcenter.com*

NurseOne

http://www.nurseone.com/

This company offers online continuing education courses aimed to improve or refresh the knowledge base of nurses. While these courses are available for free through the Internet, with payment of $10 per unit and satisfactory completion of tests, an official CEU certificate will be mailed.

Nursing Education Resources

http://daphne.palomar.edu/Library/subjects/nursinged.htm

Includes continuing education and nursing education resources, clinical simulations, reference tools, employment information, periodicals and links to general nursing sites.

Student Nurse

http://studentnurse.hypermart.net/

Website and electronic magazine for student nurses.

Osteopathy

See also: Osteopathy.

Colleges of Osteopathic Medicine

http://www.aacom.org/sch98.htm

Directory of American colleges of osteopathic medicine.

Osteopathic Medicine

http://www.oucom.ohiou.edu/OsteoMed.htm

Describes the philosophy of osteopathy, and the profession's roots.

Peterson's Osteopathic Medical Schools List

http://www.petersons.com/graduate/select/635020se.html

Links to different schools that offer programs in osteopathic medicine.

Pharmacology

See also: Drugs/Pharmacology.

A Career in Pharmacology

http://www.pharm.sunysb.edu/undergraduate/career.html

A short, inspiring statement inviting people to consider pharmacology as a career choice.

Pharmacology Departments World-Wide

http://www.kfunigraz.ac.at/ekpwww/linkinst.html

The list currently contains the names of 809 departments, institutes and laboratories from 58 countries world-wide, and includes links to the homepages of 470 of these departments.

Pharmacology and Toxicology

http://www.pharmtox.med.uwo.ca/career/career.html

Great resource discussing pharmacology and toxicology as career choices.

Schools of Pharmacy in the U.S.

http://www.li.net/~edhayes/rxschool.html

This list of schools of pharmacy includes addresses and phone numbers.

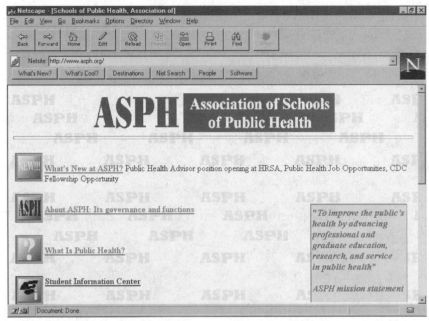

Association of Schools of Public Health. http://www.asph.org/

World List of Schools of Pharmacy

http://www.cpb.uokhsc.edu/SoP/SoPListHomePage.html

In addition to a list of schools, this site offers a link to a collection of pharmacology contininuing education sites.

Public Health

See also: Public Health.

American Public Health Association

http://www.apha.org/

Resources for public health officials. Provides information on continuing education opportunities, job openings, legislation, and more.

Association of Schools of Public Health

http://www.asph.org/

Describes the ASPS and its activities, what public health is, and provides information for students.

The Medicine/Public Health Initiative
http://www.sph.uth.tmc.edu/mph/

Includes news, links, editorials and discussion on the M/PH initiative, which seeks to fuse the fields of medicine and public health.

Student Movement of the Medicine/Public Health Initiative
http://www.studentmphi.org/

The mission of this consortium of student groups is to provide a forum for student discussion, action, and collaboration on matters related to public health and medical education, practice, and research.

Why Choose a Graduate Degree and Career in Public Health?
http://www.asph.org/career.htm

"Because you can make a difference." Site discusses the mission of public health service, and links to pages describing career opportunities.

HEALTH CARE POLICY & ECONOMICS

> *Covered in this chapter*: *Analysis & Research; Advocacy Groups; Economics; Glossaries; Government; Health Care Reform; International Issues; Links & Other Resources; Publications & Collections; Statistics & Data.*
>
> *Related chapters*: *Biomedical Ethics; Disabilities; Health Administration; Insurance & Managed Care; Public Health.*

Analysis & Research

Alpha Center

http://www.ac.org/

Nonprofit, non-partisan health care policy center offering information and analysis. Online publications, state information, updates and resources may be accessed at this site.

C. Everett Koop Institute

http://www.dartmouth.edu/acad-inst/koop/

The Institute designs and implements strategies to enhance the health of individuals, families and communities. It does this by encouraging initiatives, providing leadership if desired, and researching ways which human networks can encourage the abilities and commitment of individuals dedicated to the promotion of health. Site describes the Institute's programs, projects and events; and offers resources, contacts and news briefs. Another project still under development is the Koop Village, a web-based conference and discussion center that will address important health care issues.

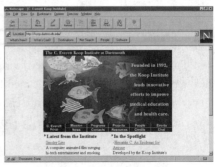

C. Everett Koop Institute. http://www. dartmouth.edu/acad-inst/koop/

Center for Health Care Strategies, Inc.

http://www.chcs.org/CHCS/welcome.htm

CHCS is a nonprofit, non-partisan policy and resource center affiliated with the Woodrow Wilson School of Public and International Affairs at Princeton.

Center on Budget and Policy Priorities

http://cbpp.org/

Non-partisan research organization and policy institute that focuses on analysis of government policies and programs, especially those affecting low and middle-income populations. The Center's reports and papers are available here.

Kaiser Family Foundation Health Policy

http://www.kff.org/archive/health.html

The Kaiser Family Foundation is an independent philanthropic society that focuses on major health care issues. It runs its own research and communication programs, often working with other groups, and makes small grants in an effort to provide reliable, non-biased health care information. This site contains reports on Medicaid and Medicare.

RAND Health

http://www.rand.org/organization/health/

Describes the health-research activities of RAND, a think-tank. Its studies are both international and domestic in scope.

Advocacy Groups

See also: Health Care Reform, later in this chapter.

The Coalition for Medicare Choices

http://www.medicarechoices.org/

This group fights to preserve the right of Medicare beneficiaries to choose health plans that meet their specific medical and economic needs. The site presents important issues regarding Medicare choices, Congressional actions and contacts, an overview of the Medicare+Choice program, and news.

Families USA Foundation

http://www.familiesusa.org/

Grassroots network that advocates for the availability of high quality, affordable health and long-term care for all Americans. To this end, you can find news releases, publications, position statements and job openings on this site.

Health Care Liability Alliance

http://www.hcla.org/

National advocacy coalition representing physicians, hospitals, blood banks, liability insurers, health device manufacturers, health care insurers, businesses, producers of medicines, and the technology industry. They are dedicated to "rescuing" the nation's health care system from what they consider to be "an out-of-control legal system that is severely damaging the delivery of health care and hurting patients."

National Health Care for the Homeless Council

http://www.nhchc.org/

Over the last five years, 5.7 million different people in the United States have been homeless for some length of time. The Council exists to help bring about reform of the health care system to best serve the needs of people who are homeless.

National Organization of Physicians Who Care

http://pwc.org/

This nonprofit organization wishes to preserve the traditional doctor-patient relationship and to ensure quality health care. It contains news and articles on Medicare reform.

NHeLP: National Health Law Program, Inc.

http://www.healthlaw.org/

Offers health care advocacy for low-income people.

Physicians Committee for Responsible Medicine

http://www.pcrm.org/

This is a nonprofit organization that promotes preventive medicine through innovative programs, encourages higher standards for ethics and effectiveness in research, and advocates broader access to medical services.

Project Vote Smart

http://www.vote-smart.org/

This group tracks the voting records, issue positions, and other information on over 13,000 political leaders including the president, members of Congress, governors and state legislators.

Economics

Health Economics and Finance Research Web Sites

http://www.medsch.wisc.edu/adminmed/econ-www.htm

List of links to government sites, organizations, discussion groups, data and other sites containing research papers and articles, legislation and legislative analysis of health economics concerns.

Health Economics: Places to Go

http://www.medecon.de/hec.htm

Ansgar Hebborn has selected sites to do with health economics, health policy, managed care, public health and other areas in the form of associations, databases, education and training, discussion and mail lists, journals, institutions and more.

Health Policy, Economics, and Practice Management Resources

http://www.psych.org/other_orgs/health_econ.html

The American Psychiatric Association provides several links to important health policy and economics websites.

HealthEconomics.com

http://www.healtheconomics.com/

Health economics, medical and pharmacy resources are broken down into categories, which include: associations, consulting/services, databases, education/ universities, employment, government, journals and publications, libraries and more.

WebEc: Health and Welfare

http://www.helsinki.fi/WebEc/webeci.html

Brief descriptions with links to health economics collections, institutions, publications and related sites. Scope is international.

Glossaries

Glossary for Healthcare Standards

http://dmi-www.mc.duke.edu/dukemi/acronyms.htm

Text file provides a brief explanation of the many acronyms in health care.

Glossaries of Health and Medical Care Terms

http://weber.u.washington.edu/~mhs/mhsgloss.html

Links to several online health, managed care and medical glossaries.

Government

Agency for Health Care Policy and Research

http://www.ahcpr.gov/

The AHCPR is the lead federal agency charged with supporting research designed to improve the quality of health care, reduce its cost, and broaden access to essential services. Site provides information on the organization, grants, clinical and consumer health information, research findings, news, and much more.

FedWorld Information Network

http://www.fedworld.gov/

This service of the U.S. Department of Commerce allows you to search through the bureaucracy of the federal government. FedWorld's goal is to provide a comprehensive central access point for searching, locating, ordering and acquiring government and business information. Over 20 different federal government databases are available for browsing.

Health Care Financing Administration

http://www.hcfa.gov/

The Health Care Financing Administration (HCFA) manages the Medicare, Medicaid, and Child Health Insurance programs. This site provides access to information on these programs, as well as to information on the Balanced Budget Act, health care research, laws and regulations, public affairs, and local information. There are separate pages for beneficiaries, plans and providers, students, researchers and state representatives. All are accessible from this site.

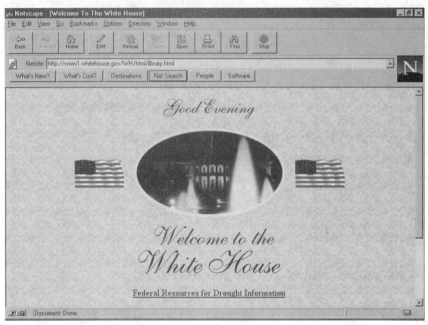

The White House. http://www1.whitehouse.gov/

Information for State Health Policy

http://www2.umdnj.edu/shpp/homepage.htm

This site is intended to help health care policy makers, state officials, health care employees, health providers, insurers, consumers and others to locate Model Reports and Standards for health statistical information and, in general, to be aware of the Information for State Health Policy Program.

National Health Security Plan

http://metalab.unc.edu/nhs/NHS-T-o-C.html

Executive Summary that includes President Clinton's 1993 health care reform plan and supporting documents.

Occupational Safety and Health Administration

http://www.osha.gov/

OSHA and state partners work to establish and enforce protective standards in the work place that will promote public safety. It supports a numer of offices with inspectors, as well as complaint discrimination investigators, engineers, physicians, educators, standards writers and others. This site details OSHA operations and standards, provides examples of OSHA success stories, presents news, regulations and other resources, as well as statistics and inspection data.

THOMAS

http://thomas.loc.gov/

"In the spirit of Thomas Jefferson," this is a service of the U.S. Congress that provides legislative information for the public via the Internet.

White House/White House Virtual Library

http://www1.whitehouse.gov/WH/html/library.html

The library contains press releases, radio addresses, photographs, executive orders, and web pages for the White House and staff, as well as links to all governmental sites and some historic national documents. Searchable.

Health Care Reform

See also: Advocacy Groups, earlier in this chapter.

The American Prospect's Health Care Reform

http://epn.org/prospect/health.html

Collection of articles on health care reform from this bimonthly magazine. Although it does not support any candidates but rather hopes to stimulate thoughtful discussion of important issues, the magazine generally reflects moral and political views that are broadly identified with the liberal and progressive positions.

Citizens for a Sound Economy: Health Care Reform

http://www.cse.org/cse/health.html

Explains this organization's perspective on health care reform, which is adamently opposed to President Clinton's plan.

Council for Affordable Health Insurance

http://www.cahi.org/

This organization is made up of companies and individuals who promote a free-market approach to health care reform, believing this is the way to preserve freedom of choice and quality of care while addressing the issue of affordability.

Health Care Reform

http://www.heritage.org/library/index/i1.html

From the Heritage Foundation's library. Articles are available mostly in *.Pdf or online format.

Health Care Reform: A Bibliography

http://www.usc.edu/isd/doc/libraries/guides/health_care.html

This bibliography provides access to a selection of government publications concerning health care reform. Most of the documents deal with recent efforts to reform the health care system of the United States, but a few deal with pre-1980 proposals for health care reform. Searchable.

National Center for Policy Analysis: Health Issues

http://www.public-policy.org/~ncpa/pi/health/hedex1.html

As well as health care reform, there are examinations, analysis, and debate of other health care issues, such as managed care, managed competition, Medicare, Medicaid, medical savings accounts, and health care delivery in other countries. NCPA is a nonprofit policy research institute.

National Coalition on Health Care

http://www.americashealth.org/

This site says that the Coalition is the largest non-partisan group working to improve America's health care. Quality, cost and coverage issues are currently central concerns. The Coalition is comprised of businesses, labor unions, religious groups, primary care providers, and educators. Site explains the Coalition's mission and some of its programs, which are still forming.

Physicians for a National Health Program

http://www.pnhp.org/

Organization has a membership of approximately 7,000 and provides anyone interested with fact sheets, discussion, newsletter and more. Site offers information on how people can get a speaker to present, as well as how to organize a town hall meeting.

International Issues

Health Reform Online
http://www.worldbank.org/healthreform/
Provides information for health care managers, analysts and decision-makers who want to learn more about the economics and financing of health care delivery in developing countries. Includes a "targeted search" engine of selected sites.

Partnerships for Health Reform
http://www.phrproject.com/
This is the U.S. Agency for International Development's project supporting health reform in developing countries.

Links & Other Resources

Health Care Information Resources on the Web
http://www.xnet.com/~hret/statind.htm
These resources were collected by the *Health Services Research* journal. Includes federal and state government resources, hospital resources, educational health resources, and other sources of health data.

Health Hippo
http://hippo.findlaw.com/
Collection of policy and regulatory materials related to health care.

Health Policy and Medical Education Enterprises
http://www.LonePear.com/
Access to the Health Policy Leadership Institute, and to the Center for Comparative Health Policy Studies.

Health Policy Cyberexchange
http://www.hpolicy.duke.edu/cyberexchange/
Examines health policy from all angles. Includes a section which identifies key health policy issues within broad areas of public health, health promotion, health protection, environmental health and preventive services. Links to the health in-dustry, research organizations, literature searches, and U.S. government branches.

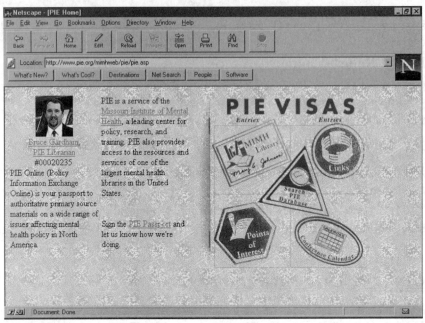

PIE Online. http://www.pie.org/mimhweb/pie/pie.asp

Idea Central's Health Policy Links

http://epn.org/idea/hciclink.html

Links to websites and information on the national health policy, state health policy, public health, health policy foundations, managed care, and other areas.

PIE Online: Policy Information Exchange

http://www.pie.org/

"Passport" to primary source materials on issues affecting mental health policy in North America. It is a service of the Missouri Institute of Mental Health, and provides access to reports and data on mental health issues.

Publications & Collections

Atlantic Unbound

http://www.theAtlantic.com/atlantic/election/connection/healthca/healthca.htm

Health care articles that have appeared in the *Atlantic Monthly*, and related health care policy links.

Electronic Policy Network

http://epn.org/

Articles and reports on health care policy and related issues.

Health Affairs

http://www.projhope.org/HA/

View the full text of the current issue, search the index for back articles, and find out how to subscribe to this health policy and managed care journal.

Health Economics

http://www.york.ac.uk/inst/che/he.htm

Journal publishes articles on all aspects of health economics: theoretical contributions, empirical studies, economic evaluations and analyses of health policy from the economic perspective. You can request a sample copy and learn how to subscribe at this site.

Health Policy

http://epn.org/idea/health.html

Virtual magazine. Articles appear full-text and address issues of health care reform, health insurance, Medicare, managed care and more.

Health Services Research

http://www.xnet.com/~hret/hsr.htm

Bimonthly journal of the Association for Health Services Research. Contains a ten-year index by subject and author, as well as articles and abstracts from more recent issues.

Statistics & Data

HRC's Online Health Policy Network

http://mtfuji.ari.net/cgi-shl/dbml.exe?Template=/cfpro/chrc/hds/hdssrch1.dbm

Links to websites containing online health data, policy reports, facts and figures, organizational resources, and other useful health care information. From the Center for Health Research and Communications, Inc.

Dartmouth Atlas of Health Care in the United States
http://www.dartmouth.edu/~atlas/
Describes the geographic distribution of health care resources in the U.S.

Health Care Data and Surveys
http://www.ahcpr.gov/data/
Main subject areas include the medical expenditure panel survey, health care cost and utilization project, HIV and AIDS cost and utilization, and medical informatics standards. From the Agency for Health Care Policy and Research.

Health Policy Information
http://www.uwex.edu/ces/flp/health/
Provides health policy information for the general consumer. It includes updates on health care issues, as well as a background on the current health care system and entitlements, basic vocabulary, frequently asked questions, and links to related sites.

National Center for Health Statistics
http://www.cdc.gov/nchswww/default.htm
Users can browse the publications and statistical tables, download selected public-use data files, conduct online database queries and searches, track progress toward Healthy People 2000 Objectives, or access FASTATS from A-Z. The site also contains information about each NCHS survey and data system, special programs and activities, upcoming seminars, conferences, and training, as well as links to other sites.

Social Statistics Briefing Room
http://www.whitehouse.gov/fsbr/health.html
Data and information in chart form showing the nation's vital statistics (birth rate, mortality rate, life expectancy), access to health services, health status, health care expenditures and other health-related information.

UCLA Center for Health Policy Research
http://www.healthpolicy.ucla.edu/
This Center at the University of California at Los Angeles conducts research, provides policy analysis and data as a public service to policy makers and community leaders, and offers educational opportunities to students. Site presents data, publications, research areas and public services.

HEART & VEINS / CARDIOVASCULAR

Anatomy

Cardiovascular Pathology Index

http://www-medlib.med.utah.edu/WebPath/CVHTML/CVIDX.html#1

There are 130 different high-quality images of the heart and veins. These include images demonstrating the normal heart, heart with artherosclerotic disease, mycardial infarction, dissection of the aorta, endocarditis, pericarditis, myocarditis, neoplasia, congenital heart disease, cardiomyopathies and other arterial and venous diseases.

Cut to the Heart

http://www.pbs.org/wgbh/nova/heart/

A companion to the NOVA series of the same name, this site shows images of diseased hearts, provides an overview of how the heart works, and shows you how blood rushes through the heart. It includes resources and "amazing heart facts."

The Heart: An Online Exploration

http://sln.fi.edu/biosci/heart.html

Informative and entertaining site geared to children allows them to explore the heart, following blood through vessels. Other heart health information is available. Accompanying resource materials.

Angina

Angina and Heart Attack
http://www.chebucto.ns.ca/Health/CPRC/angin_mi.html
Describes angina, the temporary chest pain that occurs when the heart does not receive enough blood, and identifies where it occurs and how long it usually lasts.

Angina: Patient Information
http://lib-sh.lsumc.edu/fammed/pted/angina.html
Answers some fundamental questions about angina pectoris.

Angina Pectoris Treatments
http://www.americanheart.org/Heart_and_Stroke_A_Z_Guide/anginat.html
Brief description of the drugs and invasive procedures used to treat angina.

Facts about Angina
http://www.medscape.com/govmt/NHLBI/patient/Angina.html
What it is, how it is diagnosed, how it is treated, and related facts.

Aneurysms

Aneurysm and AVM Support
http://www.westga.edu/~wmaples/aneurysm.html
Includes a number of narratives from patients, and direct e-mail connection to "Talk to a Physician" (e.g., neurosurgeon, vascular surgeon, or interventional radiologist). Discusses aortic aneurysms, arteriovenous malformations, and brain aneurysms.

Aneurysm Information Project
http://www.columbia.edu/~mdt1/
Research papers, lectures and support on aneurysms, which occur when a blood vessel dilates and threatens to rupture. There are also answers to frequently asked questions about aneurysms.

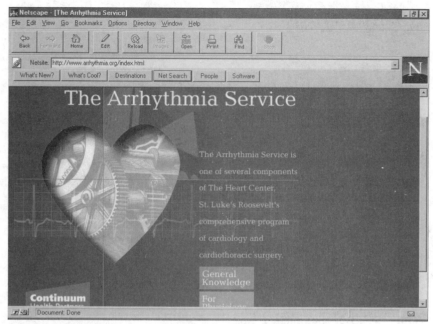

The Arrhythmia Service. http://www.arrhythmia.org/

Aortic Aneurysm: 3-D Visualization and Measurement

Http://everest.radiology.uiowa.edu/nlm/app/aorta/aorta.html

Includes an overview of aortic aneurysms, images and a patient scan protocol.

Arrhythmia

Arrythmia

http://www.icorp.net/cardio/categories/arrythmiaarticles.htm

Contains a number of articles on arrythmias.

The Arrhythmia Service

http://www.arrhythmia.org/

General knowledge and knowledge for professionals. Includes what it is, how it is diagnosed and how it is treated. Online chat for physicians.

Cardiac Arrythmias

http://icarus.med.utoronto.ca/week13/cardary.htm

Links to websites and online articles.

Atherosclerosis

Atherosclerosis

http://www.letsfindout.com/subjects/body/rficad__.html

    Basic explanation of this disease which results from a narrowing of the arteries due to build-up of plaques.

Atherosclerosis and Thrombosis Index

http://www-medlib.med.utah.edu/WebPath/ATHHTML/ATHIDX.html

    Images of arteries and veins, healthy and damaged.

How Atherosclerosis Develops

http://www.full-health.com/artery.htm

    Images and description of normal artery and an artery exhibiting a buildup of plaque. Links to related text on arterial buildup.

What Is Atherosclerosis?

http://www.americanheart.org/Heart_and_Stroke_A_Z_Guide/athero.html

    Describes this condition.

Cholesterol

Cholesterol

http://www.mayohealth.org/mayo/9306/htm/choleste.htm

    Hypertext article on cholesterol helps to sort through some of the confusing messages by providing basic information.

The Cholesterol Myths

http://home2.swipnet.se/~w-25775/

    Text cautions that what you have may have heard about cholesterol is not completely true.

Doctor's Guide to Elevated Cholesterol

http://www.pslgroup.com/ELEVCHOL.HTM

Information, news and resources on high cholesterol and what to do about it.

High Cholesterol

http://www.heartinfo.com/reviews/hchol.htm

Dozens of links to sites addressing cholesterol. They are evaluated on various qualities and the content of these sites is described.

Live Healthier, Live Longer: Lowering Cholesterol for the Person with Heart Disease

http://rover.nhlbi.nih.gov/chd/

Site explains coronary heart disease and how to lower one's cholesterol level, provides a resource library, and answers frequently asked questions.

Low Cholesterol Diet

http://www.gicare.com/pated/edtot24.htm

These patient pages describe why a low cholesterol diet is helpful, describe special considerations for those at risk for heart disease, and provide sample menus.

Clinical Trials

See also: Clinical Trials.

Cardiology/Vascular Disease

http://www.centerwatch.com/studies/listing.htm#Section1

Clinical trials directory from CenterWatch.

Clinical Trials: Heart and Vascular

http://www.telemedical.com/Telemedical/crt2.htm

Select this entry to get to a database of clinical trials for the heart and vascular system.

Congenital Heart Anomalies

3-D Visualization of Congenital Heart Disease
http://everest.radiology.uiowa.edu/nlm/app/cnjheart/cnjheart.html

Includes a CHD overview, patient scan protocols, case studies, MRI images, related websites and more. For medical professionals.

CHASER: Congenital Heart Anomalies Support, Education and Resources
http://www.csun.edu/~hfmth006/chaser/

Congenital heart defects occur in approximately 1 of every 100 live births. CHASER offers parents, professionals and patients with congenital heart anomalies the resources that may help them to deal with the financial, educational, medical and emotional issues they may encounter.

Congenital Heart Disease Online Handbook
http://www.execpc.com/~markc/congring.html

Great resource that describes the different congenital heart diseases (CHD), offers definitions and abreviations, and provides information on CHD surgery and medications.

Congenital Heart Disease Resource Page
http://www.csun.edu/~hcmth011/heart/

Support groups, web resources, and information on specific congenital coronary syndromes and disorders.

The Congenital Heart Disease Webring
http://www.adventureangling.com/chd/webring.htm

You can go to any one of the CHD websites from this site, or add a link. Also allows you to search these sites, join a genetic study, or chat with others.

Coronary Artery Disease

Ask NOAH about Heart Disease

http://www.noah.cuny.edu/heart_disease/heartdisease.html

Lots of material to understand what heart disease and stroke are. Site also contains sections on prevention, care and treatment, and resources.

Cardiovascular Center: The Daily Apple

http://thedailyapple.com/level2/cv-hmdv3.htm

Contains a variety of news and articles on heart disease, heart conditions and heart and cardiovascular health.

Coronary Artery Disease

http://www.heartsite.com/html/coronary _artery_disease.shtml

Graphic-rich and elementary explanation of atherosclerosis, angina and coronary artery disease.

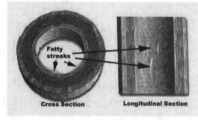

Coronary Artery Disease.
http://www.heartsite.com/html/coronary_ artery_disease.shtml

General Education Site for Cardiovascular Diseases

http://www.med-edu.com/

For physicians and other health care providers, this site offers reviews, quizzes and technical advice; for patients, their families and the general public, it provides discussions of different cardiovascular diseases in lay-person's language.

Heart Disease

http://heartdisease.about.com/

Loads of links and feature articles on cardiology and heart disease, broken down by topic. Includes different heart diseases, diagnostic tests, risk factors, transplantation, journals, online forums, and much more.

Heart Disease

http://www.largnet.uwo.ca/shine/health/heartdis.htm

Quick facts and information on the different kinds of heart diseases, as well as tests and treatments.

Heartsite.Com
http://www.heartsite.com/
Information for patients being treated for a heart-related condition. Includes explanation of the heart's function, heart diseases, treatment, tests for diagnosis and evaluation. Multimedia lecture with sound.

Heart Smart World: Guide to Coronary Heart Diseases and Treatment Information
http://www.heartsmartworld.com/
Contains essays on heart care, heart stents, and women and heart disease, plus an option to buy electronic books on these subjects.

Patient Information: Heart Disease and Stroke
http://www.medscape.com/Home/Patient/directories/HeartDiseaseAndRStroke.html
Many articles from different sources discussing angina, cholesterol, coronary heart disease, hypertension, stroke and more.

Understanding Coronary Heart Disease
http://www.geocities.com/HotSprings/1652/geninfo.html
Explains health risks, bypass operations and angioplasty.

Diet & Exercise

Exercise (Physical Activity)
http://www.americanheart.org/Heart_and_Stroke_A_Z_Guide/exercise.html
Recommendations on exercise and health from the American Heart Association (AHA). It is the AHA's Scientific Position that physical inactivity is a high risk factor of coronary artery disease.

Healthy Heart Exercise
http://sln.fi.edu/biosci/healthy/exercise.html
Advice on starting an exercise program for heart-health. Includes kinds of exercises, guidelines for beginners, and what to consider when selecting a health club.

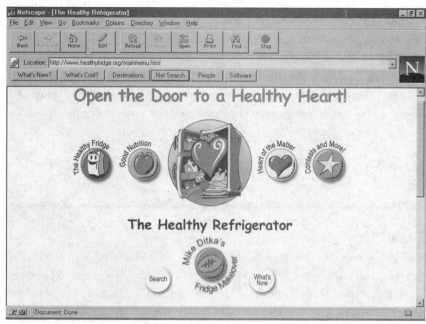

The Health Refrigerator. *http://www.healthyfridge.org/mainmenu.html*

The Healthy Refrigerator

http://www.healthyfridge.org/mainmenu.html

Give your fridge a "makeover" and help your heart at the same time.

Just Move!

http://www.justmove.org/

Online exercise diary, fitness news, database and more. Created by the American Heart Association, this site is designed to encourage people to exercise.

Discussion Groups

Cardio-Consult Discussion Group

http://pharminfo.com/conference/cconslt.html

E-mail group for cardiovascular professionals to discuss case studies, research and clinical experiences. To subscribe, send e-mail to: *LISTSERV@ SHRSYS.HSLC.ORG* with the message: "SUBSCRIBE CARDIO-CONSULT *Firstname Lastname.*"

Curious Heart Discussion Group

http://www.curiousheart.com/discussion/index.html

Instructions on joining this discussion group and on how to post messages relating to heart disease, treatment, prevention, your experiences, questions, answers, comments or any information that others might want to know about. Site also contains links, frequently asked questions, and text on "the heart in plain English" (the basics, heart disorders, and tests for the heart).

Heart Surgery Forum

http://www.hsforum.com/

For cardiothoracic professionals, this site includes forums, articles and links.

Jon's Place

http://www.geocities.com/Heartland/Hills/2571/jonsplace.htm

This site was created by a man suffering from cardiomyopathy and presents a patient's perspective on heart disease. It includes a description of the symptoms and other information, a moderated heart failure forum, and access to e-mail lists.

Online Forums and Discussion Groups in Heart Disease/Cardiology

http://heartdisease.miningco.com/msubforum.htm

Quite a few e-mail discussion groups and online forums are described. Some of the lists are for patients, some are for professionals. They cover different aspects of cardiology, such as pediatric heart disease, cardiac surgery, transplantation and perfusion.

Heart Attack (Myocardial Infarction)

Cardiac Rehabilitation and Prevention

http://www.jhbmc.jhu.edu/cardiology/rehab/patientinfo.html

Information on heart attacks, including exercise, nutrition, smoking, stress, heart health, physical activity and more.

Heart Attack and Atherosclerosis Prevention Update: Part I

*http://www.MedicineNet.com/Script/Main/Art.asp?li=MNI&d=208&cu=3133
7&w=0&ArticleKey=9749*

Describes atherosclerosis, angina, and heart attacks. Information on preventing a heart attack and coronary atherosclerosis. You can also link to Part II, which is entitled: "Improving Your Blood Cholesterol Level."

Heart Attack Basics

http://www.heart-surgeons.com/basics.htm

Includes a description of the tests and procedures used to diagnose patients with heart disorders.

Heart Attack Guide

http://www.heartinfo.org/news/htattksymp012299.htm

Heart function, symptoms of a heart attack, emergency care, tests, treatments and related articles.

Heart Attack (Myocardial Infarction)

*http://www.MedicineNet.com/Script/Main/Art.asp?li=MNI&d=238&cu=1658
3&w=0&ArticleKey=379*

Power points, illustration and text describing the circumstances of a heart attack, i.e., the death of heart muscle due to the loss of blood supply.

HeartAttacks.Com

http://www.heartattacks.com/

Heart attack prevention, diagnosis and treatment links.

You've Had a Heart Attack - What Now?

http://staff.washington.edu/bmperra/heart_help.html

What do you need and want to know about your safety and well-being?

Heart Health

Cardiac HealthWeb

http://www.bev.net/health/cardiac/

Features "Ask the Cardiologist" database and direct question submission. Also contains health news and resources to help you to assess your risk for heart disease.

Cardiovascular Information for Patients and the General Public

http://www.nhlbi.nih.gov/health/public/heart/index.htm

From the National Heart, Lung and Blood Institute, topics include high blood pressure, cholesterol, obesity, heart attack, other heart and Latino resources.

Cardiovascular Institute of the South

http://www.cardio.com/

This is a library of reports on cardiovascular topics. Article categories include arrhythmia, cardiac treatment, heart frequently asked questions (FAQs), hypertension, preventing heart disease, peripheral vascular disease, research, women and heart disease, stroke, and "words of caution."

Heart Care Index

http://www.advocatehealth.com/healthinfo/articles/heartcare//index.html

How your heart works, common problems, reducing your risk for heart disease, treatment options and recovery.

Heart Information Network

http://www.heartinfo.org/

Loads of information, including: articles on cardiovascular diseases, a drug database, CPR instructions, frequently asked questions (FAQs) about heart disease, heart products and services, heart attack guide, heart failure guide, hypertension guide, news, nutrition guide, risk assessment, and an "Ask Us" area for e-mail question submission and response from qualified physicians.

Heart Preview Gallery

http://sln2.fi.edu/biosci/preview/heartpreview.html

Learn all about the heart, read through and add your own heart-healthy recipe, ponder the heart in culture and poetry, listen to heartbeats, watch open heart surgery, view heart images, and check out links. Made to be an interactive tour.

Synapse's Heart Sounds

http://www.medlib.com/spi/coolstuff2.htm

Listen to normal heart sounds, "innocent murmurs," and defective heart sounds.

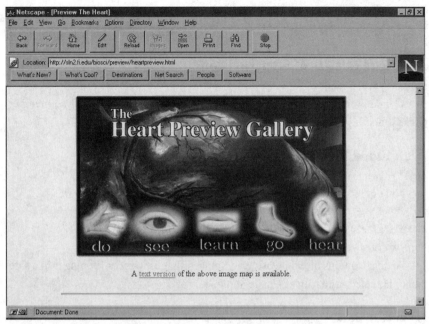

The Heart Preview Gallery. *http://sln2.fi.edu/biosci/preview/heartpreview.html*

Heart Murmurs

Heart Murmur

http://www.healthlinkusa.com/141.htm

Links to websites which may include treatments, diagnosis, prevention, support groups, e-mail lists, message boards, personal stories, risk factors, statistics, research and more. Heart disease risk factors, heart damage protection and answers to questions such as, "What causes a heart murmur?"

Heart Murmurs

http://www.aomc.org/HOD2/general/heart-HEART-4.html

Information on heart murmurs and when they might be a concern.

Three Criteria Key to Referral for Heart Murmur

http://patient.medscape.com/IMNG/PediatricNews/1998/v.32.n11/pn3211.08.01.html

The general pediatrician most needs to refer heart murmurs where there is also a click, a hyperactive precordium, or an abnormal ECG, reports this article from *Pediatric News.*

Hypertension (High Blood Pressure)

American Society of Hypertension

http://www.ash-us.org/

Contains information relating to the Society's mission, as well as member benefits and highlights from their annual scientific meetings.

High Blood Pressure Quiz

http://www.mayohealth.org/mayo/9808/htm/highblood/index.html

Nine questions that determine what you know about blood pressure.

How to Keep Your Blood Pressure Under Control

http://medicalreporter.health.org/tmr0595/hypertens0595.html

Article explains blood pressure and makes suggestions for keeping it in a safe range. Directed primarily at a male audience.

Hypertension

http://www.mayo.edu/hypertension/hyper1.htm

Patient and clinical information from the Mayo Clinic's Division of Hypertension.

Hypertension Articles

http://www.cardio.com/categories/hypertensionarticles.htm

A collection of online articles about high blood pressure, assembled by the Cardiovascular Institute of the South. You can also access information on other heart health subjects from this site.

Hypertension Information Center

http://pharminfo.com/disease/cardio/HT_info.html

From PharmInfoNet, this site contains information and background, research, articles, discussion group archives, and information on drugs used to treat high blood pressure.

Hypertension Network

http://www.bloodpressure.com/

Information about the latest research on hypertension, risk factors and lifestyle issues, basic questions and answers, discussion forums, physician registry, glossary and product description.

Possible Clue to High Blood Pressure in African-Americans

http://www.biomed.lib.umn.edu/hmed/980619_hbp.html

Citation for an article which shows that black Americans respond differently than whites do to nitric oxide, a body chemical which relaxes blood vessels during times of stress. This may explain why blacks are more prone to have high blood pressure than whites.

Primary Care Teaching Module: Treatment of Hypertension

http://www.med.stanford.edu/school/DGIM/Teaching/Modules/HTN.html

Outline of an online course.

Primary Pulmonary Hypertension

http://www.nhlbi.nih.gov/health/public/lung/other/pph.htm

Text of a report about Primary Pulmonary Hypertension, a rare lung disorder.

The Puzzle of Hypertension in African-Americans

http://www.sciam.com/1999/0299issue/0299cooper.html

This feature article shows that genes do not explain the high rate of hypertension in black Americans, for although African-Americans have a high rate of hypertension (35% of adults!), Africans do not. Instead, it must be due to external factors, which the article considers.

Organizations

American College of Cardiology

http://www.acc.org/

Patient education and clinical information for clinicians, as well as American College of Cardiology program and membership facts.

American Heart Association

http://americanheart.org/

Includes American Heart Association (AHA) information, heart diseases and treatments, stroke prevention and recovery, risk assessment, news, and the *Heart and Stroke Guide from A-Z*. A great heart reference for professionals, patients, families and the general public.

The Mended Hearts, Inc.
http://www.mendedhearts.org/

Support and help for heart disease patients and their families. Contains healthy heart articles and information on local chapters, national activities, and the Mended Hearts' visiting program.

National Heart, Lung and Blood Institute
http://www.nhlbi.nih.gov/index.htm

This site describes the NHLBI's research and educational activities, and provides cardiovascular, lung, blood and sleep disorders information for patients, the general public and health care professionals.

National Stroke Association
http://www.stroke.org/

Stroke prevention, treatment, rehabilitation, research and support. Also includes a quiz, and links to additional resources.

Society of Cardiovascular and Interventional Radiology
http://www.scvir.org/

These physicians favor interventional or minimally invasive procedures. This website offers member information, grant guidelines, and educational materials for health care professionals, and provides patient information.

The Vascular Disease Foundation
http://www.vdf.org/

Site offers Foundation news, a discussion of peripheral arterial disease and important issues, and links to related sites and sites that can help you assess risk factors for disease.

Pacemakers

Ask the Mayo Expert
http://www.mayohealth.org/mayo/askphys/qa971226.htm

Questions about pacemakers are answered by a Mayo Clinic physician.

How Pacemakers Work and Why They Are Needed

http://www.cardio.com/articles/pacemakr.htm

Describes some of the basic types of pacemakers and how they work.

Intermedics Twenty Questions about Pacemakers

http://www.imed.com/twentyqu.html

Answers key questions and discusses what to expect from pacemaker surgery, and what to expect as a pacemaker wearer.

Right in Rhythm

http://www.hoag.org/TYHTodaysPace.html

General information on pacemakers, plus "Pacemakers Myths and Facts."

Publications

eHeart

http://heart.bmjjournals.com/

View the current issue of *Heart* online (formerly the *British Heart Journal*), search the archives, check out their resources and receive "customised @lerts."

HeartWeb

http://webaxis.com/heartweb/

Online peer-reviewed cardiology journal with original contributions and regular departments. In addition, there is HeartWeb continuing medical education, online multimedia presentations, free MEDLINE access, database and search engine.

Journal of the American College of Cardiology

http://www-east.elsevier.com/jac/Menu.html

View the table of contents with abstracts, and the full text of selected articles for the current month. Search the archives, and find out about ordering information.

The Online Journal of Cardiology

http://www.mmip.mcgill.ca/heart/index.html

Medical teachings, patient wellness and caregiver resources. Includes peer review articles and abtracts, medical software and more.

Raynaud's

Facts about Raynaud's Phenomenon

http://www.nhlbi.nih.gov/health/public/blood/other/raynaud.htm

Online pamphlet from the National Heart, Lung and Blood Institute.

Raynaud's Disease Home Page

http://www.atlantic.edu/Raynaud/rayhompg.htm

General information, including symptoms and treatment, as well as resource links, questions and personal stories about patients who suffered from Raynaud's disease.

Raynaud's Foundation

http://members.aol.com/raynauds/

Information about the Foundation and about Raynaud's phenomenon, a circulatory disorder that causes a loss of blood flow to the fingers, toes, nose and/or ears.

Raynaud's Syndrome

http://www.onhealth.com/ch1/resource/conditions/item,707.asp

Introduction, symptoms and treatment.

Resources for Professionals

American Heart Association Scientific Statements

http://www.americanheart.org/Scientific/statements/

Scientific reports, advisories, guidelines, executive summary and recommendations issued from the American Heart Association with the American College of Cardiology for those who treat patients with heart conditions. Subjects covered start with: angioplasty, anticoagulants, antioxidants, arrhythmias, aspirin, blood pressure, children, cholesterol, and congenital heart defects. Index includes much more.

CARDIAX

http://www.med.umich.edu/lrc/cardiax/cardiax.html

CARDIAX is a computer-aided instructional program of 20 planned cases in basic cardiology. It uses text, digital images, audio and videos to teach cardiac diagnosis.

Cardiology Compass

http://www.cardiologycompass.com/

Extensive compilation of cardiovascular information resources. Well organized. Includes a large section on education resources.

Cardiology INDEX

http://www.ability.org.uk/cardiolo.html

Long list of sites, alphabetized. Also includes chat rooms.

Medscape Cardiology Home Page

http://www.medscape.com/Home/Topics/cardiology/cardiology.html

Today's cardiology news, treatment updates, practice guidelines and articles.

MedWebPlus's Cardiology Sites

http://www.medwebplus.com/subject/Cardiology.html

Many links to heart-related sites for clinicians, patients and the general public.

NHLBI Publications for Health Professionals

http://www.nhlbi.nih.gov/health/pubs/pub_prof.htm

A great number of NHLBI publications are available for health professionals at this site. Includes reports, studies and facts on asthma, blood, cholesterol, the heart, heart attacks and more, from the clinician's perspective.

WebDoctor: Cardiology Links

http://www.gretmar.com/webdoctor/Cardiology.html

Resources for medical professionals. Includes general resources, associations and societies, clinical practice guidelines, multimedia teaching files, pediatric cardiology, journals and computers in cardiology.

Risk Factors

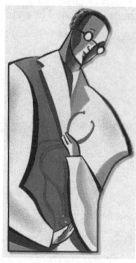

Coronary Heart Disease Risk Caclulator.
http://www.betterhealth.com/sponsors/zocor/calculator.html

Coronary Heart Disease Risk Calculator
http://www.betterhealth.com/sponsors/zocor/calcul ator.html

Input some personal data to find out your risk of heart disease.

CPRC Pages
http://www.chebucto.ns.ca/Health/CPRC/ contents.html

Discusses the risk factors that often lead to the development of atherosclerosis and coronary heart disease.

Early Warning Signs of a Heart Attack
http://www.columbia-utah.com/heartattack.html

If you notice one or more of these signs, site suggests that you get help right away.

Healthy Heart Index
http://www.thirdage.com/features/healthy/heart/

Answer a set of questions to determine your risk for heart disease.

Personality and Heart Attacks
http://medhlp.netusa.net/news/HC/00176132.htm

Those with the personality known as "Type A" have long been known to be at greater risk for heart attack, but this interview reveals that "Type D's" are also three times more likely than "non-D's" to suffer from a heart attack.

Risk Factors and Coronary Heart Disease
http://www.americanheart.org/Heart_and_Stroke_A_Z_Guide/riskfact.html

Scientific position statetment from the American Heart Association.

Takeheart Health Check

http://www.takeheart.co.uk/

Provides an estimate of the likelihood of your developing coronary heart disease, together with advice on how best to reduce this risk given your particular circumstances.

Why You Shouldn't Worry about Things Like Sex

http://www.mayohealth.org/mayo/9609/htm/triggers.htm

Although the risk of heart attack in the two hours following sexual intercourse doubles, it is still a very tiny risk.

Your Risk of a Heart Attack

http://www.miamiheartresearch.org/risk.html

Learn more about the eight major risk factors for heart attack.

Stroke

American Stroke Association

http://americanheart.org/Stroke/index.html

A division of the American Heart Association, the ASA seeks to be a complete source for information on stroke. It describes risk factors, warning signs, conditions and treatments, recovery, statistics and more.

Heart and Stroke A-Z Guide

http://www.americanheart.org/Heart_and_Stroke_A_Z_Guide/

Consumer information from the American Heart Association.

The Internet Stroke Center

http://www.neuro.wustl.edu/stroke/

Updated information about stroke care and research for health care professionals, patients and their family members. Includes many links.

On Being Struck by a Stroke

http://www.strokesurvivor.org/

A personal story and Internet links. Includes information on a stroke survivor discussion group.

Professional Stroke Links

http://www.neuro.wustl.edu/stroke/prof-links.htm

Site lists organizations, professional societies, journals and more.

Stroke

http://dna2z.com/projects/stroke/index.html

A teaching presentation designed for patients, their families, and for members of a stroke rehabilitation team.

Stroke Education

http://www.mayo.edu/cerebro/education/stroke.html

From the Mayo Clinic, this site explains what stroke is, and covers stroke warning signs, symptoms, treatment, effects, recovery and prevention.

Stroke Support & Information

http://members.aol.com/scmmlm/main.htm

Here is an opportunity to share your experiences and to find information about stroke treatment, rehabilitation and job resources. You can also find out about a stroke support chat group and e-mail support for caregivers.

Treatments for Heart Disease

About Angioplasty and Bypass Surgery

http://www.merck.com/disease/heart/cheartdis/angioplasty.html

Discusses these two popular invasive treatments for coronary disease.

Angioplasty Questions and Answers

http://www.scvir.org/patient/pibs/angiopl.htm

This procedure is explained by the Society of Cardiovascular and Interventional Radiology.

Bypass Surgery, Coronary Artery

http://www.americanheart.org/Heart_and_Stroke_A_Z_Guide/bypass.html

Describes coronary artery bypass surgery.

Drugs for Treating Cardiovascular Disease

http://www.heartinfo.org/resources/drugs.htm

Check out what your doctor has prescribed for you.

Minimally Invasive Heart Surgery

http://www.americanheart.org/Scientific/statements/1996/1115.html

The American Heart Association's medical/scientific statement discusses limited access (or minimally invasive) coronary artery surgery.

The Noninvasive Heart Center

http://www.heartprotect.com/

The Center has been successful at treating heart disease noninvasively; i.e., through low-blood pressure drugs, beta blockers, calcium channel blockers, nitrogylcerine diuretics, ACE-inhibitors and other drugs. This group believes information proves that noninvasive tests are extremely sensitive in the early detection of heart disease, and that bypass surgery and angioplasty are rarely needed.

Survival Rates Found to Be the Same for Heart Attack Patients Treated with Primary Angioplasty and Drug Therapy

http://www.heartinfo.org/primangioart.htm

Comments on the debate: "This study is an extremely important one which addresses an ongoing debate in medicine, i.e.: should people with a heart attack be given a 'clot-busting' medication or [be] taken immediately for catheterization to open up the coronary artery with a balloon?"

What to Expect, Short and Long Term, Following Bypass Surgery

http://www.cardio.com/articles/bypass.htm

General information on this major surgery.

Varicose Veins

MediData Varicose Vein Information

http://www.medi-data.co.uk/

What varicose veins are, why they occur, how to test for them and different methods of treating them.

Patient Information on Varicose Veins

http://members.aol.com/gvg97/vvinfo.htm

Presents varicose vein causes, treatment (especially surgical), recurrence and links to related sites.

Varicose Veins

http://healthy.net/library/Books/Healthyself/varicoseveins.htm

Self-care tips for those who suffer from this condition.

Varicose Veins and Pregnancy

http://digitalstarlight.com/tnpc/parentalk/pregnancy/preg30.html

Suggestions as to what to do to avoid varicose veins during pregnancy.

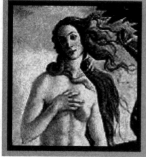

VEINSonline.com
http://www.veinsonline.com/

VEINSonline.com

http://www.veinsonline.com/

Information about venous disorders for the general public. This site offers physician referral and before and after photos, as well as answers to frequently asked questions about varicose veins, spider veins and the treatment options available.

Vessel Disorders

http://www.bu.edu/cohis/cardvasc/vessel/vessels.htm

Learn about heart problems and blood vessels: e.g., *What can go wrong with the arteries? What can go wrong with the veins?*

Vascular & Circulatory Disorders

American Venous Forum

http://www.venous-info.com/1avf.htm

This is an academic forum for physicians interested in research, education, and clinical investigation in the field of venous diseases. It provides clinical information, links, continuing medical education opportunities, a newsletter and a "case of the month."

Angioweb

http://www.angioweb.fr/english/index.html

This website is devoted to angiology resources for researchers, clinicians, doctors and students. It provides medical meeting information, newsgroups and mailing lists, databases, medical journals, vascular sites and medical societies, as well as teaching and professional training materials.

Circulatory Diseases

http://heartdisease.about.com/msubcirc.htm

Overviews of several circulatory diseases, including temporal arteritis, deep vein thrombosis, leg ulcers, Raynaud's, varicose veins and peripheral vascular disease.

Dr. S.'s Vascular Disease & Hyperhidrosis Web Page

http://www.dnai.com/~szarnick/

The latest information about various treatment options for venous, arterial and sympathetic disorders.

Mayo Gonda Vascular Center

http://www.mayo.edu/cv/wwwpg_cv/gonda/gonda_hp.htm

Information on this Center and its services, with links to articles for patients.

Vascular Disorders

http://dmoz.org/Health/Conditions_and_Diseases/Vascular_Disorders/

This web search engine has a number of links to different sites on vascular diseases, vascular surgery, vascular testing, varicose veins and related conditions.

Vascular Surgery Answers

http://www.visi.com/~irm/

Introduces you to the basics of circulatory disease, diagnosis and treatment options, in plain English.

Women and Heart Disease

Facts about Heart Disease and Women
http://www.pharminfo.com/disease/cardio/HD_women.html

Heart disease is not a "male thing," in fact, according to this site, "one in ten American women 45 to 64 years of age has some form of heart disease, and this increases to one in five women over 65. Another 1.6 million women have had a stroke."

The Healthy Heart Handbook for Women
http://www.nih.gov/health/chip/nhlbi/heart/

Identifies factors that especially make a woman at higher risk for heart disease.

Heart Disease: A Different Story for Women Than for Men?
http://pharminfo.com/pubs/ccr/ccr1_49.html

CardioConsults article that summarizes a paper published in the *Archives of Internal Medicine*.

Take Wellness to Heart
http://women.americanheart.org/

The American Heart Association's site that addresses women's heart disease and stroke concerns.

HISTORY OF MEDICINE

African-Americans in Medicine

Dr. Charles R. Drew

http://www.pluggedin.org/toolkit/projectsandgraphics/blackhist/drew.html

Biography of the first doctor to do a blood transfusion and to initiate storage of blood in "blood banks."

Faces of Science: African Americans in the Sciences

http://www.lib.lsu.edu/lib/chem/display/faces.html

List and biographies of African-Americans who have contributed to medical and other sciences.

History of African-Americans in White

http://coe.ohio-state.edu/edpl/courses/bgordon/nurses.html

Text about African-Americans in nursing. Also offers suggestions on using the material as a course for young students.

Medical Breakthroughs

http://www.kcstar.com/krt/bdoctors/bdoctors.htm

Profiles of three important African-Americans who made contributions to the medical sciences.

African-Americans in Science, Medicine and Technology

http://sun3.lib.uci.edu/~afrexh/ProfileList.html

Brief biosketches of several African-Americans in the health field.

Ancient Greek & Roman Medicine

The Aesclepion
http://www.indiana.edu/~ancmed/intro.HTM
Web page devoted to the study of ancient medicine.

Ancient Greek Medicine
http://members.tripod.com/~JFrazz9/med.html
Discusses Hippocrates, and the Hippocratic oath.

Ancient Medicine Hypertexts
http://web1.ea.pvt.k12.pa.us/medant/hyprtxts.htm
Hypertext translations of significant ancient medical texts, including those written by Hippocrates and Galen.

Antiqua Medicina: From Homer to Vesalius
http://www.med.virginia.edu/hs-library/historical/antiqua/anthome.html
An online exhibition prepared in conjunction with the colloquium, "Antiqua Medicina: Aspects in Ancient Medicine," held at the University of Virginia.

Medicine in Ancient Greece
http://viator.ucs.indiana.edu/~ancmed/greekmenu.HTM
Scholarly papers covering such topics as: the foundations of Hippocratic medicine, illness of maidens, temple cures, and midwives in the Roman world.

Anesthesia

Anesthesia History
http://www.asahq.org/asarc/hotlinks/history.html
From the American Society of Anesthesiology, this page provides links to a variety of online resources dealing with the history of anesthesiology.

Anesthesia History Files
http://www.anes.uab.edu/aneshist/aneshist.htm
Links and information.

Childbirth

Brief History of Nurse-Midwifery in the U.S.
http://www.acnm.org/focus/history.htm
"The profession of nurse-midwifery was established in the early 1920's as a response to the alarming rate of infant and maternal mortality in the U.S." Information from the American College of Nurse-Midwives.

Cesarean Section - a Brief History
http://www.nlm.nih.gov/exhibition/ cesarean/cesarean_1.html
The material at this site was originally included in a brochure accompanying an exhibit at the National Library of Medicine. Along with interesting text, it shows some ancient woodcuts and prints.

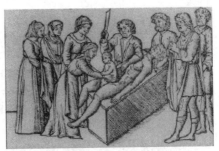

One of the earliest depictions of a Cesarean birth. At: **Cesarean Section - A Brief History**. *http://www.nlm.nih.gov/exhibition/ cesarean/cesarean_2.html*

Some Obstetrical History
http://www.umanitoba.ca/outreach/manitoba_womens_health/hist1.htm
The subtitle to this site is: "Dying to Have a Baby: the History of Childbirth."

Chinese & Asian Medicine

Chi Med: The History of Chinese Medicine Web Page
http://www.albion.edu/fac/hist/chimed/
This site is managed by an international group of scholars who study ancient Chinese medicine, and it includes a directory of libraries, a collection of electronic resources, bibliographies, syllabi, news and events.

History of Traditional Chinese Medicine
http://www.mic.ki.se/China.html
Includes many links to Chinese medical history, and some links to sites about other Asian medical traditions.

Tibetan Medicine Links and Resources
http://dharma-haven.org/tibetan/tibetan-medicine-resources.htm
Contains lots of links for study and for health.

Traditional Chinese Medicine
http://www.healthy.net/clinic/therapy/Chinmed/index.html
Includes a history of acupuncture and other resources.

Dentistry & Surgery

Cyber Museum of Neurosurgery
http://www.neurosurgery.org/cybermuseum/summary.html
Leaders, tools and breakthroughs in brain surgery.

Dental History
http://www.catalog.com/dentist/denhis.html
Site contains articles which have been excerpted from the book, *World of Invention or World of Scientific Discovery*. It discusses the history of the dental drill, false teeth, tooth extractions, toothbrushes, and more.

A History of Surgery
http://www.medinfo.ufl.edu/other/profmed/slides/pm021599/index.html
Presented in the form of a slide show.

Medical Antiques: Instruments for Surgery and Dentistry
http://medicalantiques.com/
Lots of photos and articles. With good reason, the beginning of this site has the following message: "be thankful you live in today's medical world."

Egyptian Medicine

History of Ancient Egyptian Medicine
http://www.mic.ki.se/Egypt.html
Long list of links from the Karolinska Institute.

The Medicine of Egypt
http://www.teleport.com/~sp indel/Egypt/EgyptPAge.html
The ancient Egyptians were one of the first peoples to have physicians. Site discusses the history of medicine in ancient Egypt, with images.

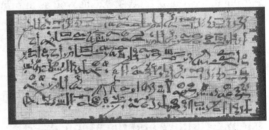
Ancient Egyptian papyrus discussing treatment of wounds. At: The Medicine of Egypt. http://www.teleport.com/~spindel/Egypt/EgyptPAge.html

Medicine
http://emuseum.mankato.msus.edu/prehistory/egypt/dailylife/medicine.html
Discusses Egyptian medicine, and even provides recipes for some ancient cures.

Florence Nightingale

Florence Nightingale
http://www.dnai.com/~borneo/nightingale/
Country Joe McDonald's tribute to Florence Nightingale.

Florence Nightingale Museum
http://www.florence-nightingale.co.uk/
Museum devoted to the founder of modern nursing.

Selection of Letters Written by Florence Nightingale
http://www.kumc.edu/service/clendening/florence/about.html
Contains 37 letters written in Florence Nightingale's own hand. Links to other resources.

Islamic Medicine

Articles and Links on Islamic Medicine and Science
http://muslimsonline.com/science/
Includes an article entitled, "Muslim Scientists, Mathematicians and Astronomers 700 to 1500 A.D.," as well as information addressing Islamic views on important medical issues.

Classical Islamic Biomedicine
http://www.mic.ki.se/Arab.html
Dozens of links to sites about Islamic medicine and sciences.

Islamic Culture and the Medical Arts
http://www.nlm.nih.gov/exhibition/islamic_medical/islamic_00.html
This is the online version of a brochure accompanying a National Library of Medicine's exhibit in celebration of the 900th anniversary of the oldest Arabic medical manuscript in the library's collections.

Libraries & Museums

Bakken Library and Museum
http://bakkenmuseum.org/
The Bakken Library and Museum is devoted to teaching and understanding the history, cultural context, and applications of electricity and magnetism to the fields of science and medicine.

History of Medicine Division
http://www.nlm.nih.gov/hmd/hmd.html
The National Library of Medicine provides a number of collections, images, exhibits and seminars, as well as profiles in science and frequently asked questions.

Images from the History of Medicine
http://wwwihm.nlm.nih.gov/
Nearly 60,000 photographs, artwork and printed texts drawn from the large collection at the NLM History of Medicine Division. Search for images or browse.

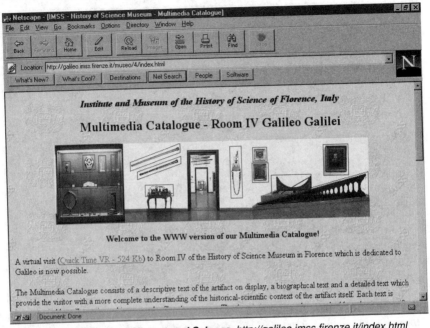

Institute and Museum of History and Science. http://galileo.imss.firenze.it/index.html

Institute and Museum of History and Science
http://galileo.imss.firenze.it/index.html

Homepage of this institute and museum located in Florence, Italy. Includes online exhibitions, news, research activities and publications, along with multimedia tours of the museum, general information and links.

Johns Hopkins University: The Historical Collection
http://www.welch.jhu.edu/ihm/

This site provides access to the library of the Institute of History of Medicine, electronic and other reference sources, and information on the Department of History of Science, Medicine and Technology.

Museum of the History of Science
http://info.ox.ac.uk/departments/hooke/

There are a number of online exhibits at this site (e.g., "The Geometry of War: 1500-1750"), as well as information on the museum, the museum newsletter and an image library.

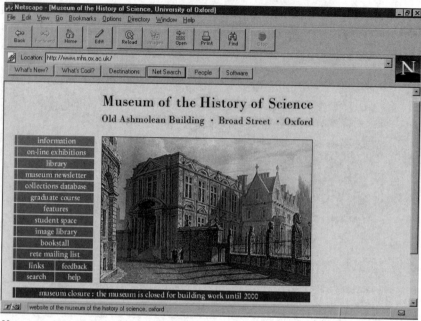

Museum of the History of Science. http://info.ox.ac.uk/departments/hooke/

Online Medical Heritage Center

http://bones.med.ohio-state.edu/heritage/

Includes a searchable list of archives, Center stats and Internet links, as well as a newsletter.

The Truman G. Blocker, Jr. History of Medicine Collections

http://www.utmb.edu:80/galveston/universities/utmb/mml/blocker.html

Site contains links as well as images of library holdings, which include rare books, archives and manuscripts, visual materials, and artifacts.

Yale Historical Medical Library

http://info.med.yale.edu/library/historical/

This libarary contains a large collection of rare medical books, journals, pamphlets, manuscripts, photographs and other artifacts.

Links and Other Resources

Galaxy's History of Medicine

http://www.galaxy.com/galaxy/Medicine/History.html

Collection of links to articles, books, collections and more.

HISTLINE

http://www.nlm.nih.gov/pubs/factsheets/histline.html

This is the National Library of Medicine's database that indexes U.S. and foreign publications on the history of health-related professions, sciences, specialties, individuals, institutions, drugs, and diseases in all parts of the world and all historic periods.

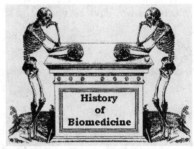

History of Biomedicine

http://www.mic.ki.se/History.html

Good starting point to jump to other sites about medicine and health care from ancient times to the present day.

History of Biomedicine.
http://www.mic.ki.se/History.html

History of Science, Technology and Medicine

http://www.asap.unimelb.edu.au/hstm/hstm_ema.htm

E-mail lists and newsgroups.

Medical History on the Internet

http://www.anes.uab.edu/medhist.htm

Great list of links to medical history sites and specialties, from Acupuncture to Women's Health.

MedWebplus's History of Medicine

http://www.medwebplus.com/subject/History_of_Medicine.html

Links to over 300 Internet sites related to the history of medicine.

Overview of HealthCare's History

http://www.infinityheart.com/overview.html

Timeline begins in 1846 with the convention in New York that later became the American Medical Association.

Primary Care Internet Guide to Medical History
http://www.uib.no:80/isf/guide/history.htm

Long list of web resources includes mail lists, libraries, documents, and museum links.

Scientific and Medical Antiques Links
http://www.utmem.edu/personal/thjones/sci_ant.htm

A collection of information relating to scientific and medical antiques. It includes telescopes, astronomy, microscopes, scales, electrical and magnetic items, calculating, surveying, navigation, meteorology, maps, globes, sliderules, astronomy, surgical instruments, bloodletting, pharmaceuticals and medical chests, electrotherapy devices, and more.

Native Americans

Aztec Medicine
http://northcoast.com/~spdtom/a-med.html

The table of contents for this online text links you to sections on the Aztec diet, medicines, mental health, practitioners and deities. Also offers a bibliography and index.

Health and Disease in the New World
http://marauder.millersv.edu/~columbus/data/art/MICOZZI1.ART

Text of article discussing the decimation of indigenous Americans due to health problems accompanying the arrival of European settlers.

"If You Knew the Conditions"
http://www.nlm.nih.gov/exhibition/if_you_knew/if_you_knew_01.html

Exhibition showing the history of health care to Native Americans.

The Roots of North American Medicine
http://www.YvwiiUsdinvnohii.net/articles/medroots.html

A peek into the health knowledge base of the Native Americans.

Organizations

American Association for the History of Medicine

http://muse.jhu.edu/journals/bulletin_of_the_history_of_medicine/information/AAHM.html

Information on how to receive this organization's *Bulletin*.

History of Science Society

http://depts.washington.edu/hssexec/

This is the world's largest society dedicated to understanding science, technology, medicine, and their interactions with society in a historical context. Anyone may join. Among the resources at this site are a history of science and technology database, and strategies on teaching the topic.

Pharmacy

History of Pharmacy Museum

http://www.pharmacy.arizona.edu/museum/index.html

Even if you can't visit the real thing at the University of Arizona, you can take a virtual tour of this museum. It houses a collection of over 60,000 bottles, original drug containers, books, store fixtures, and artifacts from Arizona's territorial days.

Marvin Samson Center for the History of Pharmacy

http://pharminfo.com/gallery/pcps.html

A selection of antique pharmacy jars and murals kept at the Philadelphia College of Pharmacy and Science.

Psychology

Freud Museum of London
http://www.freud.org.uk/

Take a virtual tour of 20 Maresfield Gardens, Hempstead: the home of Sigmund Freud and his family when they escaped from Austria in 1938. Freud's library and study have been preserved to be the way they were when he was alive.

History of Psychology
http://www.WPI.EDU/~histpsy/

Journal published by the American Psychological Association.

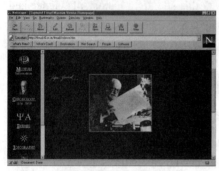

Sigmund Freud Museum Vienna
http://freud.t0.or.at/freud/index-e.htm

Museum information, exhibits, media library and information on Freud. An online service of the Sigmund-Freud-Society.

Sigmund Freud Museum Vienna.
http://freud.t0.or.at/freud/index-e.htm

Publications

19th Century Scientific American Online
http://www.history.rochester.edu/Scientific_American/

You can access past issues from as far back as August 28, 1845.

History of Science, Technology and Medicine Electronic Journals
http://www.asap.unimelb.edu.au/hstm/hstm_jou.htm

Dozens of journal links are provided.

Radiology

X-Ray Century

http://www.cc.emory.edu/X-RAYS/century.htm

Looking back to December 1, 1896. Contains book information as well as articles from other editions of the _X-Ray Century_ originally published in the 1890's.

Unusual Sites

History of the Condom and Technical Developments

http://www.durex.com/study/history.html

This site is interesting, but also commercial.

Museum of Contraception

http://www.salon1999.com/07/features/contra.html

Description of one writer's visit.

Museum of Questionable Medical Devices

http://www.mtn.org:80/quack/

See the museum holdings, which include items such as the foot operated breast enlarger pump and "violet ray devices," learn stories of "great American quacks," and much more. It is "the largest collection of medical chicanery and mayhem ever assembled under one roof."

Women in Medicine

4000 Years of Women in Science

http://www.astr.ua.edu/4000WS/4000ws.html

Includes biographies, references and images. The list emphasizes women of the past, most pre-20th century.

Clara Barton Homestead

http://www.cr.nps.gov/nr/travel/pwwmh/ma41.htm

Clara Barton was the founder and first president of the American Red Cross.

Distinguished Women of Past and Present: Health and Medicine

http://www.netsrq.com/~dbois/health.html

Collection of profiles of famous women in health and medicine.

The History of Women and Science, Health and Technology

gopher://gopher.adp.wisc.edu/11/.browse/.METAGLSHW/

A bibliographic guide.

Women in Healing and the Medical Professions

http://www.umanitoba.ca/outreach/manitoba_womens_health/wominmed.htm

Although men's names predominate in the history of medicine, more than half of the people involved in health care have always been women. This article discusses women's contributions to medicine.

HIV/AIDS

Advocacy

ACT-UP New York
http://www.actupny.org/

This group seeks to stop AIDS by actively desiminating information, by demonstrating and by uniting people. Site provides AIDS scientific, political and social news and research, and recent ACT-UP activities. Links to ACT-UP organizations based in other U.S. and foreign cities.

AIDS Action
http://www.aidsaction.org/

This organization advocates for greater "responsible federal policy for improved care and services, robust medical research and effective prevention" of HIV/AIDS. It is a network of 3200 community-based organizations.

ArtAIDS
http://www.illumin.co.uk/artaids/

"A creative website commemorating and celebrating the fight against AIDS." It features art that expresses the individual's experience with AIDS.

Estate Project for Artists with AIDS
http://artistswithaids.org/

Uses digital technology to document and present the artwork created by artists living with HIV, or who have been lost to AIDS. View the virtual collection and curated exhibition. You need Internet Explorer as your browser to view the art.

Gay Men's Health Crisis on the Web
http://www.gmhc.org/

Internet home for the New York-based group at the forefront of AIDS advocacy and support. This site offers AIDS news, support, resources, prevention and advocacy.

Mother's Voices United to End AIDS
http://www.mvoices.org/index_new.html

Advocates for improved AIDS prevention efforts, medical treatment and research towards a cure.

Antibody Testing

HIV Home Test Information
http://www.koool.com/hivtest.html

Details on this home test which is available for purchase. Simply prick your finger to obtain a drop of blood to complete the test.

HIV Testing
http://www.gmhc.org/stopping/testing.html

This online brochure explains what test results mean and discusses the advantages and disadvantages of being tested for HIV.

HIV Testing: The Body
http://www.thebody.com/testing.html

News, links and information on HIV antibody testing. A valuable feature is that items are dated and the source is identified.

HIV Testing: Museum of Science and Industry
http://www.msichicago.org/ed/AIDS/hivtst1.htm

This site encourages students to gain experience with professional lab results and guides them to actually interpret lab results. It describes the ELISA and Western Blot blood serum tests, provides sample results, instructions for teachers, and worksheets and handouts for students.

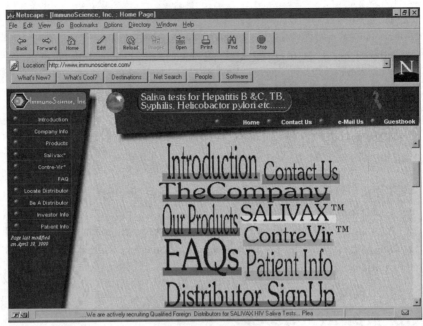

ImmunoScience, Inc. *http://www.immunoscience.com*

HIV/AIDS Diagnosis

http://www.jeffersonhealth.org/diseases/inf_diseases/aidsdiag.htm

Basic information on HIV testing and AIDS.

Home Access

http://www.homeaccess.com/hiv/main.html

At-home testing kit information, and links to related sites.

Home Pharmacy

http://www.homehivtest.com/

Three- and seven-day HIV test results, pre- and post-test counseling, and condom purchasing.

ImmunoScience, Inc.

http://www.immunoscience.com/

Site from the makers of SALIVAX HIV test, which uses saliva to test for HIV. Patient information includes a long list of links.

Testing for HIV

http://www.HIVpositive.com/f-TestingHIV/TestingMenu.html

Information on HIV testing and viral load testing; counseling checklist for physicians; FDA approved HIV tests.

Clinical Trials

See also: Clinical Trials.

ACTIS: AIDS Clinical Trials Information Service

http://www.actis.org/

Information on federal and private clinical research trials for adults and children with HIV/AIDS. Provides a long list of other sites which discuss AIDS clinical trials.

General Resources

AEGIS

http://www.aegis.com/

"The largest HIV knowledgebase in the world." Fully indexed and searchable. Includes a daily summary of AIDS news, articles, statistics, life cycle, and library.

AIDS FAQ/Gopher

gopher://gpagopher.who.ch/11/aidsfaq/

Frequently asked questions, in ten different files, from sci.med.aids, the international newsgroup on Acquired Immune Deficiency Syndrome.

AIDS Resource List

http://www.teleport.com/~celinec/aids.shtml

Includes regional, national and international sites covering many aspects of HIV/AIDS.

AIDS Virtual Library

http://planetq.com/aidsvl/index.html

This page addresses the social, political, and medical aspects of AIDS, HIV, and related issues.

The Body: A Multimedia AIDS and HIV Information Resource
http://www.thebody.com/index.shtml

This site provides the basics on AIDS and AIDS prevention, treatment updates, and research efforts. It also covers conferences and quality-of-life issues, and offers AIDS forums, questions and answers, and information on how to get support from AIDS organizations and hotlines. Search engine helps to sort through the enormous amount of information here.

CAPS: Center for AIDS Prevention Studies
http://www.epibiostat.ucsf.edu/capsweb/

CAPS program information includes prevention fact sheets, bibliographies, sections on how to develop new prevention programs, a survey for use in needs assessment, abstracts of selected relevant articles, and an overview of current behavior research on risk-taking. Links to other sites.

CDC Divisions of HIV/AIDS Prevention
http://www.cdc.gov/nchstp/hiv_aids/dhap.htm

Part of the National Center for HIV, STD and TB Prevention. Site highlights include: statistics, fact sheets, frequently asked questions, publications and slides.

Critical Path AIDS Project, Hypertext Edition
http://www.critpath.org/

A very valuable source of HIV and AIDs information, this site offers treatment and prevention information for researchers, service providers, activists and persons with AIDS (PWAs). It presents news bulletins, research, clinical trials and alternative health treatments, as well as descriptions and links to organizations and publications. This group also has a 24-hour hotline and publishes a newsletter.

Deadly Medicine
http://www.nmia.com/~mdibble

Assemblage of articles that discuss the transmission of HIV/AIDS through blood transfusion and products.

HIV/AIDS Information
http://www.cdcnpin.org/hiv/start.htm

Offers numerous publications, resources, databases, and AIDS news.

HIV/AIDS Information: Putting the Pieces Together
http://www.mcphu.edu/~AIDSinfo/

This is a workshop manual that covers alternative treatments, caregiving, drug therapy, housing, law, nutrition, psychological and spiritual aspects of HIV/AIDS. The manual is designed to function both as a "how to" guide that would be used in conjunction with the workshop, and as a reference resource on HIV/AIDS.

HIV Insite
http://hivinsite.ucsf.edu/

From the University of California at San Francisco's AIDS Research Institute. Daily information on medical and social aspects of AIDS, as well as prevention and resources. Also has state-by-state information on AIDS and HIV subjects and key topics. Includes articles, news, opinions, documents, abstracts, bibliographies and contacts. Some topics include adolescents, medical marijuana, women with AIDS, AIDS in prison, and needle exchange programs.

HIV/AIDS Internet Information Index
http://www.arens.com/hiv/

Directory of HIV/AIDS resources on the World Wide Web. Includes patient care, advocacy organizations, drug, research and clinical trials information; journals and publications; government agencies; research centers and physician links.

HIV/AIDS Program: Links
http://www.metrokc.gov/health/apu/links.htm

Selected sites from the huge number of HIV/AIDS resources available online.

JAMA HIV/AIDS Information Center
http://www.ama-assn.org/special/hiv/

News, literature library, treatment center with guidelines and reviews, educational resources for patients and professionals, prevention facts and policy updates.

Marty Howard's HIV/AIDS Home Page
http://www.smartlink.net/~martinjh/

Important and thorough information. Marty invites you to chat with him directly, and provides links to informational sites, mailing lists, regional and commercial sites; as well as to material on support groups, clinical trials, medications, and Social Security disability.

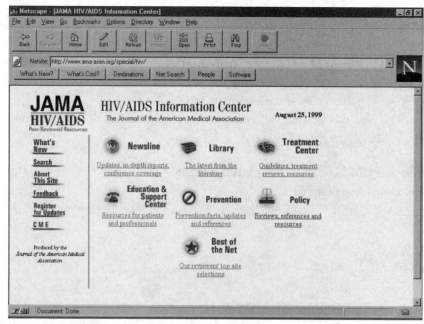

JAMA HIV/AIDS Information Center. http://www.ama-assn.org/special/hiv/

Medscape: HIV/AIDS

http://www.medscape.com/Home/Topics/AIDS/AIDS.html

Peer-reviewed clinical articles and literature reviews. Great source for recent AIDS news, treatment updates, conference summaries, symposia and more. Some items offer continuing medical education (CME) credits.

MedWebplus's Acquired Immunodeficiency Syndrome

http://www.medwebplus.com/subject/Acquired_Immunodeficiency_Syndrome.html

Many links. Includes facilities, organizations, nomenclature specialties, travelling, women's health and much more.

NOAH: AIDS & HIV Resources

http://www.noah.cuny.edu/illness/aids/aidsrsrc.html

Advocacy, medical institutions, government organizations, education, AIDS in daily life, and many Internet links.

Yahoo!'s AIDS/HIV Links

http://www.yahoo.com/Health/Diseases_and_Conditions/AIDS_HIV/

Yahoo! directory is well-organized and easy to use.

Glossaries

AIDS Glossary of Medical, Statistical and Clinical Research Terminology

http://www.teleport.com/~celinec/glossary.htm

Long list that explains different acronyms, drugs, definititions and terminology, from Abdomen to Zovirax.

Glossary of HIV/AIDS-Related Terms

http://www.hivatis.org/glossary/

"Abacavir" to "zinc finger inhibitors"; updated in June, 1999.

History

History and Origins of AIDS & HIV

http://www.avert.org/historyi.htm

"The first cases of AIDS occurred in the USA in 1981, but they provide little information about the source of the disease. There is now clear evidence that the disease AIDS is caused by the virus HIV. So to find the source of AIDS we need to look for the origin of HIV." Informative and precise comments on what is known about the history and origins of AIDS and HIV, as well as a more detailed description of its medical history since 1981.

So Little Time: An AIDS History

http://www.aegis.com/topics/timeline/default.asp

Interesting site traces that the history of AIDS from 1926, when some scientists believe HIV spread from monkeys to humans, to the present. In 1997, 6.4 million deaths (total) had thus far been attributed to AIDS, and the approximate number of HIV-positive people world-wide was 22 million. In 1998, 665,357 new cases of AIDS were diagnosed in the U.S.

International Scene

AIDS Coordination Bureau
http://www.kit.nl/ibd/html/acb.htm

The site of this consortium of nonprofits from the Netherlands contains a document database and maintains a collection of materials dealing with various aspects of HIV/AIDS in developing countries. Among material included are policy papers and directives from international and national organizations, articles, project descriptions and reports, newsletters and periodical publications, conference papers, manuals and guidelines for setting up educational and counseling programs.

AIDS Economics Home Page
http://www.worldbank.org/aids-econ/

Focus of this page is on the public economics of HIV/AIDS prevention and treatments. To this end, it provides special feature reports, announcements, news and papers, most of which were created by the World Bank. See also *http://www.worldbank.org/html/extdr/hivaids/default.htm*, which summarizes the World Bank's response to HIV/AIDS.

HIV.NET
http://hiv.net/hiv/intern/us.htm

The English language version of the European Information Center for HIV and AIDS. Analysis of the European AIDS epidemic, selected abstracts, conference reports and mailing lists. Literature screening service checks 48 scientific journals.

UNAIDS
http://www.us.unaids.org/

The Joint United Nations Programme on HIV/AIDS offers fact sheets, statistics, searchable database, news, and conference information. Partners include UNICEF (U.N. Children's Fund), UNDP (U.N. Development Programme), UNFPA (U.N. Population Fund) UNDCP (U.N. International Drug Control Programme), UNESCO (U.N. Educational, Scientific and Cultural Organization), WHO (World Health Organization) and the World Bank.

Needle Safety

North American Syringe Exchange Network
_http://www.nasen.org/NASEN_II/index.html_

List of syringe exchange programs, HIV/AIDS information, safe sex information, drug policy and drug treatments, and a mailing list.

Project SERO (Syringe Exchange Resources Online)
http://projectsero.org/

Comprehensive online information about needle exchange and its role in preventing the spread of HIV and AIDS, hepatitis and other blood-borne diseases. There is an overview of needle exchange as well as testimonies, a library/news archive, and information on research, statistics and legal issues.

Safe Injection/Vein Care Page
http://www.safeworks.org/Injection/

Images and text carefully demonstrate the safest way to shoot up, if you are going to do so anyway.

Safe Works AIDS Project
http://safeworks.org/

Needle exchange, condoms and safe sex distribution program in Minneapolis/ St. Paul area. Links to sites on the web about needle-exchange programs, by region. A lot of information on how to set up an exchange program.

Safer Injection Manual
http://cures-not-wars.org/junkie/inject.html

Site provides advice on the way to prevent injection-related diseases.

Newly Diagnosed

The Basics
http://www.aegis.com/ni/topics/basics.asp

Advice and information for those who have just found out they are HIV positive.

Testing HIV Positive: What You Should Know

http://www.thebody.com/tdoh/testpos.html

Basic information for those who have been told they are infected with the human immunodeficiency virus.

HIVpositive.com

http://www.HIVpositive.com/index.html

Site addresses issues for those who have HIV. Includes a great deal of information on the virus and AIDS, including Centers for Disease Control statistics and a glossary of terms, nutrition concerns, treatment, pain, opportunistic infections, testing, women and children with HIV, caregivers, drug advisories, resources and assistance, money issues, news, and help in finding a doctor.

On Learning You're HIV Positive

http://www.thebody.com/learning.html

Lots of information for those who have just been diagnosed. Includes articles on choosing a physician, how to tell others about your test results, and how to prevent an opportunistic infection. Also offers hotlines and other services.

Organizations

The Family AIDS Network

http://www.familyaidsnet.org/

Nonprofit organization of AIDS activist Mary Fisher. The Family AIDS Network concentrates its efforts towards AIDS prevention. You can find the latest information on HIV/AIDS news and other resources at this site.

International Association of Physicians in AIDS Care

http://www.iapac.org/

Dialogue and discussion of AIDS issues.

National AIDS Fund

http://www.aidsfund.org/

The primary purpose of the National AIDS Fund is to provide the resources necessary for local AIDS leaders to fight the disease in their communities. Its grants help provide care and services, and the Fund seeks to prevent new infections through education, advocacy, and research.

Office of AIDS Research
http://www.nih.gov/od/oar/

The National Institutes of Health (NIH) Office of AIDS Research plans, coordinates, evaluates, and funds all of the NIH AIDS research projects.

Yahoo! AIDS/HIV Organizations
http://dir.yahoo.com/Health/Diseases_and_Conditions/AIDS_HIV/
Organizations/

Directory to hundreds of organizations. Many of these are regional.

Pathology
See also: Pathology.

San Francisco General Hospital Department of Pathology
http://kersch.ucsf.edu/

Site presents five different case studies related to AIDS. Images are provided, along with a microscopic description, diagnosis and discussion.

Textbook of AIDS Pathology
http://medlib.med.utah.edu/WebPath/TUTORIAL/AIDS/AIDS.html

Includes many images.

Public Policy & Ethics
See also: Needle Safety, earlier in this chapter.

Canadian HIV/AIDS Legal Network
http://www.aidslaw.ca/

Articles and reports discuss the legal, ethical and human rights issues raised by HIV/AIDS.

HIV/AIDS Legislation
http://www.ncvc.org/infolink/info64.htm

Discusses issues raised by the HIV testing of incarcerated individuals.

Information and Resources on HIV-Related Legal, Ethical and Human Rights Issues

http://www.aidslaw.ca/biblio/sites.htm

A long list of links with descriptions, broken down into a variety of subjects.

JAMA Ethics and Policy Update

http://www.ama-assn.org/special/hiv/policy/policy.htm

Collection of opinions and commentary on HIV/AIDS policy, including a review of such key issues as testing, reporting, confidentiality, privacy, disability and discrimination.

Project Inform's Advocacy and Policy Page

http://www.projinf.org/org/advopoli.html

Project Inform provides HIV/AIDS treatment information and advocacy. Site offers action alerts and press releases, and information on managed care and Medicaid HIV/AIDS issues.

Public Policy: HIV/AIDS Around the World

http://www.iapac.org/arndworldpp.html

Articles about the HIV/AIDS situation in Cuba, England, Germany, Mexico, Romania, and Venezuela.

San Francisco AIDS Foundation: Public Policy and Advocacy

http://www.sfaf.org/policy/

Discusses the government's response to AIDS, and offers *HIV Policy Watch*, a monthly publication. Also provides brief updates on ongoing HIV policy issues such as legislation and funding, state and federal HIV prevention efforts, HIV surveillance, needle exchange, the status of various federal health care reform initiatives, housing advocacy, and more.

Publications

AIDS Online

http://www.aidsonline.com/

View the latest issue online, and obtain ordering information. Full text versions available with Adobe Acrobat Reader. A publication of the International AIDS Society.

AIDS Reader

http://www.medscape.com/SCP/TAR/public/journal.TAR.html

A peer-reviewed, clinical journal devoted exclusively to HIV disease and its complications.

AIDSWEEKLY PLUS

http://www.newsfile.com/x1a.htm

Order a sample copy or check out current issue. Subscription information.

Alert! News about AIDS

http://www.mcs.net/~garyh/alert.html

AIDS newsletter from a Christian group.

HIV/AIDS Publications

http://sis.nlm.nih.gov/pagedpub.htm

Describes HIV/AIDS publications of the National Library of Medicine.

Internet Grateful Med/AIDSLINE

http://igm.nlm.nih.gov/

Grateful Med through the Internet. Online computer file containing references to published literature on HIV and AIDS. Indexes journals from biomedical, epidemiological, health care administration, oncologic, social and the behavioral sciences. Citations and abstracts to articles, monographs, meeting papers, government reports, newspaper articles and theses, from 1980 to the present. Online access is free, but there is a charge for each search.

Journal of AIDS/HIV

http://www.medical-library.org/j_aids.htm

This monthly journal includes information in outline-format on general care and opportunistic infections. Also includes a medical library and links to other online journals. While some articles require registration, others do not.

Morbidity and Mortality Weekly Reports on AIDS

http://www.cdc.gov/nchstp/hiv_aids/pubs/mmwr.htm

Monthly publication from the Centers for Disease Control. Abstracts are available online, and full text is, too, if you download Adobe Acrobat Reader.

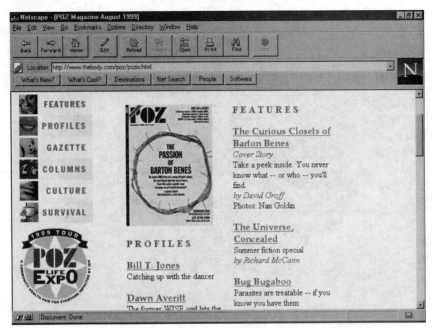

POZ Magazine. *http://www.thebody.com/poz/pozix.html*

Positive Nation - Web Edition

http://www.positivenation.co.uk/

Monthly print and electronic magazine offers features, regular articles and news updates. Strives to represent all people affected by HIV and AIDS in the U.K.

POZ Magazine

http://www.thebody.com/poz/pozix.html

Magazine for HIV-positive people. Includes features, profiles, culture, regular columns, news and survival issues.

Research

AmFAR: American Foundation for AIDS Research

http://www.amfar.org/

Nonprofit agency dedicated to AIDS biomedical and clinical research, AIDS prevention, and a sound AIDS-related public policy.

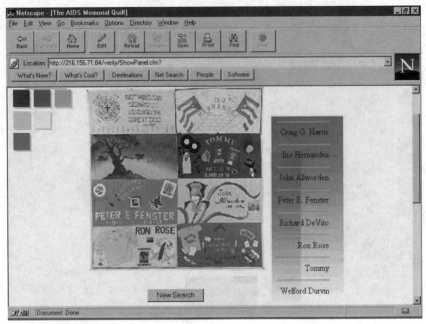

AIDS Memorial Quilt. http://www.aidsquilt.org/

AVERT: AIDS Education and Research Trust
http://www.avert.org/

AIDS education and research trust offers information, United Kingdom statistics, news and publications.

CDC Statistics on New AIDS Cases in the U.S. Per Year
http://www.sunlabs.com/~shirriff/java/statsgraph.html

Graph shows the adolescent/adult causes of AIDS up to 1998.

HIV Sequence Database
http://hiv-web.lanl.gov/

HIV genetic sequence data collection, annotation, analysis and publication.

HIV/AIDS Surveillance
http://www.cdc.gov/nchstp/hiv_aids/surveillance.htm

Statistics and reports from the Centers for Disease Control and Prevention.

JAMA HIV/AIDS Information Site

http://www.ama-assn.org/special/hiv/hivhome.htm

Resources for physicians, other health professionals and the public. Offers clinical updates, news, articles and information on social and policy issues. Links to the National Library of Medicine's AIDS databases, and continuing medical education credit for physicians.

Support

AIDS Memorial Quilt

http://www.aidsquilt.org/

The AIDS Memorial Quilt is an enormous patchwork quilt of 3-by-6-feet panels (the size of a human grave), each devoted to the memory of a person who died from AIDS. This site discusses how to make and submit a panel. Search for names and view over 41,000 panels.

AIDS Project Los Angeles

http://www.apla.org/apla/

Site offers AIDS information and resources The mission of APLA is to improve lives of people affected by HIV disease by providing direct services; reducing the incidence of HIV infection through risk-reduction education; and advocating for fair and effective public policy.

Day One

http://www.aegis.com/topics/dayone/

Site to help people who have just discovered they are HIV-positive starts by giving you five pointers that it calls "Big Deals."

HIV/AIDS Support Groups

http://www.ama-assn.org/insight/spec_con/hiv_aids/supptgrp.htm

Contact information and description of national HIV/AIDS organizations and resources, state and local HIV/AIDS hotlines, and treatment resources.

HIV-SUPPORT

http://www.web-depot.com/hemophilia/hiv-support.info

Guidelines to joining in this electronic support group for people with HIV or AIDS. Both emotional support and medical advice are shared.

sci.med.aids

http://www.aids.wustl.edu/

General information on this newsgroup. Links to frequently asked questions.

Spiritual Support for AIDS

http://www.thebody.com/cgi/faith.html

You can ask an experienced Reverend and/or a Catholic priest spiritual questions dealing with AIDS, or you can read what others have asked and the responses they received.

Treatment

See also: Clinical Trials.

AIDS Alternative Treatment

http://www.critpath.org/alt.htm

This site provides a long list of links and information on alternative, complementary and unconventional treatments for AIDS.

AIDS Treatment Data Network

http://www.aidsinfonyc.org/network/

Lots of material on AIDS and AIDS treatment options. Includes a directory of clinical trials; simple fact sheets on treatments, conditions, and tests; a drug index; *Treatment Review*, the Network's newsletter; information on AIDS in Spanish, glossaries of drugs and of terms; description of alternative treatments; and links.

AIDS Treatment News/Internet Directory

http://www.aidsnews.org/

Reports on experimental and standard AIDS treatments.

AIDS Treatments

http://www3.hmc.edu/~mwright/bio/treatments.html

Discusses two families of drug treatments: reverse transcriptase inhibitors and protease inhibitors.

AIDSTRIALS and AIDSDRUGS

http://www.nlm.nih.gov/pubs/factsheets/aidstdfs.html

Fact sheet about these two NLM databases.

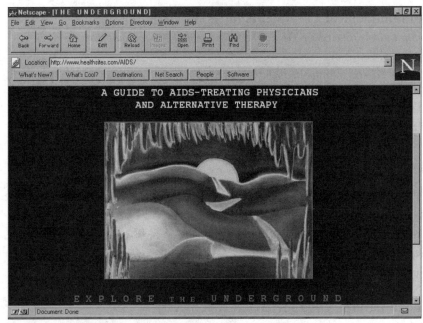

The Underground. *http://www.healthsites.com/AIDS/*

Exercise and HIV

http://www.qcfurball.com/cat/aids/exercise.html

Article stresses the importance of lean body mass for preserving the AIDS patient maintains a high quality of life and longer length of survival.

HIV/AIDS Treatment Information Service

http://www.hivatis.org/

Information on federally-approved treatment guidelines for HIV and AIDS.

HIV Health Library Index

http://www.aac.org/hivtreat/index/intro.html

A subject index to HIV/AIDS treatment literature.

Immunet

http://www.immunet.org/immunet/home.nsf/page/homepage

Treatment information on HIV/AIDS; updates, resources and a forum.

Immunological Treatments for HIV/AIDS
http://hivpositive.com/f-Treatment/5-Treatments/f-Immunology/Immunology Menu.html

Details on immunological treatments for AIDS.

Talking Treatment: Community AIDS Treatment Exchange
http://www.catie.ca/treatment.nsf/by+category

Search earlier discussions, add a new message, or view messages by category, topic, author, or date.

The Underground
http://www.healthsites.com/AIDS/

Contains a searchable database of AIDS physicians, lets you learn about alternative therapies and doctors who will practice them. You can send in your success story, chat with others and check out their list of AIDS links.

Yoga Group: Yoga for HIV/AIDS
http://www.yogagroup.org/

Provides free yoga classes and information to those with HIV/AIDS. You can read about the programs offered or read articles and check out which postures are recommended for HIV/AIDS patients.

Women and HIV/AIDS

Basic Resources for Women and HIV/AIDS
http://www.hivpositive.com/f-Resources/f-17-NewslettersInfo/wompath.html

Newsletters, press releases, selected materials, organizations, electronic bulletin boards and Internet resources devoted to women with HIV/AIDS.

Facts about Women and HIV/AIDS
http://www.safersex.org/women/women.cdc.html

From the Centers for Disease Control and Prevention, this factsheet provides a lot of numbers, but unfortunately only covers up to 1995.

PANWHA Fact Sheets on Women and HIV/AIDS
http://www.apa.org/ppo/hivfact.html

There are two sheets: one discusses women with HIV/AIDS and substance abuse, and the other questions whether AIDS policies address women's lives realistically.

Women and HIV/AIDS Information
http://www.fas.harvard.edu/~minnella/ws375.html

Straightforward list of links that includes frequently asked questions.

Women's AIDS Network
http://www.womens-aids-network.com/

Provides a monthly newsletter and educational forums; and information on referrals as well as a resource library.

The Women's Place
http://www.geocities.com/HotSprings/Villa/2998/

Links and information especially geared toward women with AIDS.

HOSPICE CARE

Related chapters: *Aging/Gerontology; Biomedical Ethics; Death & Dying; Pain & Pain Management.*

All About Hospice: A Consumer's Guide

http://www.nahc.org/Haa/guide.html

Describes the purpose and philosophy of hospice, the range of services most often provided, methods of payment, how to locate and evaluate a hospice provider, and the hospice patient's bill of rights.

American Academy of Hospice and Palliative Medicine

http://www.aahpm.org/

All about the Academy, membership and events. Links to other hospice and palliative care sites.

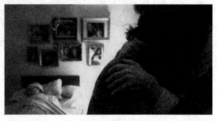

Choosing a Good Death

http://www.boston.com/globe/special reports/1996/june/hospice/home.htm

One woman's story about her decision to receive hospice care.

Choosing a Good Death.
http://www..boston.com/globe/specialreports/1996/june/hospice/home.htm

Five Wishes

http://www.agingwithdignity.org/awd/five_wishes.html

You can download the Five Wishes document that helps you express how you want to be treated if you are seriously ill and unable to speak for yourself. Unlike many living wills, it addresses personal, emotional and spiritual needs, as well as medical needs.

Frequently Asked Questions about Hospice

http://www.teleport.com/~hospice/faq.htm

Twenty questions with answers from Hospice Web.

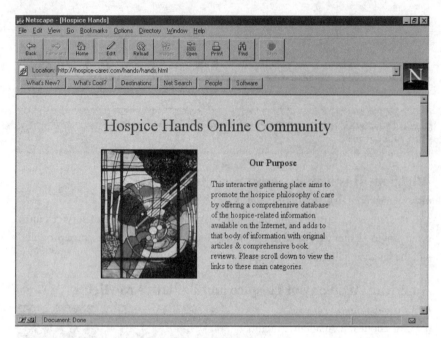

Hospice hands. *http://hospice-cares.com/hands/hands.html*

Homecare Online

http://www.nahc.org/home.html

Service of the National Association for Home Care. Includes home care and hospice locator, consumer materials and Association information.

Hospice and Palliative Care

http://www.acsu.buffalo.edu/~drstall/hospice.html

For patients, caregivers and health professionals. Contains a list of bookmarks to euthanasia, grief counseling and hospice and palliative care sites, a list of online discussion groups, and some thoughtful reflections and practical tips.

Hospice and Palliative Care Resources

http://wings.buffalo.edu/faculty/research/bioethics/hospice.html

A list of resources with information for consumers and for clinicians.

Hospice Foundation of America
http://www.hospicefoundation.org/

General information on hospices and specific information about the Foundation. Learn about hospices and how to find a hospice, and read publications, books, and stories about hospice situations.

Hospice Hands Online Community
http://hospice-cares.com/hands/hands.html

Lots of information, including a hospice primer that discusses the philosophy of hospice and how to provide spiritual, psychosocial and physical care, as well as bereavement and volunteer services. Site also has a hospice chat room and several forums, an e-mail list, library of resources, employment pages, and links.

HospiceNet
http://www.hospicenet.org/

Resources for patients, families and caregivers. Services include how to find a local hospice team. Patient information on pain management and self-help, pain relievers, how to talk with children, and more. Finally, there are also a number of bereavement resources, including advice, suggestions, affirmations and words of comfort.

Medicare Hospice Benefits
http://www.zianet.com/connealy/hospice/medicare.html

Basic questions with answers on the Medicare Hospice Benefit and on hospice care in general.

National Hospice Organization
http://www.nho.org/

Provides the basics of hospice, information on the organization and how to locate a hospice. Also provides a discussion forum, links and publications.

Zen Hospice Project
http://www.zenhospice.org/

Projects, articles, reading lists and a newsletter.

INFECTIOUS DISEASES

E. Coli

E. Coli Genetic Stock Center
http://cgsc.biology.yale.edu/

Database of *E. coli* information, including *E. coli* genotypes, gene names, properties, linkage maps, and gene product information. Direct queries of database are possible.

E. Coli Genome Project
http://www.genetics.wisc.edu/

Site created by the E. Coli Genome Center at the University of Wisconsin at Madison, whose project goal is to completely sequence the *E. coli* genome and several *E. coli* phages. FTP files showing the sequence that has been decoded thus far may be downloaded.

EcoCyc: Encyclopedia of E. Coli Genes and Metabolism
http://ecocyc.PangeaSystems.com/ecocyc/ecocyc.html

Databank describing the genes and intermediary metabolic activity of *E. coli*. Written for the scientific community.

Ebola

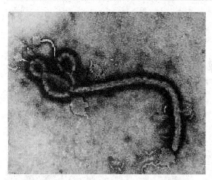

*The Ebola Virus. At: **Dr. Frederick A. Murphy Talks about the Ebola Virus.** http://www.accessexcellence.org/WN/ NM/interview_murphy.html*

Dr. Frederick A. Murphy Talks About the Ebola Virus

http://outcast.gene.com/ae/WN/NM/int erview_murphy.html

Dr. Murphy was the first to view Ebola through an electron microscope.

Ebola Outbreaks - Updates

http://www.bocklabs.wisc.edu/ outbreak.html

Citations for articles and other documents relating to recent Ebola outbreaks, as collected from World Health Organization (WHO), Centers for Disease Control and Prevention (CDC), CNN, AP Newswire, Reuters news service, and other sources. Links to documents appearing on the web.

Ebola Recommended Reading List

http://www.bocklabs.wisc.edu/ebola.html

Lists documents about the Ebola virus. Collected from scientific journals, news publications, various television media, Centers for Disease Control (CDC) reports and books.

Ebola Virus Links on the Web

http://www.iohk.com/UserPages/amy/ebola.html

Information on Ebola from health authorities, scientists and others. Also provides links to three related newsgroups.

Fact Sheets: Ebola Hemorrhagic Fever

http://www.cdc.gov/ncidod/dvrd/spb/mnpages/dispages/ebola.htm

General and straightforward information about the Ebola virus offered in question and answer format.

Kerry Townsend's Homepage

http://www.ru.ac.za/departments/journ/awol/ebola.html

Short news article on the Ebola virus and virus outbreaks, written by Kerry Townsend of Rhodes University in South Africa.

Map of Zaire

http://www.lib.utexas.edu/Libs/PCL/Map_collection/africa/Zaire.GIF

This map of Zaire (Congo) identifies Kikwit, the city where Ebola re-appeared in 1995. It is a large *.gif image.

Newest Occurrences of Ebola

http://www.uct.ac.za/microbiology/ebopage.html

The latest on Ebola outbreaks, as well as lists and links to ProMED articles, popular print media, and World Health Organization (WHO) releases providing news updates and general information on the virus.

Emerging Diseases

Anatomy of an Epidemic

http://library.advanced.org/11170/

Very beautiful site contains links and general disease information and information on specific epidemics. Fascinating animated maps demonstrate the spread of epidemics. There are also quizzes, disease discussion, and a glossary of key words.

Communicable Disease Surveillance and Report

http://www.who.int/emc/index.html

This division of the World Health Organization (WHO) surveys disease outbreaks around the world and provides news and health advice for travellers. Site includes a list of diseases covered, an index of outbreaks reported, the *Weekly Epidemiological Record*, safety guidelines for labs and for transport of infectious material, reports on anti-infective drug resistance, and fact sheets.

Emerging Infections Information Network

http://info.med.yale.edu/EIINet/

Uses state-of-the-art technology to promote discussion of emerging infections world-wide. Describes seminars and runs weekly theme-based forums.

Emerging Infectious Diseases Resource Link

http://www.cdc.gov/ncidod/id_links.htm

General and specific information on emerging diseases. Includes links to related websites, *Emerging Infectious Diseases Journal*, online newsletters and other publications.

Program for Monitoring Emerging Diseases (ProMED) Electronic Discussions

http://www.healthnet.org/programs/promed.html

Global system of early detection and timely response to disease outbreaks that was proposed by the Federation of American Scientists. You can subscribe to nine different mail groups here.

ProMED: Program for Monitoring Emerging Diseases

http://www.fas.org/promed/

ProMED was formed by the Federation of American Scientists to establish global monitoring of emerging diseases. It also operates as an information source and subscription mailing list for scientists, public health officials, journalists and laypeople.

General Resources

Bad Bug Book

http://vm.cfsan.fda.gov/~mow/toc.html

This FDA site is oriented to laypeople and offers information on foodborne pathogenic microorganisms and natural toxins.

Bugs on the Web

http://bugs.uah.ualberta.ca/webbug/index.htm

Links to articles on different aspects of microbiology.

CDC Homepage

http://www.cdc.gov/

This homepage for the Centers for Disease Control and Prevention offers health information, publications, traveler's information, training and employment, as well as data collection and statistics.

CDC Wonder

http://wonder.cdc.gov/

Start here to access CDC reports, text- and numeric-based public health data.

CELLS Alive!

http://www.cellsalive.com/

This beautiful and user-friendly site contains commentary and images of microbiology in action. Includes scanning electron microscope photographs and computer animation of how cells fight infection, and how viruses and bacteria behave.

Centre for the Epidemiology of Infectious Diseases

http://www.ceid.ac.uk/

This site from the Department of Zoology, University of Oxford, offers technical information on infectious diseases, including publications, research, news, seminars, and a dictionary of epidemiology.

Communicable Disease Fact Sheets for Consumers

http://www.health.state.ny.us/nysdoh/consumer/commun.htm

Addresses basic questions on over 50 different infectious organisms and communicable diseases.

Communicable Diseases Fact Sheets

http://www.charm.net/~epi1/diseases.html

The Maryland Department of Health has prepared fact sheets on a large number of diseases.

Epidemic: The World of Infectious Diseases

http://www.amnh.org/exhibitions/epidemic/

This educational site accompanies a special exhibit at the American Museum of Natural History, and "tells stories about infectious diseases." It seeks to explain how the combination of ecological/environmental changes, evolution and culture create disease-producing conditions.

Epidemiology

http://www.epibiostat.ucsf.edu/epidem/epidem.html

Covers infectious diseases and provides epidemiological information and numerous links world-wide.

General Resources for Infectious Diseases

http://128.95.122.195/inpho/diseases/infectious/general.html

Institutions, references and articles on emerging diseases and surveillance efforts.

Global Health Network

http://www.pitt.edu/HOME/GHNet/

An international alliance of health experts assembled from government, global organizations, businesses and academia, the Global Health Network develops programs for the world-wide prevention of disease. Available in eight different languages.

Infectious Diseases Links

http://www.medmark.org/inf/

Long list of links from MedMark.

Infectious Diseases Links

http://128.205.200.103/id/ID_Links.html

Starting point to launch into search for information on infectious diseases. Links to government sites and organizations.

Medical Microbiology Home Page

http://biomed.nus.edu.sg/microbio/home.html

This site for medical doctors, medical students and scientists was created by microbiologist Raymond Lin and is full of links to other microbiology sites, journals, and organizations.

Microbial Underground (U.S.)

http://www.lsumc.edu/campus/micr/mirror/public_html/index.html

A companion site to The Microbial Underground (U.K.). It offers a collection of web pages with medical, micro- and molecular biological links, created as part of a project to build an online course in medical microbiology. You can find everything relating to microbiology on the Internet, including news, websites, courses, newsgroups, bulletin board services, culture and stain data, and online publications.

OUTBREAK

http://www.outbreak.org/cgi-unreg/dynaserve.exe/index.html

An online information source addressing the emerging diseases. Offers an overview of emerging diseases, articles on specific diseases and recent outbreaks, as well as a glossary of related terms. It also provides a world-wide collaborative database of disease outbreaks.

Virtual Library of Diseases

http://www.nfid.org/library/

This site created by the National Foundation for Infectious Diseases offers fact sheets and clinical updates as well as links to infectious diseases resources on the Internet, including information on Acquired Immunodeficiency Syndrome (AIDS), hepatitis and Ebola.

WHO's *Weekly Epidemiological Record*

http://www.who.int/wer/index.html

Distributed every week, this free electronic publication contains epidemiological information on cases and outbreaks of all diseases listed under the International Health Regulations, as well as on other infectious diseases and health problems. Requires Acrobat Reader to receive electronically.

World Wide Web Communicable Diseases Resources

http://www.open.gov.uk/cdsc/links.htm

Links to mailing lists, public health and disease sites across the globe.

Immunizations/Vaccinations

See also: Children's Health/Pediatrics - Immunizations; Public Health - Travel Recommendations.

Adult Immunization Overview

http://www.cdc.gov/nip/schedule/adult/default.htm

Vaccines and toxoids recommended by age. General information, indications, contraindications, and comments.

Childhood Immunization Schedule

http://www.cdc.gov/nip/pdf/child-schedule.pdf

PDF format.

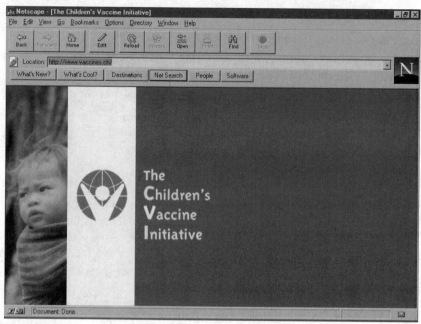

The Children's Vaccine Initiative. http://www.vaccines.ch/

Childhood Vaccinations

http://www.noah.cuny.edu/healthyliving/ushc/childimmuniz.html

Addresses the risks of getting immunized as well as the risk of not getting immunized. Suggests which immunizations children should receive, and offers a recommended schedule for immunization of healthy infants and adults that is easy to understand.

The Children's Vaccine Initiative

http://www.vaccines.ch/

Global program to promote childhood vaccinations.

Clinician's Handbook of Preventive Services

http://text.nlm.nih.gov/ftrs/pick?collect=ppip&dbName=ppipc&cd=1&t=9181 46662

Start from the table of contents to find immunization information for specific diseases, including references, patient resources and recommendations. Several chapters discuss the immunization of children, other chapters discuss the immunization of adults.

Fact Sheets for Adult and Adolescent Immunization

http://www.nfid.org/factsheets/

From the National Foundation for Infectious Diseases.

Immunization Action Coalition

http://www.immunize.org/

Information on the Coalition and its publications, *NEEDLE TIPS* and *Vaccinate Adults!* Ready-to-print documents about vaccines, adult immunization, Hepatitis A and B, legal issues and lawsuits. Many resources, including schedules recommending guidelines for infant, adult, child and adolescent immunizations, as well as guidelines for vaccinating pregnant women.

The Immunization Gateway: Your Vaccine Fact-Finder

http://www.immunofacts.com/

A great number of links to sites providing up-to-date vaccine and immunization information on the Internet. Information ranges from the general to specific, and covers items parents would wish to know, as well as public health professionals. Links to different state immunization programs are also provided.

National Vaccine Injury Compensation Program

http://www.hrsa.dhhs.gov/bhpr/vicp/new.htm

Although only rarely does anyone have an adverse reaction to a vaccine, it can happen. This program offers assistance to consumers who have suffered as a result of vaccinations. It helps them to file a claim so that they can receive compensation.

NIP: National Immunization Program

http://www.cdc.gov/nip/

NIP "provides leadership for the planning, coordination, and conduct of immunization activities nationwide."

Parents Guide to Childhood Immunizations

http://www.hoptechno.com/book42.htm

Plain text description of diphtheria, tetanus (lockjaw), pertussis (whooping cough), polio, measles, mumps, rubella (German measles), and haemophilus influenzae type b (Hib). For parents.

Six Common Misconceptions about Vaccinations

http://www.cdc.gov/nip/publications/6mishome.htm

Addresses some misconceptions parents and others may have about the safety of vaccination, and explains why they are misconceptions.

Vaccination Requirements and Health Advice

http://www.who.int/ith/english/welcome.html

Publications from the World Health Organization on travel medicine.

Vaccine Safety: What You Need to Know

http://www.cdc.gov/nip/vacsafe/

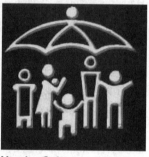

The National Immunization Program has prepared this page to address concerns about the safety of vaccinations. It provides fact sheets, and answers questions such as: What are vaccines made of? How are they licensed? Are side effects monitored?

Vaccine Safety.
http://www.cdc.gov/nip/vacsafe/

Vaccine Weekly

http://www.newsfile.com/x1v.htm

News briefs and article summaries are offered on vaccine-related research topics world-wide. Full access to the text of articles is available with subscription.

Vaccines and Diseases News

http://www.biol.tsukuba.ac.jp/~macer/NBBV.html

References to books, research articles and other published and governmental texts discussing vaccines and related topics. Compiled by the Eubios Ethics Institute.

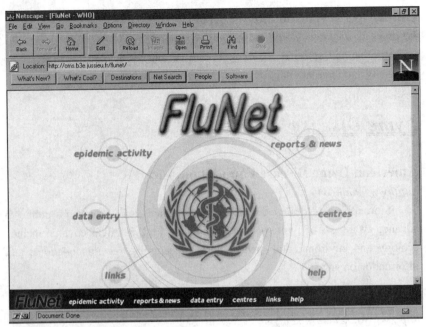

FluNet. http://oms.b3e.jussieu.fr/flunet/

Influenza

FluNet

http://oms.b3e.jussieu.fr/flunet/

This is the World Health Organization's information system to monitor influenza activity by acting as a central database for coordinating a global surveillance. It offers maps and graphs of recent outbreaks, weekly reports, and a "global situation summary." Its mission is to be able to give early alerts of epidemics and thereby improve public health by allowing for epidemic preparation and control.

Influenza Bibliography

http://www.nimr.mrc.ac.uk/Library/flu/

Lists recently published journal articles on influenza. Includes general and clinical articles, articles on prevention and control, epidemiology, epizootiology, immunology, pathology, influenza genetics and viruses. Updated 6 times each year.

Influenza Prevention and Control

http://www.cdc.gov/ncidod/diseases/flu/fluvirus.htm

Vaccine and antiviral information; and current influenza surveillance both nationally and internationally.

Lyme Disease

American Lyme Disease Foundation, Inc.

http://www.aldf.com/

Informative site designed for both professionals and the general public to advance awareness of Lyme disease throughout the U.S. Areas covered include ecology and environmental management, precautions, recommendations, and information on vaccines.

Ask Noah About: Lyme Disease

http://www.noah.cuny.edu/lyme/lyme.html

In-depth outline of links are arranged to answer the following questions: *What is Lyme disease? How is it treated?* and *What are the potential complications?* Lots of good information.

Dawnie's Lyme Disease Site

http://www.geocities.com/HotSprings/Spa/6731/

This page was created by a patient suffering from Lyme disease. It contains information, links, Lyme stories, and support.

Lyme Disease

http://www.uri.edu/artsci/zool/ticklab/Lyme.html

Attractive site offering general information on Lyme disease and the biomonics (i.e., life cycle and spread) of black-legged deer ticks. Provides links to other relevant sites and research studies. Site is maintained by The Rhode Island Tick Pickers at the Tick Research Laboratory, University of Rhode Island.

Lyme Disease

http://www.cdc.gov/ncidod/diseases/lyme/lyme.htm

You can download this public information brochure or read it online.

Lyme Disease Chat

http://www.x-l.net/chat/

This is the place to discuss issues relative to tick-borne disease, including mutual support and friendship.

Lyme Disease Foundation, Inc.

http://www.lyme.org/index2.html

National nonprofit medical health care agency dedicated to finding solutions to tick-borne disorders. Lots of information on Lyme diseases, ticks, as well as on Lyme research, education and the prevention of tick-borne diseases.

Lyme Disease Information Resource

http://www.x-l.net/Lyme/index.html

Clearinghouse for information about Lyme disease. Offers many links and information on conferences, meetings, organizations, clinical studies and research.

Lyme Disease: Introduction

http://www.cdc.gov/ncidod/dvbid/lymeinfo.htm

Information from the Centers for Disease Control and Prevention describes Lyme disease natural history, epidemiology, risk factors, diagnosis, prevention and vaccine recommendations.

The Lyme Disease Network Online

http://www.lymenet.org/

Keep up on the events and activities of the Lyme community, including the latest research study results and treatment recommendations, illustrations of ticks, contact information for Lyme disease support groups, and links to related websites.

#Lyme

http://www.sky.net/~dporter/lymeirc.htm

Internet chat for Lyme disease support occurs Tuesdays and Fridays at 10 p.m. (EST). Information at this site.

Malaria

Doctors' Answers to "Frequently Asked Questions": Malaria
http://www.druginfonet.com/faq/faqmalar.htm

Site addresses drug-related questions on malaria.

Frequently Asked Questions about Malaria
http://www.outbreak.org/cgi-unreg/dynaserve.exe/Malaria/faq.html

Answers to common questions about _Plasmodium_ and malaria.

Malaria: An Online Resource
http://www.rph.wa.gov.au/labs/haem/malaria/index.html

Regularly updated site provides good malaria information. Includes diagnosis, prevention, treatment, history and self-assessment area with case studies.

Malaria Database
http://www.wehi.edu.au/MalDB-www/who.html

Information resource for scientists working in malaria research. Includes malaria genome sequencing, nucleotide and protein information and jobs available in the field.

Malaria Discuss Mail Server
http://www.wehi.edu.au/MalDB-www/discuss/listserv.html

Search the archives of this discussion group or peruse frequently asked questions. To subscribe, send an e-mail to: _listserv@wehi.edu.au_ and in the body of the message, type "subscribe malaria (_preferred personal name_)."

Malaria for Travelers
http://www.travelhealth.com/malaria.htm

General overview and historical perspective on this disease, as well as malaria reports for different regions of the world.

Malaria Prevention and Control
http://www.who.int/ctd/html/malaria.html

This site is maintained by WHO/Division of Control of Tropical Diseases, and it offers malaria statistics, disease control activity advice and updates, and links to additional resources.

Organizations

International Society for Infectious Diseases
http://www.isid.org/
Organization comprised of scientists from all over the globe who share and discuss their work.

National Center for Infectious Diseases
http://www.cdc.gov/ncidod/
Information about the prevention and control of traditional, new, and re-emerging infectious diseases in the United States and around the world.

National Foundation for Infectious Diseases Homepage
http://www.nfid.org/
The NFID site provides infectious diseases fact sheets, clinical updates, information on adult immunization, additional web sources, brochures, and a newsletter entitled *The Double Helix*.

National Institute of Allergy and Infectious Diseases
http://www.niaid.nih.gov/
This Institute provides grants and support to scientists conducting research to better diagnose, treat and prevent the many infectious, immunologic and allergic diseases that afflict people world-wide. Site provides overview of the Institute and its programs, grant information, publications and access to the four different divisions.

Parasitology

American Society of Parasitologists Links
http://www-museum.unl.edu/asp_image/links.html
Provides links to societies, institutions and journals of parasitological interest.

Bacterial Infections and Mycoses
http://www.mic.ki.se/Diseases/c1.html
Information on specific diseases, bacterial organisms, eye infections, skin diseases, fungi, and zoonoses, as well as links to numerous related web resources.

Karolinska Institute's Linkages to Parasitic Sites

http://www.mic.ki.se/Diseases/c3.html

Connections to images and research studies on particular parasites and the diseases they cause, as well as to other parasitology sites on the Internet.

Parasites, Parasites, Parasites

http://ascaris.med.tmd.ac.jp/

Site offers information on parasitic infections for clinicians, the opportunity to offer your diagnosis, link to related websites and tour the Meguro Parasitological Museum in Cyberspace.

The Parasitology Images List

http://www.life.sci.qut.edu.au/LIFESCI/darben/paramast.htm

Dozens of images of medically important parasites, including protozoa, nematoda, platyhelminthes, arthropods and miscellaneous images.

Parasitology Page

http://www.pasteur.fr/Bio/parasito/Parasites.html

A narrated list of sites specifically related to parasitology and molecular biology. Includes journals, institutes, global organizations and government sites.

A Selection of Parasite Journals

http://www.rz.uni-duesseldorf.de/WWW/MathNat/Parasitology/paen_jou.htm

Journals of parasitology and related specialties.

Plague

CDC Plague Information Page

http://www.cdc.gov/diseases/plague.html

Information about the disease for the public and for health care workers. Includes description, diagnosis, treatment, spread, vaccines and prevention.

Frequently Asked Questions on the Plague

http://www.outbreak.org/cgi-unreg/dynaserve.exe/Plague/faq.html

Good information on the plague, including types, symptoms, transmission and treatment.

Medieval Sourcebook

http://www.fordham.edu/halsall/source/boccacio2.html

This is a description of the Black Death, as described by the author of *The Decameron*, Giovanni Boccaccio (1313-1375).

Plague

http://www.ento.vt.edu/IHS/plague.html

Well-organized presentation on the plague, including information on causal agents, vectors, forms, and life cycle in humans. Also offers histories of past plague epidemics. Part of a virtual presentation on "Insects and Human Society" delivered by Dr. Tim Mack of the Entomology Department at Virginia Tech.

Plague and Public Health in Renaissance Europe

http://jefferson.village.virginia.edu/osheim/intro.html

Hypertext archive offers narratives, medical counsel, government records, religious and spiritual writings and images documenting the arrival, impact and response to the bubonic plague in Western Europe from 1348-1530. Created by the Institute for Advanced Technology in the Humanities.

The Plague: Buboes, Masses and Kinases

http://pestilence.uchicago.edu/

Lecture with accompanying images and references. Includes historical and artistic representations of the Black Death, and a description of the bacterium that caused it.

Plague Fact Sheet

http://www.cdc.gov/ncidod/dvbid/plagfact.htm

Basic information on the clinical features of the plague in its different forms.

Prevention

Compliance Control Center

http://users.aol.com/comcontrol/comply.html

Discusses the benefits of proper handwashing in preventing the spread of infection.

Foodborne Illness Education Information Center
http://www.nal.usda.gov/fnic/foodborne/foodborn.htm

Food safety discussion, government links, database, and publications.

Infection Control/Emerging Concepts
http://www.ic-ec.com/

Provides information, training materials and consultation about communicable diseases in order to help the health care worker, protect the patient and promote compliance with applicable legal requirements.

Office of Disease Prevention and Health Promotion
http://odphp.osophs.dhhs.gov/default.htm

Fact sheets, publications, and links. ODPHP provides leadership in stimulating, coordinating, and unifying national disease prevention and health promotion strategies among federal, state, and local agencies and major private and voluntary organizations.

Publications

Bug Bytes
http://www.ccm.lsumc.edu/bugbytes/

Bi-weekly online publication on infectious diseases.

Emerging Infectious Diseases
http://www.cdc.gov/ncidod/eid/index.htm

Peer-reviewed, online journal published by the National Center for Infectious Diseases. Index and abstracts of articles in present and past issues. Articles may be downloaded. Spanish language version also available.

Infectious Disease News
http://www.slackinc.com/general/idn/idnhome.htm

This electronic publication devoted to infectious diseases offers articles and bulletins, as well as online forums, seminars, and a chat room.

Infectious Disease Newsletter

http://www.zilker.net/~medair/newslet.html

An electronic newsletter summarizing recent research on epidemiology and infectious disease treatment as published in journals in the field. Article titles and summaries are provided, as well as links to related sites.

Journal of Infectious Diseases

http://www.journals.uchicago.edu/JID/

Official journal of the Infectious Diseases Society of America. Access to the electronic edition of this journal, as well as to information on the print version. Browse the latest issue and other available issues.

Morbidity and Mortality Weekly Report

http://www2.cdc.gov/mmwr/

The online version of *MMWR*, a weekly publication based on Centers for Disease Control and Prevention data as reported by state health departments. Contains provisional weekly disease morbidity and mortality data, disease information, reports, news, and survey results.

Traveler's Health

International Society for Travel Medicine

http://www.istm.org/

Composed of physicians, nurses and public health professionals around the world, ISTM advocates and facilitates education, service, and research activities in the field of travel medicine, including preventive and curative medicine within specialties such as tropical medicine, infectious diseases and more. Site offers news, publications, a travel clinic directory, links and more.

State Department Travel Warnings & Consular Information Sheets

http://travel.state.gov/travel_warnings.html

Travel warnings are issued when the State Department recommends that Americans avoid visiting a certain country.

Travel Health Online

http://www.tripprep.com/index.html

Profiles on more than 200 countries, including immunization recommendations, contact information on travel medicine providers around the world, and facts about various health concerns related to travel.

Travelers' Health

http://www.cdc.gov/travel/

Users select their region of travel and receive a summary of health risks, precautions and vaccinations recommended for travelers. Graphical Travel Map allows you to point to the region of the world you will be visiting to receive health information on that area.

Tuberculosis

Ask NOAH About: Tuberculosis

http://noah.cuny.edu/tb/tb.html

Site offers basic information on tuberculosis and AIDS-related tuberculosis, including care and treatment.

Division of Tuberculosis Elimination

http://www.cdc.gov/nchstp/tb/

For the general public, patients and health care providers. This site provides information on tuberculosis prevention and eradication, including frequently asked questions (FAQs), and access to an online newsletter and the Tuberculosis Information Management System (TIMS), a software program allowing entry into and queries to a national database on the administration of TB prevention, surveillance and control programs.

Multidrug-Resistant Tuberculosis (MDR-TB) Annotated Bibliography

http://uhs.bsd.uchicago.edu/uhs/topics/resist.tb.bib.html

Bibliographical and MEDLINE information accompany a summary of each article. List of articles is grouped by the following topics: reviews, epidemiology and high risk groups, diagnosis, treatment strategies and outcomes, public health, the law, and editorials.

National Tuberculosis Center

http://www.umdnj.edu/~ntbcweb/

This Center was founded in response to the resurgence of tuberculosis in the U.S. Site provides a brief history of TB, TB frequently asked questions, TB transmission and pathology, diagnosis, treatment and infection. Maintained by the New Jersey Medical School National Tuberculosis Center, of the University of Medicine and Dentistry of New Jersey.

The Return of TB

http://www.pbs.org/saf/4_class/45_pguides/pguide_302/4532_tb.html

A guide for teachers from PBS.

TB/HIV Research Laboratory

http://www.brown.edu/Research/TB-HIV_Lab/

Offers an overview of Brown University's TB/HIV Research Laboratory and current projects, and provides information on all aspects of tuberculosis, from famous people who died from TB, to clinical data on the disease.

TB Clinical Policies and Protocols

http://www.cpmc.columbia.edu/tbcpp/cover.html

Information for health care professionals.

tb.net: The Global TB Network

http://www.south-asia.com/ngo-tb/

Collection of resources on the disease, and also about training programmes, conferences, computer software, organizations, databases and related material.

Tuberculosis and Airborne Diseases Weekly

http://www.newsfile.com/x1t.htm

"The latest" information on TB control, programs, drug resistance, vaccines and related topics. Abstracts of articles in current and past issues are available; full text is accessible only with subscription.

Tuberculosis Resources

http://www.cpmc.columbia.edu/resources/tbcpp/

Tuberculosis patient information, a description of tuberculosis protocols and related resources.

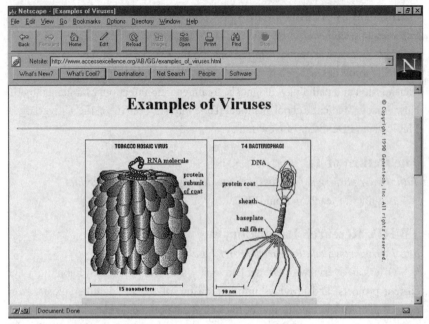

Examples of Viruses. http://www.accessexcellence.org/AB/GG/examples_of_viruses.html

WHO Tuberculosis Site
http://www.who.int/gtb/

News alerts, publications, activities, and World Health Organization programs devoted to eliminating tuberculosis.

Virology

All the Virology on the WWW
http://www.tulane.edu/~dmsander/garryfavweb.html

Very thorough list of links includes institutes, servers, societies and organizations, publications, government resources, patents and technology, online courses and virus images. Helpful and complete table of contents.

The Big Picture Book of Viruses
http://www.tulane.edu/~dmsander/Big_Virology/BVHomePage.html

A catalog of electron microscopsy and computer assisted images of viruses, as well as information on their taxonomy, a list of virus families and individual viruses, a guide to virus structure, online virology tutorials and other links.

Examples of Viruses

http://www.accessexcellence.org/AB/GG/examples_of_viruses.html

Illustration of three viruses: the tobacco mosaic virus, the T4 bacteriophage, and the Human Immunodeficiency Virus (HIV).

Pathology and Virology Center

http://www-sci.lib.uci.edu/~martindale/MedicalPath.html

Martindale's Health Science Guide offers world daily reports on travel warnings and immunization updates, as well as multimedia web courses on virology and pathology, databases, case and teaching files.

Ray's Virology Home Page

http://fiona.umsmed.edu/~yar/home.html

Ray provides his lecture notes covering arboviruses to viral zoonoses, as well as links to CDC fact sheets and selected virus sites.

Virology Newsgroup Archive

http://www.bio.net:80/hypermail/VIROLOGY/

Post your own query or article, or read the latest in virology, sorted by subject or by date.

Virology Websites: The Ultimate List

http://www.virologyweb.com/

Alphabetical listing.

Virus Diseases

http://www.mic.ki.se/Diseases/c2.html

The Karolinska Institute in Sweden has provided users with a long list of virology web links. Everything from lecture notes, tutorials, and student papers, to U.S. FDA and Department of Health information sheets. The list of sites that focus on specific viruses and virus-caused diseases is extensive.

INSURANCE & MANAGED CARE

Chronic Care

Chronic Care
http://www.chroniccare.com/

This site features an educational "system" or game, called Chronic Care Challenges, which allows the visitor to learn about and begin to understand the problems experienced by the chronically ill.

Chronicnet
http://www.chronicnet.org/

Provides information on managing chronic illnesses. Contains listings of national and local organizations, statistics on chronic care, and links to caregivers and organizations developing new programs to deal with the chronically ill.

National Chronic Care Consortium
http://www.ncccresourcecenter.org/

Homepage for the National Chronic Care Consortium, which believes the health care industry's primary purpose has changed from providing acute care to providing chronic care. The Consortium's mission is to improve delivery of chronic care services. Includes links to other organizations.

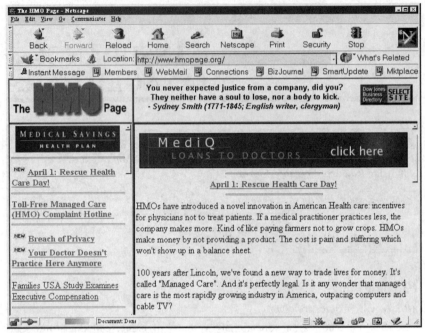

The HMO Page: http://www.hmopage.org/

Consumer Advocacy & Information

Center for Patient Advocacy

http://www.patientadvocacy.org

A coalition that fights for patients' rights. This site discusses managed care reform issues, and provides helpful information for people with insurance problems. Visitors are also able to send e-mail to their representatives and senators from this site.

Consumer Coalition for Quality Health Care

http://www.consumers.org

Nonprofit organization which seeks to provide consumer protection and quality improvement in health care. Website features a Quality Watchline, where visitors can e-mail their problems or complaints regarding health plans, health care providers or health care facilities.

Empower! The Managed Care Patient Advocate

http://www.comed.com/empower

A place where members of managed care health plans can come to discuss their opinions, problems and difficulties, and hopefully get results. The site's goal is to empower patients to speak up for better health care. Provides an interactive discussion forum for patients, doctors and employers.

Healthscope

http://www.healthscope.org/

Consumer advice for Californians and others on how to evaluate and choose a health care plan.

Navigating the Health Care System

http://www.eqp.org

Site to help patients understand their health care plans and deal with common problems and questions that arise when joining a plan. Includes a checklist detailing consumer's rights and responsibilities. Site produced by Employer Quality Partnership, a coalition of several employer associations.

OpenSeason

http://www.openseason.com/

An interactive site featuring information on health and health insurance.

Society for Healthcare Consumer Advocacy

http://www.shca-aha.org/

Offers information on how patients can untangle billing problems, deal with living wills, and confront doctors and health care organizations about abuses.

Ethics

See also: Biomedical Ethics.

AMSO-Ethics and Managed Care

http://www.amso.com/ethics.html

Site covers the ethical dilemmas of managed care, and attempts to help physicians manage managed care in order to run their practices better.

The Bioethics Consultation Group
http://www.bioethics-inc.com/

An interdisciplinary group of professionals in ethics, medicine, law, nursing and theology, the Group offers training and support of corporate and hospital ethics committees, clinical case review, and assistance in developing health policy options for government and private institutions.

Center for Healthcare Ethics
http://www.chce.org/

The Center promotes ethical behavior in managed care and other health care organizations by enabling ethics committees and health care professionals to educate themselves and become advocates for improving patient care. This page presents a forum for discussion and assistance, and provides lots of links.

Institute for Ethics
http://www.ama-assn.org/ethic/ethinsti.htm

Established by the AMA in 1997, the Institute performs research in the area of bioethics, publishes scholarly papers, and runs educational programs on the subject. Managed care is one of the four emphasized topics for research.

Glossaries

What is Managed Care? A Glossary
http://www.wnet.org/mhc/Info/Guide/Resglossary.html

A glossary of managed care terms.

HMOs

The HMO Group
http://www.hmogroup.com/index.html

Formerly The HMO Group, now called The Alliance of Community Health Plans, the Group consists of over 30 practice-based HMOs that exchange data and ideas.

The HMO Page

http://www.hmopage.org/

A site to educate consumers to the evils of HMO's, to give consumers the information they need in order to fight back for quality health care, and to help them make good health care decisions. Page features links to a toll-free managed care complaint hotline, and e-mail to Congress. Information on Medical Savings Accounts, and a special segment that documents the "Managed Care Atrocity of the Month."

How to Fight Your HMO

http://www.bright.net/~ewp/fight_your_hmo.html

Authored by a patient who had trouble with her HMO, this site provides specific information on how to fight your HMO if you disagree with a decision or are dissatisfied with its performance.

Long Term Care

Long Term Care Reimbursement

http://www.Longtermcare.com/partnership.htm

Contract billing organization offering its services primarily to skilled nursing facilities which deal with long-term care.

VSB Corp

http://www.vrsc.com/

VSB Corp. helps people with life-threatening illnesses sell all or part of their existing life insurance policies. Such people can use the financial resources to pay for treatment, living expenses, or other financial burdens that have resulted from the illness.

Managed Care

Aetna U.S. Healthcare
http://www.aetnaushc.com/

This large health insurance company's website contains consumer information including its EZenroll program, help with finding a doctor, and information on health topics.

AHCPR Research about Managed Care Organizations
http://www.ahcpr.gov/research/

Information from the Agency for Health Care Policy and Research, which is part of the U.S. Department of Health and Human Services. The agency does research to help improve the quality of, reduce cost of and improve access to health care.

Business of Medicine/Managed Care
http://www.acponline.org/journals/news/busman.htm

Information and tips for physicians on how to conduct their practice as a successful business.

The Families USA Fdn. Managed Care Information
http://www.familiesusa.org/managedcare+u/

Site examines proposed and pending managed care legislation in terms of its effects on consumers. Sign a national petition urging Congress to pass a Managed Care Bill of Rights.

Managed Care Information Center
http://www.themcic.com/mcweb.html

Provides management information to health care executives, including subscription-based newsletters and directories with information about pending legislation and marketing tips. Site features extensive links to websites for health plans, health care associations, government agencies and other managed care sites.

Managed Care Interface Magazine
http://www.www.medicomint.com

This magazine covers health care policy decision making, health care delivery systems, pharmacoeconomics and pharmacy practice issues for health care management and executives.

Managed Care Magazine
http://www.managedcaremag.com/

Describes itself as an independent guide for physicians and health plan executives on capitation, contracting, physician compensation, disease management, NCQA accreditation & HEDIS, ethics, practice management, formulary development, and other health insurance matters. Site includes table of contents for current issue, archives search, and briefs of recent managed care news.

Managed Care Resources
http://www.acponline.org/mgdcare/mgdcare.htm

A free service for members of the American College of Physicians and for the American Society of Internal Medicine. It provides physicians with information about managed care so that they can make informed choices about how it will affect their practice.

Managed Care Sites
http://www2.umdnj.edu/gpph/

Students in the graduate program of Public Health at Rutgers University in New Jersey built this site, which provides information on and links to other managed care sites that they felt were useful or relevant.

MedConnect Managed Care Forum
http://www.medconnect.com/finalhtm/managedcare/managedhome.htm

Hosted by MedConnect, an online hub for physicians and other health care professionals. Visitors must register in order to access this forum.

UCG Health Information Group
http://www.ucg.com/health/index.htm

UCG is a publishing company offering books and directories, newsletters, conferences and electronic publications. Their health care publications cover such wide-ranging topics as Medicare reimbursement, health care information systems and accreditation. Order the publications here on their website.

Your Money and Your Life: America's Managed Care Revolution

http://www.wnet.org/mhc/index.html

Funded by the Robert Wood Johnson Foundation, this is a Web companion piece to the PBS report of the same name. It offers information and a discussion forum on managed care issues.

Medicaid

Center for Health Care Strategy

http://www.chcs.org/

Find information about the Medicaid Managed Care Program, which is trying to make managed care work for Medicaid recipients who have chronic illnesses.

HCFA Medicaid Information

http://www.hcfa.gov/medicaid/medicaid.htm

Information for both health care professionals and the general public about the Medicaid program, eligibility and benefits.

Medicaid Managed Care

http://www.chcs.org/mmcp.htm

More and more states are forcing Medicaid patients into managed care situations to reduce costs. This program (funded by the Robert Wood Johnson Foundation) seeks to ensure all new managed care arrangements meet the needs of Medicaid beneficiaries who have chronic health and social problems. The website takes requests for grants to fund model development studies and policy studies.

Medicaid Managed Care Fact Sheets

http://nhelp.org/pubs/mc1996fact.html

Samples of fact sheets prepared by the National Health Law Program regarding Medicaid managed care. The fact sheets can be ordered.

National Health Law Program (NHeLP) Publications

http://nhelp.org/publications.shtml#med

Publications available for sale that provide information on Medicaid and other health programs.

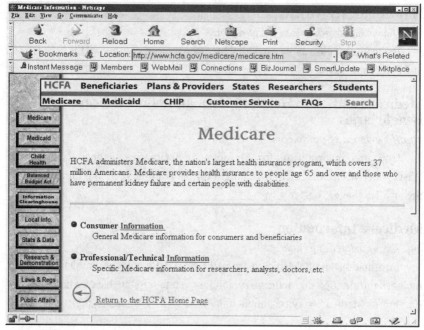

HCFA MedicareInformation: http://www.hcfa.gov/medicare/medicare.htm

Overview of the Medicaid Program

http://www.hcfa.gov/medicaid/mover.htm

Provides eligibility information, services offered and links to more information about the Medicaid program.

Medicare

Facts On... Medicare

http://epn.org/library/agmedi.html#r-f01

From the Electronic Policy Network, this site provides basic information on Medicare.

HCFA Medicare

http://www.hcfa.gov/medicare/medicare.htm

Information for consumers as well as professionals on Medicare, from the Health Care Financing Administration (HCFA), the government agency that oversees the program.

How Medicare Works

http://www.house.gov/wise/medicare.htm

Basic information explaining how Medicare works, courtesy of the U.S. House of Representatives.

Medicare and You: Helpful Information for Medicare Beneficiaries

http://www.medicareinfo.com/

Contains information for Medicare beneficiaries, especially those in Wisconsin and Illinois. Includes changes for the coming year, and information in Spanish language.

Medicare Information

http://ssa.gov/mediinfo.htm

Information about Medicare from the Social Security Administration site. Includes information on Medicare premiums, a state-by-state list of who to contact for various Medicare services, and a link to the HCFA Medicare site.

Physician Resources

Healtheon

http://www.healtheon.com/

An Internet solutions company whose focus is to network health care providers, insurers, consumers, suppliers and diagnostic labs on the web. Offers an electronic data interchange (EDI), and is developing other services.

WebMD

http://www.webmd.com

Site features a Health & Wellness Forum for consumers with health information and breaking news. However, its real purpose is to serve its physician members by providing accredited CME, an extensive library of medical research and information, and most importantly practice management tools such as direct online links to major insurance providers that save physicians time and money with insurance verifications.

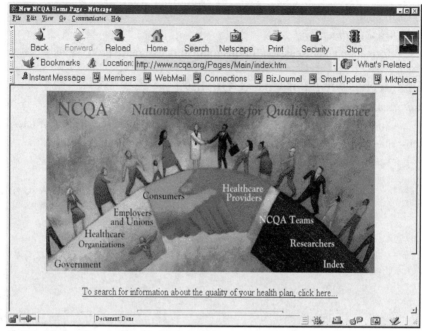

National Committee for Quality Assurance: http://www.ncqa.org/

Quality Assurance

Joint Commission on Accreditation of Healthcare Organizations
http://www.jcaho.org/

The JCAHO accredits more than 19,000 health care institutions in the U.S. and other countries in order to improve the quality of public health care. The organization's website allows hospitals to find out about accreditation requirements, and also allows the general public to file complaints against institutions if they did not receive quality care.

National Committee for Quality Assurance
http://www.ncqa.org/

An independent, nonprofit organization dedicated to assessing and reporting on the quality of managed care plans, including health maintenance organizations. Accreditation and performance measurements are addressed.

QualiNET
http://www.qualinet.com/

Information and discussion forums for quality assurance professionals.

Quarterly Journal of Cost & Quality
http://www.cost-quality.com/

A journal for health care industry executives. Sample current feature articles, subscribe, and link to other websites on managing costs in health care.

KIDNEYS / NEPHROLOGY & UROLOGY

> *Covered in this chapter: Dialysis; General Topics; Hemolytic Uremic Syndrome; Kidney Stones; Nephrotic Syndrome; Organizations; Pathology; Polycystic Kidney Disease; Publications.*
>
> *Related chapters: Cancer/Oncology; Transplantation.*

Dialysis

Dialysis Discussion Group
http://cybermart.com/aakpaz/support.html

The Dialysis mail list was created in June, 1995 by Dan Flasar for the benefit of dialysis patients. It offers a discussion group created for dialysis patients and their families who are trying to gain technical information, as well as benefit from the experience of others. It is sponsored by the Washington University at St. Louis (WUSTL). To subscribe, send e-mail to: *listproc@mail.wustl.edu* and in message body type: "subscribe dialysis *Yourname*." AOL users must type "subscribe" in the subject header of the e-mail; in other cases it may be left blank.

Dialysis Online! Message Boards
http://www.he.net/~brumley/renal/boards.html

Threaded message boards for health care professionals treating end-stage renal disease (ESRD) and other kidney diseases and failure.

Hypertension Dialysis Clinical Nephrology
http://www.medtext.com/hdcn.htm

An official education program of the American Society of Nephrology. The site serves physicians and nurses who treat patients with renal disease, and provides them with information on renal disorders and their treatment, as well as information on hypertension, dialysis, and clinical nephrology. Includes frequently asked questions and answers, summaries of news and recent articles, and information on relevant medical products, services and drugs.

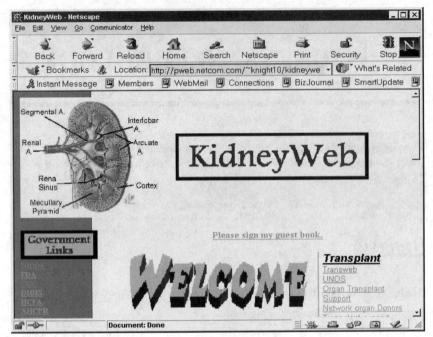

KidneyWeb, describes itself as a "one-stop shop to kidney dialysis and other related sites".

KidneyWeb

http://pweb.netcom.com/~knight10/kidneyweb.html

A site designed for both health care providers, as well as kidney patients and their families. At this site, you can search for kidney dialysis units by zip code and be linked to dialysis equipment companies. Also includes extensive links to transplant resources, government organizations, journals, associations, and other renal disease information.

General Topics

Acute Renal Failure

http://anatomy.adam.com/mhc/top/000501.htm

On this page, the A.D.A.M. interactive curriculum teaches the basics of kidney function, and the causes, prevention and treatment of acute renal failure. Links provide information to other curriculum lessons such as hypoparathyroidism or testing for urine pH.

Alport Syndrome Home Page
http://www.cc.utah.edu/~cla6202/ASHP.htm

This site covers Alport Syndrome, a hereditary disease that affects renal functioning as well as hearing, vision and other body systems. The site offers forums for chat and message boards, as well as information about the Alport Study at the University of Utah.

The Canadian Pediatric Kidney Research Centre
http://www.cheori.org/kidney.htm

The CPKRC is part of the Children's Hospital of Eastern Ontario Research Institute. This site coordinates communication and research efforts devoted to fighting pediatric kidney disorders across Canada.

Diabetes and Kidney Disease
http://www.diabetes.org/ada/c70f.html

This site, sponsored by the American Diabetes Association, explains why diabetes damages kidneys. Written for patients and their families, it discusses symptoms and treatment of diabetic kidney disease, and various forms of dialysis.

Emory University Renal Division
http://www.cc.emory.edu/RENAL/home.html

A clinical site which offers lectures and audio clips on renal-related conditions. Provides links to other nephrology resources on the Web, as well as access to recent publications and research activities at Emory University School of Medicine in Atlanta, Georgia.

Kidney
http://chorus.rad.mcw.edu/index/53html

Start on this page if you want to get concise information about a specific kidney disorder. Everything from acute kidney transplant rejection to xantho-granulomatous pyelonephritis. Part of CHORUS, Collaborative Hypertext of Radiology, an online service for physicians and medical students.

Kidney and Urologic Health
http://www.healthtouch.com/level1/leaflets/118277/118277.htm

This site provides a large number of "leaflets" on subjects such as urinary tract infection, incontinence, kidney stones, cysts, transplants, dialysis, benign prostatic hyperplasia and penile disorders.

National Institute of Diabetes and Digestive and Kidney Diseases

http://www.niddk.nih.gov/

Homepage for the NIDDK, which is part of the National Institutes of Health. This site provides updated information for the public, patients and health care providers about digestive, endocrine, kidney and urologic diseases, including diabetes and obesity. Searchable databases offered.

National Kidney and Urologic Diseases Information Clearinghouse

http://chid.nih.gov/subfile/contribs/ku.html

The Clearinghouse is a service of the National Institutes of Health. Authorized in 1987, it provides information about diseases of the kidneys and urologic system to people with these disorders and to their families, health care professionals, and the public. This site allows you to search a database that provides titles, abstracts, and availability information for documents on kidney and urologic diseases.

The Nephrology Research and Training Center

http://nephaux.dom.uab.edu/

The Center at the University of Alabama at Birmingham studies kidney disease and physiology, focusing on research and clinical aspects. This site describes the Center's research.

The Nephron Information Center

http://nephron.com/

A good starting place for information about the variety of kidney disease links and web resources available for both health care professionals and patients. Offers quick references for diabetic nephrology, hypertensive nephropathy, glomerulonephritis, polycystic kidney disease, interstitial nephritis, end-stage renal disease and many other kidney disorders. Also offers links to organizations, physician resources, quality improvement, and transplant information.

NIDDK Patient Recruitment

http://www.niddk.nih.gov/patient/patient.htm

Provides information about NIDDK-funded studies on kidney disease, and how to get involved.

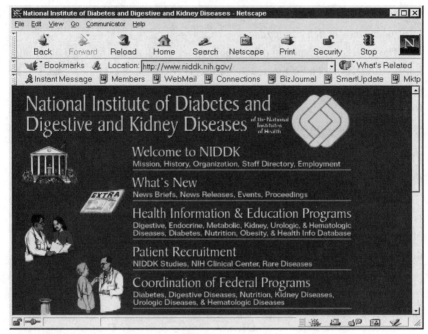

NIDDK Home Page. *http://www.niddk.nih.gov/*

Parts and Workings of the Human Kidney

http://www.clark.net/pub/nhp/med/kidney/basics.html

Learn the basic anatomy of the kidney, its role in the body, and how it works.

The RENALNET Information Service

http://www.renalnet.org/

Clearinghouse for information on the cause, treatment and management of kidney disease and end-stage renal disease (ESRD). Site serves educational, research and treatment purposes. Extensive and easy-to-use. Nephrology resources, ESRD resources, information and other links offered.

Renalworld

http://renalworld.com/

Provides "renal resources from around the globe." Contains links to information about kidney disease, the effect of earthquakes on kidney patients, transplant resources, and physician resources.

United States Renal Data System

http://www.med.umich.edu/usrds/

The USRDS is a national data system which collects, analyzes and distributes information about end-stage renal disease (ESRD) in the United States. The program is funded by the NIDDK at the NIH. A research guide offers information for using USRDS standard analysis files. Statistics provided show incidence, prevalence, treatment, transplants, outcome and demographic data on ESRD.

Urologic and Male Genital Diseases

http://www.mic.ki.se/Diseases/c12.html

A good starting place to gather information. This site was developed by Karolinska Institute, Sweden's only university for medicine. It provides a multitude of links to information about kidney, bladder, urologic, prostate and other genital diseases and conditions.

Hemolytic Uremic Syndrome

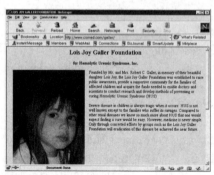

Lois Joy Galler Foundation,
http://www.comed.com/galler/

Lois Joy Galler Foundation for Hemolytic Uremic Syndrome

http://www.comed.com/galler/

This site was created to raise public awareness of HUS and to promote research on developing preventive and treatment strategies. It provides a description of HUS, its symptoms, mode of transmission, treatment, statistics and new research.

Hemolytic Uremic Syndrome, Post-Diarrheal

http://www.cdc.gov/epo/mmwr/other/case_def/hus.html

Clinical information.

Kidney Stones

Dallas Urology Associates: Kidney Stone Diagnosis and Treatment

http://www.dua.com/KSTONE.HTM

A discussion of kidney stones and their treatment, including shockwave lithotripsy and open surgical removal.

Kidney Stones in Adults

http://www.niddk.nih.gov/health/urolog/pubs/stonadul/stonadul.htm

Kidney stones are one of the most painful and common disorders of the urinary tract. This site provides good basic information on what kidney stones are, how they form, who they affect, and how they are diagnosed and treated. Also provides tips on prevention of kidney stones, and other resources.

The Kidney Stones Network Newsletter

http://www.readersndex.com/
imprint/000000d/newslett.html

Approximately one million Americans are affected by kidney stones each year. This is a quarterly newsletter with information and support groups.

Nephrotic Syndrome

Nephrotic Syndrome (Nephrosis)

http://www.rxmed.com/illnesses/nephrotic_syndrome.html

Information about this chronic kidney condition, including its causes, signs, symptoms, risk factors, prevention, treatment and prognosis.

Nephrotic Syndrome/The Parents Place

http://privat.schlund.de/k/kidney-children/nsindex.htm

Nephrotic syndrome is not a disease, but a set of signs and symptoms including protein in the urine, low blood protein, and swelling. It occurs in about 2 out of 100,000 children. This page offers links to other sites for more information on the syndrome, as well as private users' pages for parents with children affected by the syndrome.

Organizations

American Association of Kidney Patients
http://www.aakp.org/aakpteam.html

The AAKP is a nonprofit, membership-based national voluntary health organization providing education, support and advocacy to kidney patients and their families. This site offers links to support groups, end-stage renal disease education, patient stories and treatment options.

American Nephrology Nurses Association
http://anna.inurse.com/

Homepage for the ANNA. Provides members with information about upcoming events, career opportunities and member services. Links to the ANNA journal.

Kidney Dialysis Foundation
http://www.kdf.org.sg/

A nonprofit organization based in Singapore that helps subsidize hemodialysis treatment for end-stage kidney disease patients.

National Enuresis Society
http://www.peds.umn.edu/Centers/NES/

Addresses bedwetting in children, which is not an emotional problem, but may develop into one if the child is punished.

National Kidney Foundation
http://www.kidney.org/

Provides information about kidney diseases and treatment for health care professionals and patients. Also provides information about organ and tissue donors and recipients.

Pathology

Renal Pathology Index
http://www-medlib.med.utah.edu/WebPath/RENAHTML/RENALIDX.html

Slides and diagrams illustrating pathological diagnosis of various renal diseases such as glomerulonephritis, renal cell carcinoma and polycystic kidney disease.

Polycystic Kidney Disease

Polycystic Kidney Disease
http://www.coolware.com/health/medical_reporter/kidney2.html

Article by Joel R. Cooper of *The Medical Reporter* describes this genetic disease, its symptoms and associated problems. Some links provided.

Polycystic Kidney Disease (PKD)
http://www.clark.net/pub/nhp/med/pkd.html

Describes polycystic kidney disease in terms of anatomy, symptoms, progression, prevalence, diagnosis, treatment and related questions. Glossary available, and link to the Polycystic Kidney Research Foundation.

Polycystic Kidney Disease Research Foundation Home Page
http://www.pkdcure.org/

International organization solely devoted to determining the cause, for improving clinical treatment of and discovering a cure for polycystic kidney disease. This site provides information about PKD for the public and health professionals, news about ongoing research, lobbying efforts, and links to other related sites.

Publications

American Journal of Kidney Diseases

http://www.ajkdjournal.org/index.html

The official journal of the National Kidney Foundation, this site permits a search of articles from 1981 to present, offers the atlas of renal pathology, and provides subscription information.

Digital Urology Journal

http://www.duj.com/

A peer-reviewed journal of adult and pediatric urology on the World Wide Web. Includes articles and reports, patient information, and links to other sites.

Journal of Renal Nutrition

http://www.jrnjournal.org/jrn/about.html

Quarterly journal published by the Council on Renal Nutrition of the National Kidney Foundation.

LIVER / HEPATOLOGY

Alpha 1-Antitrypsin Deficiency

Alpha 1-Antitrypsin Deficiency
http://www.alphalink.org/

Chat rooms and mailing list for patients with alpha 1-antitrypsin deficiency and their families.

Alpha 1 National Association
http://www.alpha1.org/

Informative site devoted to promoting an understanding of alpha 1-antitrypsin deficiency, a rare disease afflicting the lungs and liver of less than 100,000 Americans. Site provides information for patients and personal stories, as well as medical and research news, product information, Internet links and other resources.

Cirrhosis

The PBC Foundation
http://www.nhtech.demon.co.uk/pbc/

This organization offers support to individuals who suffer from PBC (Primary Biliary Cirrhosis) and to their families.

Primary Biliary Cirrhosis Patient Support Network
http://www.superaje.com/~pbc/index.htm

The Network was founded in 1981 and is dedicated to helping families affected by primary biliary cirrhosis by providing them with information about liver disease and related issues. Offers links to other relevant sites.

Hepatitis

CDC Hepatitis Branch
http://www.cdc.gov/ncidod/diseases/hepatitis/index.htm

Information about hepatitis types A, B, C, D, E and G, including fact sheets and frequently asked questions (FAQs). The CDC recommends that everyone be tested for hepatitis C.

Hepatitis C: An Epidemic for Everyone
http://www.epidemic.org/

Opens with an introduction from former U.S. Surgeon General Dr. C. Everett Koop on the potential for hepatitis C to become an epidemic. Provides information on the disease and its epidemic status. Features self-tests to assess your risk and test your knowledge. Contains information on managing the disease nutritionally. Site was developed by the trustees of Dartmouth College.

Hepatitis C Information Network
http://www.htinet.com/live/hepc/

Part of HealthTalk Interactive, this site allows visitors to listen to audio files that provide information about hepatitis as well as the latest news, research, and treatments. Broadcast programs were made possible through a grant from Amgen. Visitors can also sign up for an e-mail newsletter.

Hepatitis Central
http://hepatitis-central.com/vikki.html

Hepatitis C infects four times as many people as HIV, and there is no vaccine and no cure. Thus, this site was started by Vikki—who has had hepatitis C for over 30 years—to educate the public as well as health care professionals about the disease. Visitors can learn about HCV, sign up for an e-mail newsletter, and get an update on a class action lawsuit for HCV+ patients.

Hepatitis Family
http://www.bnatural.com/hepatitis-family/

A site devoted to hepatitis patients and their families to offer e-mail support, strength and love. Provides links to related sites.

Hepatitis Foundation International

http://www.hepfi.org/home.htm

This foundation seeks to create awareness of the world-wide problem of viral hepatitis, and to educate the public and health care professionals about its prevention, diagnosis and treatment. Site includes information about hepatitis, research articles, a newsletter, and links.

Hepatitis Haven

http://www.tiac.net/users/birdlady/hep.html

Site for those who have chronic hepatitis B/C that contains: links to recent news articles and scientific research; information on treatment options and drug regimens such as Infergen by Amgen; a directory of doctors and hospitals that treat hepatitis; tips for receiving social security; suggestions for support groups; and information on liver transplants.

Hepatitis Place

http://www.hepplace.com/index.html

"Someone you know has hepatitis" proclaims this site. Find information here on new research and treatment, pertinent breaking news, as well as help with applying for disability benefits from Social Security Administration.

Hepatitis WebRing

http://www.hepring.org/

Intended to be an easy and informative way to find information on the Web about hepatitis by allowing visitors to hop between hepatitis-related websites. One button even allows the visitor to jump to a random hepatitis-related site that's been listed. Invites "heppers" to list their own pages and make the ring bigger.

Hepatitis Weekly

http://www.homepage.holowww.com/1h.htm

Weekly electronic publication on viral hepatitis as well as non-A/non-B (NANB) hepatitis. News and research summaries offered, including discussions of vaccines, government regulations, transmission, incidence, prevention and treatment. Full-text is available only with subscription.

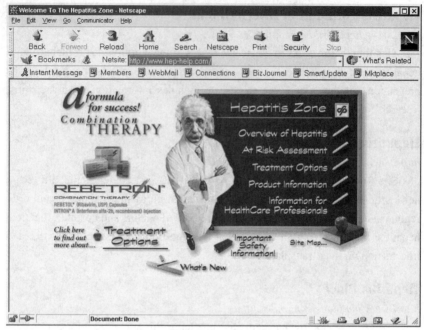

The Hepatitis Zone: http://www.hep-help.com/

Hepatitis Zone

http://www.hep-help.com/

Information about hepatitis and the combination treatment of Rebetol/Intron A. Site includes an overview of the disease, risk assessment, product information and treatment information for health care professionals.

HepNet

http://www.hepnet.com/

Learn about hepatitis in an interactive environment with education modules, slide presentations, and online quizzes. The organization also offers an e-mail subscription service to interested parties.

Issues of Injury: What is Hepatitis C?

http://www.mcn.com/ioi/1998/hep-c.htm

Issues of Injury is a medical-legal quarterly of Medical Consultants Network. This issue covers hepatitis.

Liver Disease

100 FAQs on Liver Disease
http://sadieo.ucsf.edu/alf/alffinal/toplivdisfaqs.html

Sponsored by the American Liver Foundation, this site features 100 frequently asked questions about the liver and liver disease. A few of the topics include hepatitis, gallstones, alcoholism and transplantation.

Chronic Autoimmune Liver Disease Support Group
http://members.aol.com/pbcers/liverdis.htm

A place for liver disease patients and friends to discuss medical information, medication, new research, pain management and the "ups & downs" of daily life. Features many links to other liver disease and related sites, including one to help file for disability insurance from Social Security and Medicaid.

Diseases of the Liver
http://cpmcnet.columbia.edu/dept/gi/disliv.html

Alphabetical list of dozens of liver diseases and conditions with hypertext links to relevant files. Links to current research papers in liver disease as well. Maintained by Columbia-Presbyterian Medical Center.

Highlights in Liver Disease
http://www.highlights.wellweb.com/home.html

Part of WellnessWeb, this site contains coverage of the annual meeting of the American Association for the Study of Liver Diseases. It also has some multimedia and interactive features. The visitor can listen to audio files of interviews with some of the nation's leading biomedical researchers studying hepatitis C, as well as sign up for a news service to receive notification of new coverage or developments.

Organizations

American Association for the Study of Liver Disease
http://hepar-sfgh.ucsf.edu/

Information about the Association, its membership, committees, upcoming meetings and publications. For physicians and scientists who study and treat liver diseases.

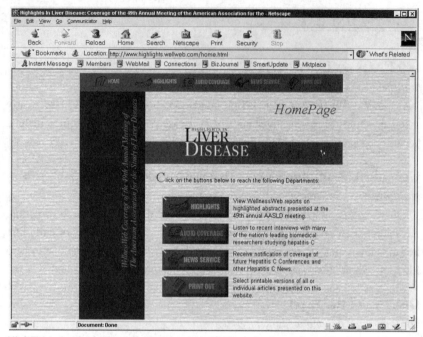

Highlights in Liver Disease: *http://www.highlights.wellweb.com/home.html*

American Liver Foundation
http://sadieo.ucsf.edu/alf/alffinal/homepagealf.html

Consumer-oriented information on the Foundation as well as on the liver and liver diseases. Includes description, disease symptoms, treatment, frequently asked questions, publications, and additional educational resources.

The American Liver Foundation Delaware Valley Chapter
http://www.netaxs.com/~emagroup/alfdelva.htm

An active chapter of the national ALF, this site provides a lot of links, especially regarding hepatitis. Also contains information on the Delaware Valley Transplant Program.

Children's Liver Alliance (CLA)
http://www.livertx.org/viewer.html

An organization dedicated to empowering children with liver disease, their families and care providers by disseminating information, providing a support network, acting as liaisons between health providers and families, and promoting organ donation and transplantation to the public. Site features a newsletter, online meetings, educational seminars and a library of information.

Hepatitis C Foundation

http://www.hepcfoundation.org/

Nonprofit, all volunteer organization that provides support and education to patients and their families. Site offers information on treatments and advice for those who are living with the disease.

Hepatitis Research Foundation

http://www.hepatitis.ca/

Provides information on hepatitis research, as well as pertinent news articles and links to related sites.

Pathology

See also: Pathology chapter.

Hepatic Pathology Index

http://www-medlib.med.utah.edu/WebPath/LIVEHTML/LIVERIDX.html

Over 60 images of normal and diseased livers and liver cells.

Pharmacy

PharmInfoNet

http://pharminfo.com/pubs/medbrief/mb3_11.html

Information about a new oral drug treatment for chronic hepatitis B.

Publications

Hepatology

http://hepatology.aasldjournals.org/

Official journal of the American Association for the Study of Liver Diseases. Site allows visitor to access archive issues, search for articles, browse table of contents and subscribe.

Liver Transplantation and Surgery

http://lts.aasldjournals.org/

Published for the American Association for the Study of Liver Diseases and the International Liver Transplantation Society. Site offers visitor access to archives, ability to search for articles, browse current table of contents, and subscribe.

Lungs / Respiratory & Pulmonary

Asthma

Allergy and Asthma FAQ Home Page
http://www.cs.unc.edu/~kupstas/FAQ.html

This site describes itself as an informal gathering of all of the net wisdom on allergies and asthma. There is a special (but not exclusive) emphasis on children's health. Site offers general information, resources, book reviews, recipes and many related web links.

Allergy and Asthma Network/Mothers of Asthmatics, Inc.
http://www.aanma.org

The AAN/MA calls itself as grassroots patient education association. This site offers organization information and activities, an online survey, general asthma and allergy information, research news, and a bulletin board of events.

Allergy and Asthma Rochester Resource Center
http://www.aarrc.com/

This site describes the Center, its staff and activities. It provides information and advice on allergy triggers and asthma medication, as well as on research studies and results. Links for both physicians and patients are provided.

Allergy, Asthma and Immunology Online
http://allergy.mcg.edu/

An information and news service for patients, their families and health professionals.

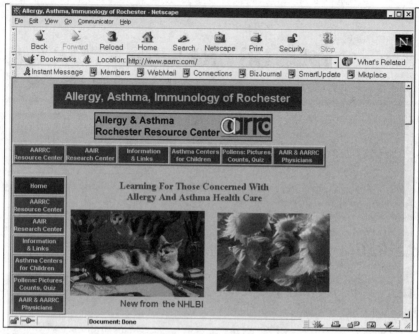

Allergy& Asthma Rochester Resource Center, http://www.aarrc.com/

American Lung Association Asthma Page

http://www.lungusa.org/asthma/index.html

Colorful site with lots of information for adults and children about asthma, as well as medications and prevention. Children's section features Bronkie, a cartoon dinosaur with asthma.

Asthma

http://www.med.virginia.edu/docs/cmc/tutorials/asthma/

Developed by the University of Virginia Health Sciences Center, Children's Medical Center, this tutorial for children and their parents provides information on asthma, including its symptoms and why it occurs.

Asthma Information Center

http://www.ama-assn.org/special/asthma/asthma.htm

From the *Journal of the American Medical Association*, this site contains asthma-related news stories, peer-reviewed research, clinical guidelines and resources for physicians, patient educational resources, as well as links to other websites devoted to asthma information and education.

The Asthma Management Model System

http://www.nhlbisupport.com/asthma/index.html

The Asthma Management Model System is a tool designed to facilitate science-based decision making and evidence-based medicine in long-term asthma management. The site consists of three main components: the Research Mode links to a variety of searchable databases; the Education Mode provides immediate access to clinical practice guidelines, an electronic library, patient education materials, and teaching/learning tools; and the Communication Mode allows the visitor to register for updates. Central to the system is the Asthma Management Model, an interactive program for analyzing the clinical problem of asthma and its long-term management. The Model was developed by an international panel of experts, and is found in the Research section.

Asthma Society of Canada

http://www.asthmasociety.com/

A national volunteer-based organization devoted to improving the quality of life for people with asthma. The website provides information about asthma, asthma management, and links to related websites.

Doctor's Guide to Asthma Information and Resources

http://www.pslgroup.com/ASTHMA.HTM

Includes the latest medical news and alerts on asthma, drug information, discussion groups and newsgroups, and related websites.

Global Initiative for Asthma

http://www.ginasthma.com

A collaboration between the National Heart, Lung and Blood Institute of the NIH and the World Health Organization. Its objectives are to increase public awareness of asthma and its health consequences, to identify the reasons for the increased prevalence of asthma, to promote study of the relationship between asthma and the environment, and to reduce asthma morbidity and mortality. The site provides updates on Initiative progress, and guides to asthma management.

Healthy Kids

http://KidsHealth.org/parent/healthy/

The Kids Health website offers a section devoted to asthma and allergies, including frequently asked questions and advice on asthma management.

National Asthma Education and Prevention Program
http://www.nhlbi.nih.gov/nhlbi/othcomp/opec/naepp/naeppage.htm

Administered by the National Heart Lung and Blood Institute to address the growing problem of asthma in the U.S., this site offers health-related information for patients and health care providers.

National Institute of Allergy and Infectious Diseases
http://www.niaid.nih.gov/

As part of the National Institute of Health, this institution has created a website that provides news, research and fact sheets on allergies and asthma, as well as on many other infectious diseases and disorders of the immune system.

Pharmaceutical Information Network:
Asthma Information Center
http://www.pharminfo.com/disease/immun/asthma/asthma_info.html

This resource for patients and physicians provides information on drugs used to treat asthma.

Teach Your Patients About Asthma
http://www.meddean.luc.edu/lumen/Medicine/Allergy/Asthma/asthmatoc.html

A clinician's guide containing ten teaching units on asthma management. It includes learning records and patient worksheets that may be printed and used by the physician and his or her patient. The guide is part of the National Asthma Education Program at the National Institute of Health.

Bronchitis

American Lung Association: Chronic Bronchitis
http://www.lungusa.org/diseases/lungchronic.html

This page of the American Lung Association website addresses the most basic questions about chronic bronchitis, including what it is, how serious it is, and treatment options.

Chronic Obstructive Pulmonary Disease

Chronic Obstructive Pulmonary Disease Patient Guide
http://www.lung.ca/copd/tofc.html

Description, lung anatomy, diagnosis and management of chronic obstructive pulmonary disease (COPD). Includes medication, coping stragies, and living with COPD.

COPD Fact Sheet
http://www.lungusa.org/diseases/copd_factsheet.html

COPD includes emphysema and chronic bronchitis, diseases characterized by obstruction to air flow. This document provides an explanation of the disease, its symptoms, statistics of who it strikes, and its treatment.

Cystic Fibrosis

Canadian Cystic Fibrosis Foundation
http://www.ccff.ca/~cfwww/intro/pub.htm

Reports, brochures and publications offer patients and their families valuable information on cystic fibrosis.

Cystic Fibrosis Foundation Home Page
http://www.cff.org/

The Foundation's mission is to find a means to cure and control cystic fibrosis. Its website provides information on the disease, recent news, on-going research, and opportunities to get involved with clinical studies, as well as other online resources of interest to cystic fibrosis patients/families.

UMHS Cystic Fibrosis Center Home Page
http://wwwhosp.umhc.umn.edu/cfcenter/

The University of Minnesota has created a guidebook for cystic fibrosis care, offering 21 chapters on diagnosis, treatment, complications, and follow-up for physicians who are treating patients with cystic fibrosis. In addition, this site offers a long list of related web links to pages created by individuals sharing personal stories, international organizations and others.

Emphysema

American Lung Association: Emphysema

http://www.lungusa.org/diseases/lungemphysem.html

Page of the American Lung Association website provides information on emphysema: what it is, how serious it is, what causes it, and how it may be treated.

Emphysema

http://www.alignment.org/emph.htm

Fact sheet on emphysema.

Organizations

American Academy of Allergy, Asthma and Immunology

http://www.aaaai.org/

Offers patient and physician education resources, as well as information about the organization and its meetings.

American Association of Respiratory Care

http://www.aarc.org/

This busy website lets members help with the association's lobbying efforts and letter-writing campaigns, gain continuing education credits, perform an online patient assessment course, and look for a job.

American Lung Association

http://www.lungusa.org/

General information and news about asthma and other lung-related problems, as well as ALA activity at the national and local levels, and legislative and medical updates.

American Thoracic Society

http://www.thoracic.org/

The American Thoracic Society is the medical section of the American Lung Association. This site provides information for medical personnel on professional education programs and conferences, relevant legislative news and press releases, as well as ATS journals and other publications.

Asthma and Allergy Foundation of America

http://www.aafa.org/

A nonprofit organization dedicated to finding a cure and controlling asthma and allergic diseases. The website offers a general store with informative books, pamphlets and videos for adults and children, educational materials for health providers, and information about local chapters and support groups.

Joint Council of Asthma, Allergy and Immunology

http://www.jcaai.org/

The JCAAI is an organization for allergists and immunologists to keep them abreast of changing socio-economic and political developments that impact their practice. The organization's site offers information, practice parameters for physicians dealing with related diseases, as well as links to other websites.

National Jewish Medical and Research Center

http://www.njc.org/

The only medical and research center in the U.S. devoted entirely to respiratory, allergic and immune system diseases. On the website, find out about patient services, treatment and research.

Respiratory Care

RC-Web

http://www.hsc.missouri.edu/shrp/rtwww/rcweb/docs/rcweb.html

Created by the University of Missouri's Respiratory Therapy Program, this page serves students, educators, physicians and others interested in respiratory care. The AARC Clinical Practice Guidelines are linked. Special feature includes a Lung Sounds page.

Respiratory Care Related Links

http://www.hsc.missouri.edu/shrp/rtwww/rcweb/docs/rtlinks.html

Alphabetical listing of over 100 sites on the web related to respiratory care and lung health, both for health care consumers and for medical professionals.

Respiratory Links Page

http://www.xmission.com/~gastown/herpmed/respi.htm

A long list of links to respiratory care and sleep disorder sites, loosely defined. Includes societies, publications, chat lines, hospitals, employment opportunities and educational sites, as well as industry and drug sites.

The RT Corner

http://www.rtcorner.com/

Website for respiratory therapy students includes online articles, exercises, chat room, e-mail forum, chest x-ray-of-the-day, links and bulletin board.

MEDICAL EQUIPMENT

Advantage Medical Electronics

http://www.advantagemed.com/

Informative website tells about the company and its products. It is in the process of developing an online catalog.

AKW Medical

http://www.akwmedical.com/

New and used medical equipment sales and service based in El Cajon, California. Website provides information about the company, a list of used equipment in stock, and links to manufacturers of new equipment.

All Imaging Systems Inc.

http://www.allimaging.com/

New and refurbished ultrasound machines, and replacement parts. Site provides information about the company, listing of reconditioned and pre-owned ultrasound systems for sale, used transducers for sale or exchange, replacement parts currently in stock, a quotation request form, and useful links.

American Medical Supplies & Equipment

http://www.amerimed.com/

Medical equipment supplier based in Miami, Florida. Site provides brief company information, product list and Web specials.

Anderson Medical Equipment Co.

http://www.Andersonmedical.com/

Medical equipment supplier based in Ohio. Site features company profile, biographies, available inventory listing, and association links.

Bio-Medical Equipment Service Co.

http://www.87.Net/BMES/

Company sells telemetry and cardiac monitoring equipment and parts, as well as repairs fiberoptic scopes, pulse oximeters, telemetry machines, and other bio-medical equipment. Company has a national scope, but is based in Kentucky.

C&A Export Co.

http://www.cnaexport.com/

International medical division carries over 150,000 new and pre-owned products and a wide variety of spare parts for brand-name monitors, ultrasounds, endoscopes and other equipment. Site lists major equipment the company carries.

Choice Medical Systems Inc.

http://www.choicemedical.com/

This company supplies diagnostic ultrasound equipment and parts. Website lists in-stock ultrasound systems, transducers, peripherals and supplies.

Dale Technology

http://www.daletech.com/

Biotechnology company's website features product listings and technical support.

Diagnostix Plus Inc.

http://www.diagplus.com/index.htm

Diagnostix Plus, Inc. buys, sells, trades, rents and supports nuclear imaging equipment and accessories. The company invites customers to trade in their old systems and accessories towards purchase/rental of new equipment.

Dominion Imaging & Recycling Inc.

http://www.DominionImaging.com/

World-wide x-ray and medical equipment sales and service based in Washington, D.C. Site provides company information, contacts, and list of the equipment they carry.

D.R.E. Incorporated

http://www.dremedical.com/

Since 1984, D.R.E. has marketed new and refurbished medical equipment, especially anesthesia equipment for the medical and veterinary markets. Site provides information about its products in both English and Spanish.

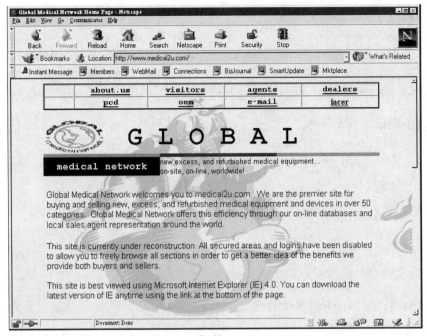

Global Medical Network: http://www.medical2u.com

Endoscopy Support Services Inc.
http://www.endoscopy.com/

Provides endoscopy equipment for medical and veterinary markets. Site offers company information, lists products and services, and even offers Web specials with photos. Features an online catalog and a used equipment inventory list which can be obtained on a subscription basis via e-mail.

General Biomedical Service Inc.
http://www.generalbiomedical.com/

Regional distributor of critical care medical equipment based in Louisiana. Site provides company information and list of products with pictures.

Global Medical Network
http://www.medical2u.com/

A site for buying and selling new and refurbished medical equipment on the Internet.

High Technology Inc.
http://www.htmed.com/

Medical equipment sales, service and consulting, especially for ultrasound, EKG monitors and laboratory equipment. Site features an equipment list with pictures; call for availability and pricing.

Imaging Associates
http://www.ImagingA.com/

Site offers information on company which sells, services and repairs ultrasound equipment and visual medicine software.

Inmark
http://www.inmarkcorp.com/

Information about the company and about the different types of x-ray equipment and software it reconditions and sells.

Integrity Medical Systems
http://www.integritymed.com/

Company offers world-wide sales, lease and rentals of refurbished medical equipment. Its website lists used equipment for sale, as well as equipment wanted.

International Association of Medical Equipment Remarketers
http://www.iamer.com/

Website representing the trade group for medical equipment dealers, leasers, refurbishers and servicers. Find out about membership and upcoming events, and link to member companies.

Kaman Medical
http://www.kamanmedical.com/

Buys and sells medical equipment at wholesale prices. Specializes in hospital liquidations. Site offers company information, inventory list and e-mail response.

Labworld Inc.
http://www.labworld1.com/

Sells remanufactured instrumentation for clinical laboratories. Equipment list and extensive company information on website.

Lancer Medical Services

http://www.medmart.com/lancer/

Company designs, manufactures, sells and services general purpose sterilizers, surgical instrument washers, pharmaceutical grade GMP sterilizers and biohazard waste retorts. Find information about the company and its products on its website.

Laser Labs

http://www.Laserlabs.com/

Lists and sells new and used lasers. Site features a free listing service for used equipment, and a weekly "hot list" of new products that have just become available.

Medelco Medical Electronics Co.

http://www.medelco.com/

Florida company specializing in preowned medical equipment, lists available merchandise and monthly specials on its site.

Medequip Engineering Services

http://www.medeq.com/

Website gives information and phone number for company, which provides new and re-manufactured operating room equipment, service and maintenance.

MedNet Locator

http://mednetlocator.com//equip.html

Direct source for buying and selling used medical equipment, especially in the fields of otolaryngology and ophthalmology.

MedPlanet

http://www.medsales.com/

Classified ads for medical products and equipment. This site seeks to help the visitor find the best medical products at the lowest prices; lists products for sale and wanted; and features an extensive medical equipment dealer list.

MedStore

http://www.medstore.com/

Listing of companies that offer new, used and refurbished medical equipment for sale, repair or recalibration.

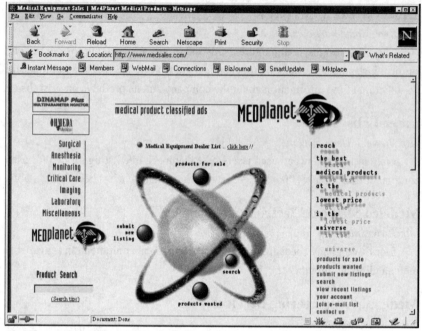

MedPlanet: *http://www.medsales.com/*

MedTech Imaging

http://www.medtechimaging.com/

Provider of quality pre-owned and refurbished ultrasound equipment. Site provides company profile, current inventory and lease options.

M.E.L.'s Place

http://www.invisionet.com/bioequip.htm

Provides pertinent Internet links for health care service and support professionals, including the names and websites of medical equipment companies and resalers.

Pioneer Medical

http://www.pioneermedical.com/

Regional company serving the southeast United States by providing medical equipment, especially respiratory, wound care and biomedical. Site provides information about the company, inventory and employment opportunities.

PMR Techmed

http://www.pmrtechmed.com/

International provider of emergency medical supplies and equipment to qualified emergency medical personnel. Site features some products, mostly defibrillators.

Prescott's Inc.

http://www.surgicalmicroscopes.com/

Company provides surgical microscopes. Its website lists equipment.

Priority Medical

http://www.prioritymedical.com/

Provider of pre-owned ultrasound equipment. Site provides information about the company and answers frequently asked questions about ultrasound.

Products Group International Inc.

http://www.productsgroup.com/

Provides ultrasound equipment and supplies to veterinary and medical markets. Site provides company information, products and services, and links to other health-related websites.

Progressive Medical International

http://www.ProgressiveMed.com/

Distributor of emergency medical equipment and supplies. Website features "hot sheet specials," which are deals offered on the Web.

Sunnico International Inc.

http://www.sunnico.com/

Company buys and sells pre-owned diagnostic imaging equipment, including MRI, CT, ultrasound, mammography and radiation machines. Site offers a listing of products available, as well as a place to list items for sale.

Surgical Image Laboratories Inc.

http://www.Surgicalimage.com/

A high-tech manufacturing and repair facility for endoscopes, the company's website offers information on the company, scope manufacturing and repair, and an online order form.

The Scope Exchange
http://www.scopex.com/

Company provides high-quality pre-owned endoscopic equipment. Site contains information about the company, inventory list, and helpful hints on flexible scope maintenance.

TLC Medical Equipment Corp.
http://www.medstore.com/tlcmedical/

Wholesale distributor and discount supplier to physicians, health care professionals, laboratories and medical institutions. Website features company information and e-mail contact form.

TriMed Inc.
http://www.trimedic.com/

Based in Miami, this medical equipment distributor continuously updates its website to include pictures and descriptions of the products it carries.

Used Equipment World Inc.
http://www.uew.com/

Website designed for buyers and sellers of used medical equipment and spare parts. Searchable database of over 5,000 items.

Whittemore Enterprises Inc.
http://www.wemed1.com/

Refurbished medical equipment. Website includes a searchable database of current inventory and an online wholesale catalog with pictures.

MEDICAL HUMOR

Addiction

Humor and Addiction
http://www.users.cts.com/crash/e/elmo/funindex.htm
  Page is part of a website dedicated to recovery for individuals in hopeless conditions of mind, body and spirit. E-mail jokes back to the author, too.

Health Care

American Association for Therapeutic Humor
http://www.aath.org/
  Organization committed to better understanding humor and laughter as they relate to health and well-being. Site provides information on membership and activities, as well as humor with its joke of the week and funny, "quotable quotes."

Emergency Medical Humor
http://home.cwnet.com/catspaw/emshumor.htm
  For the emergency room crowd, "tasteless, sick, twisted and funny material."

Health Care Humor
http://www.webcom.com/mdtaxes/humor.html
  Jokes relating to the health care industry.

Humor Page: Medical
http://www.swcbc.com/medical.html
  Lots of jokes related to health and medical topics.

The Humor Potential, Inc.
http://www.stressed.com/

Company provides seminars and products on stress reduction, mixing humor with life experiences as a coping mechanism. Its website features company information, a speaker's bureau, a store, and "laughter self tests" for fun.

The HUMOR Project, Inc.
http://www.wizvax.net/humor/

Promoting the positive power of humor and creativity in everyday life with Daily Laffirmations, funny stories, and a speaker's bureau. Also, submit stories here for "Chicken Soup for the Laughing Soul."

HUMORx
http://www.humorx.com/

Web page of nurse and therapeutic humorist Karyn Buxman, who makes presentations to business and health professionals on how to put humor into their personal and professional lives.

Jest for the Health of It!
http://www.mother.com/JestHome/

Website for company that does seminars and presentations on health and humor.

Managed Care Jokes
http://www.ncpamd.com/mcjokes.htm#

Notes, jokes and humor about managed care. For example: *Q:* How many managed care reviewers does it take to change a light bulb? *A:* Five. One to receive the authorization forms and put them at the bottom of a pile; the second to put the pile in a storage closet; the third to refuse to authorize the light bulb change because the authorization forms were never received; the fourth to process the resubmitted authorization forms; and the fifth to authorize a ten-watt light bulb because it uses less electricity.

Medical Bloopers
http://www.ep-publishing.com/bloopers.html

Website promoting a blooper-a-day desk calendar.

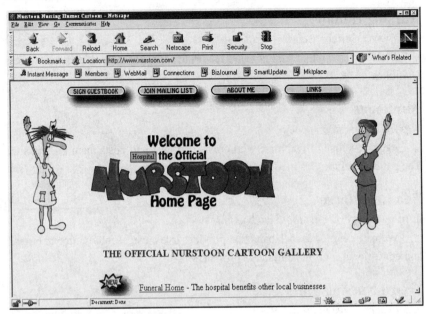

Nurstoon, *http://www.nurstoon.com/*

Medical Humor Page

http://dacc.uchicago.edu/medhumor.html

Part of the University of Chicago's Anesthesia and Critical Care Department's website. Contains anagrams and links to other health-related humor sites.

Mistaken Dictation

http://www.bargain-mall.com/medical5.htm

Funny quotes taken from actual medical records dictated by physicians. Originally published in a column written by Richard Lederer, Ph.D. for the *Journal of Court Reporting*. These and other language gems are featured in Lederer's 1997 book *Fractured English*, published by Pocket Books.

Nursing

Home Health Humor

http://www.whidbey.com/ihn/humor.html

Humorous personal stories from home health care workers.

Nursing Humor
http://www.jocularity.com/

Links to other nursing humor sites featuring brain teasers, inspirational stories, and jokes.

Nurstoons
http://www.nurstoon.com/

Page developed by a nurse who draws cartoons and posts them on this site. The gallery includes his work, as well as some guest cartoons.

Too Live Nurse
http://www.vgernet.net/toolive/who.html

Website devoted to rock band that provides live musical entertainment, humor and educational tools to health care providers.

Weird Nursing Tales
http://users.twave.net/texican/

Fun for nurses, including jokes, humor and scary "ghost" stories.

Sleep

The Lighter Side of Sleep
http://www.stanford.edu/~dement/sleephumor.html

Amusing jokes and anecdotes about sleep and the lack of it, submitted by visitors.

Weight Loss

Dieter's Guide to Weight Loss During Sex
http://www.maui.net/~jms/weight.html

Have some fun! A light-hearted guide showing the number of calories burned during sex.

MEDICAL IMAGING / TELEMEDICINE

Gamma Knife

Center for Image-Guided Neurosurgery
http://www.neuronet.pitt.edu/groups/ctr-image/welcome.html

Information about gamma knife surgery from the University of Pittsburgh, which is investigating and developing the use of this minimally invasive neurosurgical procedure to enable safer and more effective treatment for patients with brain disorders.

Medical Imaging

Andrew Barclay's Medical Imaging Pages
http://www.emory.edu/CRL/abb/

Radiology and nuclear medicine images.

Center for Human Simulation
http://www.uchsc.edu/sm/chs/

Describes the projects going on at the University of Colorado Health Sciences Center's Center for Human Simulation. The project combines human anatomy and computed three-dimensional imaging, resulting in a three-dimensional, high resolution database of human male and female anatomy (the Visible Human) as derived from direct analysis of anatomical specimens and radiological imaging.

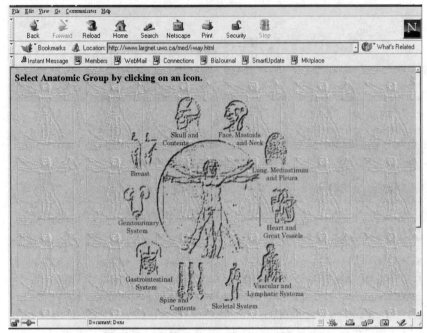

Medical Imaging Database: http://www.largnet.uwo.ca/med/i-way.html

Medical Imaging Database

http://www.largnet.uwo.ca/med/i-way.html

Click on anatomic area to access database of cases containing radiologic images, case history and diagnosis.

Medical Imaging Resources on the Internet

http://agora.leeds.ac.uk/comir/resources/links.html

A list of medical imaging resources that are available on the Internet, grouped according to geographic region, content, sources of funding and Usenet newsgroup.

National Library of Medicine Quantitative Visualization/ Teleradiology Project

http://everest.radiology.uiowa.edu/nlm/nlmhome.html

Using the Internet, the Library of Medicine hopes to educate primary care personnel in rural settings on the aspects and benefits of multimodality image processing and analysis. Rural centers that do not have the capability to analyze their image data can obtain expert consultation from the University of Iowa via the Iowa Fiber Optic Network. Trained technologists, with a team of physicians and members, will be made available to provide consultation.

The "Virtual" Medical Center: Medical Imaging Center

http://www-sci.lib.uci.edu/HSG/MedicalImage.html

Extensive links to *.MPEG movies and thousands of medical images.

Volume Slicer Applet Demos

http://www.cc.emory.edu/CRL/java/slicer/

Java-based application that allows a 2-dimensional scan of a 3-dimensional object to be re-sampled into 3 sets of images along X, Y and Z axes.

Nuclear Medicine

Cases Related to Nuclear Medicine

http://mfs.med.u-tokai.ac.jp/radiology/index.html

Offer your own diagnosis after looking at x-ray and scan images.

The Nuclear Medicine Browser

http://www.xs4all.nl/~dschonf/

Provides links to sites featuring medical images and information for oncology, radiology, positron emission tomography, and imaging manufacturers.

Radiology

Chiropractic Radiology WebPage

http://web.idirect.com/~xray/chiro.html

Make a cyber diagnosis, download vertebral screensavers, or link to other chiropractic sites.

CHORUS

http://chorus.rad.mcw.edu/

CHORUS = Collaborative Hypertext of Radiology. This site for medical students and physicians is a quick reference to more than 1,100 documents describing: diseases, radiological findings, differential-diagnosis lists ("gamuts"), pertinent anatomy, pathology, and physiology. CHORUS documents are indexed by organ system and are interconnected by hypertext link.

Radiologic Anatomy Interactive Quiz

http://www.gsm.com/resources/raquiz/

An interactive quiz regarding analysis of x-ray images.

Radiological Society of North America Launch Pad

http://www.rsna.org/

Search the RSNA database, or browse through key categories related to the radiological sciences. Many websites covering a huge variety of topics are provided, including anatomy on the web, medical ethics, nuclear medicine and telemedicine.

The Radiology Library

http://www.embbs.com/xray/xr.html

Web-based radiology teaching library containing hundreds of images. For those people who are interested in emergency computed tomography, a CT scan page has images that are between 15K-25K for faster download.

Telemedicine

The First International Telemedicine Trial to China: Zhu Ling's Case

http://www.radsci.ucla.edu/telemed/zhuling/

In April 1995, a young student from Beijing University, Bei Zhicheng, sent an SOS e-mail message through the Internet to ask for international help for a young female university student, Zhu Ling, suffering an unknown but severe disease. Bei received over 2,000 e-mail replies from 18 countries. The Internet played a very important role in saving Zhu Lin's life. This site tells about Zhu's diagnosis and treatment via the Internet.

NLM National Telemedicine Initiative

http://www.nlm.nih.gov/research/telemedinit.html

The National Library of Medicine supports 19 telemedicine projects. This site offers information on each, its purpose, and other telemedicine programs.

Telemedicine Information Exchange

http://tie.telemed.org/

These pages provide basic information on telemedicine and its applications, a brief history of telemedicine, business and product news summaries, examples of historical and current uses, and articles and abstracts from journals. Also contains a particularly thorough list of links to telemedicine-related sites from medical images to videoconferencing. A TIE forum presents experts' answers to frequently asked questions.

Telemedicine Resources

http://icsl.ee.washington.edu/~cabralje/tmresources.html

Offers a list of web resources and services related to telemedicine. The resources are broken down into four categories: general telemedicine, compression and teleconferencing standards, networking, and medical imaging.

Ultrasound

See also: Pregnancy - Ultrasound, Amniocentesis & Other Prenatal Tests.

Obstetric Ultrasound

http://www.ob-ultrasound.net/

A good site for comprehensive information about this technology and how it is used in obstetrics. Site features hypertext links and an image gallery.

Ob-Gyn Ultrasound Online

http://www2.ultrasoundedu.com/ultrasoundedu/

An interactive text and journal with teaching files, reference charts, collected abstracts, selected articles, and links to other related sites.

MEDICAL LAW

Americans with Disabilities Act

Accessibility Guidelines for Buildings and Facilities
http://www.access-board.gov/bfdg/adaag.htm

Contains technical specifications for the design and alteration of public buildings that need to be accessible under the Americans with Disabilities Act (ADA).

Americans with Disabilities Act Document Center
http://janweb.icdi.wvu.edu/kinder/

Site provides full text of the various legal documents and laws pertaining to the ADA, as well as links to pertinent sites.

Americans with Disabilities Act Home Page
http://www.usdoj.gov/crt/ada/adahom1.com

The U.S. Department of Justice maintains this site. Find information about the toll-free ADA phone line, ADA enforcement programs, ADA status reports, new or proposed regulations, and ADA Technical Assistance grants.

The Arc's Access ADA Activities
http://TheArc.org/ada/adaindx.html

The Arc (formerly the Association of Retired Citizens) site educates the public about accessibility, features links to related sites, and provides an Access Strategies Chart of functional solutions to common problems that disabled people face when trying to access businesses.

Health Insurance

COBRA Online
http://www.medlaw.com/

Online health law resource center provides information on COBRA benefits, medical malpractice, health issues, health care economics and related subjects.

Insure.com: Health Insurance
http://www.insure.com/health/

Insure.com is an online newsletter for consumers about the insurance industry. Includes a complaint finder and a lawsuit library, readers' forum, links and health insurance frequently asked questions.

National Association of Insurance Commissioners
http://www.naic.org/

Comprised of chief insurance regulators in all 50 states, the District of Columbia, and U.S. territories, the NAIC helps state regulators to protect the interest of insurance consumers, and provides a forum for developing policy which states are invited to adopt.

Social Security Online
http://www.ssa.gov/SSA_Home.html

Information and publications on Social Security entitlement programs including Medicare.

Malpractice

Online Medical Malpractice Magazine
http://www.a-r-m.org/

Published by the Association for Responsible Medicine, this patient-advocate magazine lists the malpractice records of Florida doctors, the risks associated with common medical treatments, advice on how to file a malpractice claim, and information on how to protect your self from a malpractice mistake.

Medical Law

FindLaw Internet Legal Resources
http://www.findlaw.com/
Site that features extensive links to legal resources, including health law.

Health Consumer Alliance
http://www.healthconsumer.org/
The Health Consumer Alliance is a united effort of eight legal services and health policy agencies "skilled and experienced at addressing the health problems of low-income consumers." Its site provides information about the organization, its services, and its publications.

Health Hippo
http://hippo.findlaw.com/
A collection of policy and regulatory materials related to health care. Some of the topics covered include: advance directives, the Balanced Budget Act, HIPAA, infection control standards, long-term care, Medicare Plus + Choice, health care reform and codes dealing with quality assurance in health care, to name a few. The site also features a link to the Federal Register.

Health Law Research Gateway
http://lawlib.slu.edu/healthcenter/research/research_index.htm
St. Louis University Center for Health Law Studies provides news about health law, as well as links to other resources on the Web.

The Health Law Resource
http://www.netreach.net/~wmanning/
A site for people interested in health care law. Provides resources for health care practitioners, legal professionals and the public, specifically regarding the regulatory and transactional aspects of health care law practice. Subject areas include telemedicine, bioethics, privacy, Medicare/Medicaid, fraud & abuse, and mergers & acquisitions.

The Medical and Public Health Law Site
http://plague.law.umkc.edu/
Online textbook for physicians.

Medical Protection Society
http://www.mps.org.uk/medical/

International nonprofit association offering medico-legal services to physicians. Site offers advice, case reports and links.

Medical Record Privacy
http://epic.org/privacy/medical/

Site presents laws, articles and discussion about medical privacy law and policy, and consumer advice on safeguarding medical records.

National Health Law Program
http://www.healthlaw.org/

NHeLP is a 30-year-old national public interest law firm working for "justice in health care for low-income people." This site provides information on the organization and its services, legal research to pertinent court cases, links, news headlines, and a list of consumer resources.

Psychiatry and the Law
http://ua1vm.ua.edu/~jhooper/index.html

This site is authored by the University of Alabama's Department of Psychology and Neurology and its School of Law. It provides information on legal issues that psychiatrists face, landmark legal cases in mental health law, and links to other related sites.

MEDICAL REFERENCES / RESOURCES

Computers/Internet

Healthcare Information and Management Systems Society
http://www.himss.org/

Website for a nonprofit organization representing information and management systems professionals in the health care industry. Site provides information about the organization, how to join, upcoming events, education and professional development opportunities.

Medicine by Modem
http://www.news.com/SpecialFeatures/0%2C5%2C7943%2C00.html?nd

News.com special report that discusses the benefits and cautions for both physicians and consumers who want to use the Internet for medical information. The site features related stories and links.

Consumer Health

AMA Health Insight
http://www.ama-assn.org/consumer.htm

Consumer health resource. Includes specific conditions, general health information and medical care advice.

American Board of Medical Specialties Patient Education Program
http://www.certifieddoctor.org/

Verify that your doctor is board certified, or locate a board-certified doctor.

beWell.com
http://beWELL.com

This site is divided into "healthzines": Healthy Athlete, Healthy Man, Healthy Woman, Healthy Eating, Healthy Mind, Healthy Parenting and Healthy Sexuality. It offers columns for the Healthy Traveler, and RxAlert for drug developments.

Health Information Resources
http://www.nih.gov/health/

Site describes publications, hotlines, programs and other resources, including Internet resources, that are available from the National Institutes of Health.

HealthSeek.com
http://www.healthseek.com/

Commercial, online service for health care professionals, consumers and companies providing news, information and links.

Internet Health Resources
http://www.ihr.com/

Access to information on infertility, homeopathy, health care publications and Bay-area health services.

Mayo Clinic Health Oasis
http://www2.mayohealth.org/index.htm

Top-rated site features health news and consumer resources. Includes a health library covering different conditions, a glossary, and access to various "centers" on allergies, Alzheimer's, cancer, children, heart, men, women and nutrition.

MedicineNet
http://www.medicinenet.com/

Provides information on diseases and treatments, procedures and tests, pharmacy information, medical terminology, first aid and poison control centers. Site also features news, treatment updates, and health facts. MedicineNet is published by a network of doctors for the general public.

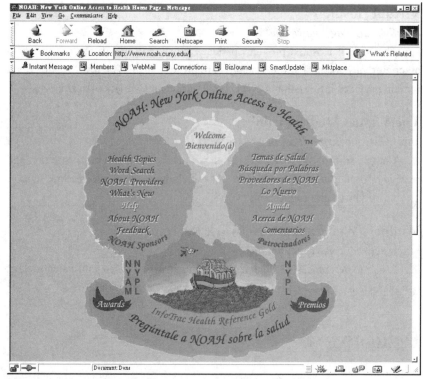

New York Online Access to Health: http://www.noah.cuny.edu/

The Merck Manual of Diagnosis and Treatment Online

http://www.merck.com:80/!!rABLW3Y3TrABLY0OmS/pubs/mmanual/

Searchable online version of this famous handbook of medical disorders and therapies.

New York Online Access to Health Main Menu

http://www.noah.cuny.edu/

Main menu is in English and in Spanish. Allows surfers to browse through health topics, or perform a word search.

Paper Chase

http://www.paperchase.com/

A medical information service available to both health professionals and the general public which provides access to MEDLINE, Aidsline, CancerLit and HealthSTAR with registration. Service is available for a monthly or yearly fee.

Virtual Hospital

http://vh.radiology.uiowa.edu/

The Virtual Hospital provides patient care support and distance learning to practicing physicians and other health care professionals. The Iowa Health Book section provides information to the general public on a variety of health issues.

The Virtual Medical Clinic

http://www.mediconsult.com/

Choose from over 50 medical topics, ranging from AIDS to Strokes; and receive information, articles and links. Also includes medical information, support groups, products, and suggestions.

Wellness Web Patient's Network References

http://wellweb.com/refer/refer.htm

Links to references of medical and general use, divided into categories of complementary medicine, conventional medicine, and nutrition/fitness.

Databases

DynaMed: Medical Information System Database

http://www.DynamicMedical.com/

A medical information database that contains over 2,000 diseases, updated daily, for use by health care providers in their work. Visitors must register to use the site, but it's free.

Firstmark Mailing Lists, Labels and Databases

http://www.firstmark.com/

Website for company that sells databases in either mailing label or telemarketing formats. The health care databases include choices of physicians, pharmaceutical companies, nurses and health care centers.

NLM Online Databases and Databanks

http://www.nlm.nih.gov/pubs/factsheets/online_databases.html

Describes 40 NLM online databases, including: AIDSDRUGS, AIDSLINE, AIDSTRIALS, CANCERLIT, HealthSTAR, MEDLINE, PDQ, TOXLINE and TOXNET.

Drug References

See also: Drugs/Pharmacology.

Healthtouch

http://www.healthtouch.com/

Find information about more than 10,000 prescription and over-the-counter medications, and access information about pharmacies in your community. The site also provides information about organizations such as the American Diabetes Association and others; and it provides health information on Medicare, women's health, diabetes, liver problems and nervous system disorders.

PDRNET.COM

http://www.pdrnet.com/

Online _Physicians' Desk Reference_ free to physicians. Also find access to MEDLINE and to PDR prescription information here.

Gateways

Achoo!

http://www.achoo.com/

Very comprehensive site featuring information about health care as well as links to health-related sites on the Web.

Alice!

http://www.columbia.edu/cu/healthwise/

Columbia University's Health Education Program includes _Go Ask Alice!_ which is an interactive question-and-answer response service.

CliniWeb

http://www.ohsu.edu/cliniweb/

CliniWeb is maintained by Oregon Health Services University and offers an index and table of contents to clinical information on the World Wide Web. Includes approximately 10,000 website links.

Diseases, Disorders and Related Topics
http://www.mic.ki.se/Diseases/index.html

Alphabetical list to links covering hundreds of diseases. From Sweden's Karolinska Institute.

Edmund's Home Page
http://www.edhayes.com/

Begun as a personal homepage by a pharmacist at Stony Brook University Medical Center, this site has grown to provide many links to different health-related sites, including medical, dental, pharmacy, nursing, bioscience, and nutrition.

Galaxy's Medicine
http://galaxy.einet.net/galaxy/Medicine.html

Links to medical information, arranged by specialty and disease. Includes academic organizations, commercial organizations, directives, government agencies and private organizations.

Hardin Meta Directory: Internet Health Sources
http://www.lib.uiowa.edu/hardin/md/index.html

Their slogan is, "We list the best sites." The "best" sites are categorized in a long list of topic areas, such as allergies, emergency medicine, ob/gyn, and surgery to name a few. The "best" sites are determined by their connection rates, which supposedly indicates a site is receiving care and attention.

Health Web
http://healthweb.org/

A cooperative effort by a number of health sciences libraries to provide organized access to evaluated, non-commercial, health-related, Internet-accessible Web resources. Links and information on a number of health and medical topics.

Health/Medical Internet Entry Points
http://www.age.ne.jp/x/akagi/healthep.htm

Colorful and animated site features links to websites for international health organizations, U.S. government health departments, health and medical databases, AIDS information, communicable disease and travel health, disaster preparedness and relief organizations, as well as news agencies and broadcast networks.

Healthfinder

http://www.healthfinder.gov/

The United States government's consumer health site. Includes links to chosen online publications, databases, support groups, organizations, government sites and other health information resources on the Web.

Inter-Links Health Resources

http://alabanza.com/kabacoff/Inter-Links/medicine.html

Links to Internet resources for information on health and medicine, including National Institutes of Health, National Library of Medicine, MEDLINE, CNN and the New York Times.

Martindale's Health Science Guide

http://www-sci.lib.uci.edu/~martindale/HSGuide.html

A multimedia health information resource that features over 56,000 teaching files, over 126,000 medical case examples, over 1,000 multimedia courses, and over 3,500 databases.

MedWorld Best Sites

http://www-med.stanford.edu/medworld/medlinks/

Selective listing of some medical websites. Divided into categories such as: patient resources, physician resources, research, clinical sciences, basic sciences, news and information, and "cool sites."

OHSU Library: Internet Resources

http://www.ohsu.edu/bicc-Library/netcat/netcat.htm

List of and links to health and medical resources on the Web.

The Six Senses Review

http://www.sixsenses.com/

Reviews health and medical websites. Sites are rated on content, aesthetics, interactivity, innovation, freshness, and character. Allows visitors to submit sites for review, and to search or browse for sites by topic.

WWW Medical Indexes

http://www.intmed.mcw.edu/MedIndex.html

Long list of medical sites and indexes gathered by the Medical College of Wisconsin.

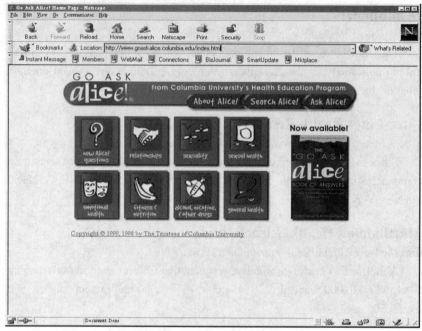

Go Ask Alice!: http://www.goaskalice.columbia.edu/index.html

Health Education

Go Ask Alice!
http://www.goaskalice.columbia.edu/index.html

Columbia University's Health Education Program offers answers to questions on different health topics. Submit questions about sexuality, sexual health, relationships, general health, emotional well-being, alcohol/drugs, and fitness and nutrition.

MEdIC: Medical Education Information Center
http://dpalm2.med.uth.tmc.edu/

A multimedia health education tool for both professionals and consumers, developed by the University of Texas, Houston Department of Pathology and Laboratory. One feature is the Health Explorer where information on a range of diseases can be found. Another feature is Education, which lists courses offered by the university for continuing medical education.

Hospitals

Council of Teaching Hospitals
http://www.aamc.org/hlthcare/teach/
  Lists hospitals in the council, both alphabetically and geographically.

HospitalWeb
http://neuro-www.mgh.harvard.edu/hospitalweb.shtml
  Lists hospitals that have pages on the Internet.

Libraries

Galen II
http://www.library.ucsf.edu/
  The digital library of the University of California at San Francisco. Search databases, literature, electronic journals and selected Internet resources.

The Internet Public Libraries
http://ipl.sils.umich.edu/svcs/greatlibs/
  Collection of library web pages with a summaries of their resources on specific topics.

Library of Congress
gopher://marvel.loc.gov:70/11/global/med/general/
  Gopher menu from the U.S. Library of Congress.

National Network of Libraries of Medicine
http://www.nnlm.nlm.nih.gov/
  Access to world-wide biomedical information for U.S. health care professionals.

U.S. National Library of Medicine
http://www.nlm.nih.gov/
  This site provides information about the Library, as well as news, access to databases and special information programs, NLM publications (fact sheets, reports and ordering information), research programs, grant information, and many links.

Medical Research

National Center for Research Resources
http://www.ncrr.nih.gov/
The Center creates and provides critical research technologies and shared resources.

Professional Resources

ACP Online
http://www.acponline.org/
The website for the American College of Physician and the American Society of Internal Medicine features a career resource center, a list of websites for internists, and articles from *Annals of Internal Medicine.*

Alphabetical List of Specific Diseases/Disorders
http://www.mic.ki.se/Diseases/alphalist.html
Alphabetical list of specific diseases and disorders with related web links.

Doctor's Guide to the Internet
http://www.pslgroup.com/DOCGUIDE.HTM
This site was designed to save physicians hours of browsing while providing them with a comfortable and friendly environment from which to derive the most value from the Internet. It provides medical news and alerts, information about new drugs or indications, a medical bookstores, and links to medical sites on the Web.

HCN: Health Communication Network
http://www.hcn.net.au/
Australian-based site containing medical databases, indexes, publishing and bibliographic information, forums and other information for paying members.

Health Professionals' Online
http://www.hpol.net/
Provides health professionals access to popular medical literature databases, drug databases, medical news, disease centers, discussion groups and directories of medical research for a monthly fee.

HealthEconomics.com

http://www.healtheconomics.com/

Site features a number of links to sites providing disease information and medical humor, and to associations, institutions and commercial medical companies, medical libraries and more.

HealthGate

http://www.healthgate.com/

Site for health care professionals organized according to the following categories: research tools, continuing medical education, health news, book reviews, and patient education. Research tools includes access to MEDLINE, CANCERLIT, AIDSDRUGS, AIDSTRIAL, HealthSTAR, and Morbidity & Mortality Weekly Report (MMWR) for free.

Journal Club on the Web

http://www.journalclub.org/

An interactive medical literature review where the host, Michael Jacobson, MD, MPH, will comment on a couple of recent articles each month, then encourage feedback from readers.

MedConnect

http://www.medconnect.com/

Interactive site offering continuing medical education and job search online, a managed care forum, medical news, and marketplace.

MedForum

http://www.migraine.com/

Medical forum for physicians, journalists and the general public. Includes peer-reviewed Internet journal *LifeLines*, information on the business of medicine, access to newsgroups, JobLine, and M.D. On Call research, which costs $300 per research request.

MedGate

http://www.medgate.com/

Company sells Occupational Health, Safety and Environmental software for health care industry. This software can be purchased on its site.

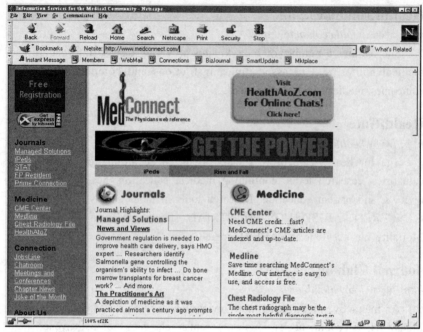

MedConnect: *http://www.medconnect.com/*

The Medical Center Web

http://www.medcenter.com/

Access to the World Congress of Cardiology in English or Portuguese.

Medical Matrix

http://www.medmatrix.org/

Use of the site requires registration, which is free. Access to clinical medicine resources online, including MEDLINE, journals, continuing medical education (CME) opportunities on the Internet, news, prescription assistance, textbooks, forums, patient information and classified ads.

The Multimedia Medical Reference Library

http://www.med-library.com/medlibrary

Resources are divided into the following categories: audio, clinical trials, journals, medical equipment auctions, medical reference libraries, medical schools, medical services, medical software, products, and professional organizations.

Net Medicine

http://www.netmedicine.com/

Site includes a CyberPatient simulator, PhotoRounds Challenge, EKG of the Month, Radiology Rounds, Pediatric Topics, patient education center and practice opportunities. Also offers free MEDLINE, and the Medfinder search engine.

Online Clinical Calculator

http://www.intmed.mcw.edu/clincalc.html

This calculator finds the Bayesian Analysis of prevalence, sensitivity and specificity; and clinical calculations of estimated blood level, body surface/body mass ratio, weight and measurement conversions. Site hosted by the Medical College of Wisconsin.

Physician's Guide to the Internet

http://www.webcom.com/pgi/

Site offers both professional and personal information for physicians. A section on Physician Lifestyles includes articles on health, family life, professional opportunities and personal finance. The site also provides access to clinical resources, CME courses, medical news, a job board and "fun stuff" which includes articles on travel, food, restaurants and wine.

Physicians' HomePage

http://php2.silverplatter.com/php/mt-lib.htm#about

Membership allows access to *MD Digests*, Internet Library, *MD Opinions* (primary care questions), *MD Drugs*, medical journals, and more. Flat rate fee is reduced for medical residents.

Physician's Online

http://www.po.com/Welcome.html

Members receive free access to MEDLINE and other medical and drug databases, an e-mail account, stock quotes, continuing medical education (CME) opportunities, physicians-only discussion groups, non-medical resources, and more. To join, you must install the Physicians' Online (POL) software (instructions provided at site).

Primary Care Baseline

http://www.med.ufl.edu/medinfo/baseline/

Contains clinical care algorithms and drug list.

WebDoctor
http://www.gretmar.com/webdoctor/home.html
Contains a peer-reviewed index of Internet medical resources, by specialty and disease. Particularly large section on rural medicine.

What's New at the American Medical Association
http://www.ama-assn.org/what_new/what_new.htm
Association updates, registration and policy information, the current month's edition of *JAMA*, conference announcements, etc.

Search Tools

Health A to Z
http://www.HealthAtoZ.com/
Search engine to seek health sites on the Internet.

Health Explorer
http://www.healthexplorer.com/
Over 3,000 health-related websites. Search by topic or keyword.

Internet Sleuth Health Database Search Engine
http://www.isleuth.com/heal.html
Search a variety of health databases by keyword or topic.

Med Bot Search Tool
http://www-med.stanford.edu/medworld/medbot/
This "Super Search" tool allows you to access information from four different indices at once, and will report findings on a single page for easy reference.

Med Hunt
http://www.hon.ch/MedHunt/
Search the Internet with this search engine from Health on the Net Foundation. Includes library, media gallery, and free MEDLINE access.

Med Web

http://WWW.MedWeb.Emory.Edu/MedWeb/

Database of medical related Internet sites that can be easily browsed by using keywords. One of the best health search engines.

OMNI

http://omni.ac.uk/

A UK gateway to biomedical resources on the Internet.

Statistics

Cancer Statistics Review

http://www-seer.ims.nci.nih.gov/Publications/CSR1973_1996/

From the National Cancer Institute. Provides incidence, mortality, and survival data from 1973 through 1996. Represents about 10 percent of the U.S. population.

Center for International Health Information

http://www.cihi.com/

This organization's purpose is to provide information on the Population, Health, and Nutrition (PHN) sector in developing countries that are assisted by USAID (United States Agency for International Development).

The Combined Health Information Database

http://chid.nih.gov/

Do a detailed or a simple search on a variety of topics, including AIDS, arthritis, cancer, diabetes, maternal and child health, and weight control. Site also has links to National Institutes of Health, Centers for Disease Control, and Health Resources and Services Administration, which is a department of Health and Human Services.

Country Health Profiles: Health in the Americas

http://www.paho.org/english/country.htm

Describes the general health trends, specific health problems and risks, and the health care resources and services available in approximately 40 countries in the Americas. From the Pan American Health Organization.

Health Insurance Statistics

http://www.census.gov/hhes/www/hlthins.html

Information comes from the U.S. Census Bureau. Topics include cross-sectional studies of health insurance coverage and children's health insurance, as well as longitudinal studies of lack of coverage.

Medicare and Medicaid Statistics and Data

http://www.hcfa.gov/stats/stats.htm

Statistics on Medicare and Medicaid.

National Center for Health Statistics

http://www.cdc.gov/nchswww/

Site for the CDC's National Center for Health Statistics. The mission of the NCHS is to provide statistical information that will guide actions and policies to improve the health of the American people. Site offers news releases, fact sheets, publications, employment opportunities, a Web search and links.

Science Based Facts on Drug Abuse and Addiction

http://www.nida.nih.gov/NIDACapsules/NCIndex.html

Site provides information on drug abuse and addiction, the health effects of specific drugs, the link between drug abuse and AIDS, and information on the National Institute on Drug Abuse(NIDA) which is part of the National Institutes of Health.

Scientific Data, Surveillance, Health Statistics, and Laboratory Information

http://www.cdc.gov/scientific.htm

Site provides data regarding death rates, sexually transmitted diseases, hazardous materials, Y2K issues, HIV surveillance, pregnancy risk assessment, and assisted reproductive technology success rates, to name a few.

Statistical Tables: Information from the Centers for Disease Control

http://www.cdc.gov/nchswww/datawh/statab/pubd.htm

Statistical information on behavioral risk factors (i.e., overweight, high cholesterol, smoking habits), chronic diseases, infant and child health, sex education and sexual activity.

Substance Abuse and Mental Health Statistics

http://www.samhsa.gov/oas/oasftp.htm

Statistics on mental health and substance abuse prevalence. Includes the preliminary results from the group's 1997 National Household Survey on Drug Abuse.

WHOSIS

http://www.who.int/whosis/

The World Health Organization's Statistical Information System provides health and health-related information about international travel and health, AIDS/HIV statistics, immunizations, and mortality statistics world-wide.

MEDICAL SCHOOL WEBSITES & INFORMATION

*Covered in this chapter: U.S. Medical Schools (by state); Canadian Medical Schools (by province); Medical Schools: Lists; General Medical Education Information; Residency. [Note that all schools listed are all accredited by the Association of American Medical Colleges (AAMC), unless they are marked with an *.]*

Related chapter: Health Care Careers & Education.

U.S. Medical Schools

Alabama

University of Alabama School of Medicine (Birmingham)
http://www.uab.edu/uasom/

University of South Alabama, College of Medicine (Mobile)
http://southmed.usouthal.edu/index.html

Arizona

The University of Arizona College of Medicine (Tucson)
http://www.medicine.arizona.edu/

Arkansas

University of Arkansas for Medical Sciences (Little Rock)
http://www.uams.edu/

California

University of California, Davis, School of Medicine
http://www-med.ucdavis.edu/

University of California, Irvine, College of Medicine
http://meded.com.uci.edu/

University of California, Los Angeles, School of Medicine
http://www.medsch.ucla.edu/

University of California, San Diego, School of Medicine
http://medicine.ucsd.edu/

University of California, San Francisco, School of Medicine
http://www.som.ucsf.edu/

Charles Drew University of Medicine & Science (Los Angeles)
http://www.cdrewu.edu/

Loma Linda University School of Medicine
http://www.llu.edu/llu/medicine/

University of Southern California, Keck School of Medicine (Los Angeles)
http://www.usc.edu/schools/medicine/

Stanford University School of Medicine (Palo Alto)
http://www-med.stanford.edu/school/

Colorado

University of Colorado School of Medicine (Denver)
http://www.uchsc.edu/sm/sm/

Connecticut

University of Connecticut Health Center, School of Medicine (Farmington)

http://www9.uchc.edu/index.html

Yale University School of Medicine (New Haven)

http://info.med.yale.edu/ysm/index.html

District of Columbia

The George Washington University Medical Center

http://www.gwumc.edu/

Georgetown University School of Medicine

http://www.dml.georgetown.edu/schmed/

Howard University College of Medicine

http://www.med.howard.edu

Florida

University of Florida College of Medicine (Gainesville)

http://www.med.ufl.edu/

Florida State University/University of Florida Program in Medical Sciences (Tallahassee)

http://www.fsu.edu/~pims/pims.html

University of Miami School of Medicine

http://www.med.miami.edu/

University of South Florida College of Medicine (Tampa)

http://www.med.usf.edu/med.html

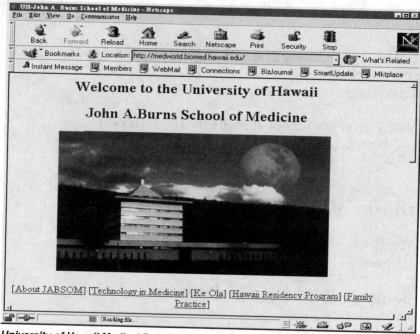

University of Hawaii Medical School. *http://medworld.biomed.hawaii.edu/*

Georgia

Emory School of Medicine (Atlanta)
http://www.emory.edu/WHSC/MED/index.html

Medical College of Georgia School of Medicine (Augusta)
http://www.mcg.edu/SOM/Index.html

Mercer University School of Medicine (Macon)
http://www.mercer.edu/musm/

Morehouse School of Medicine (Atlanta)
http://www.msm.edu/

Hawaii

University of Hawaii John A. Burns School of Medicine (Honolulu)
http://medworld.biomed.hawaii.edu/

Illinois

Finch University of Health Sciences/Chicago Medical School
http://www.finchcms.edu/

Loyola University, Chicago, Stritch School of Medicine (Maywood)
http://www.meddean.luc.edu/

Northwestern University Medical School (Chicago)
http://www.nums.nwu.edu/introtext.htm

Rush-Presbyterian-St. Luke's Medical Center (Chicago)
http://www.rush.edu/

Southern Illinois University School of Medicine (Springfield)
http://www.siumed.edu/

The University of Chicago Pritzker School of Medicine
http://pritzker.bsd.uchicago.edu/

The University of Illinois at Chicago College of Medicine
http://www.uic.edu/depts/mcam/

The University of Illinois College of Medicine at Rockford*
http://www.rockford.uic.edu/

University of Illinois College of Medicine at Urbana-Champaign*
http://www.med.uiuc.edu/

Indiana

Indiana University School of Medicine (Indianapolis)
http://www.medicine.iu.edu/home.html

Iowa

University of Iowa, College of Medicine (Iowa City)
http://www.medicine.uiowa.edu/

University of Osteopathic Medicine and Health Sciences (Des Moines)*
http://www.uomhs.edu/

Kansas

University of Kansas School of Medicine (Kansas City)
http://www.kumc.edu/som/som.html

Kentucky

University of Kentucky College of Medicine, Chandler Medical Center (Lexington)
http://www.comed.uky.edu/Medicine/welcome.html

University of Louisville School of Medicine
http://www.louisville.edu/medschool//

Louisiana

Louisiana State University Medical Center (New Orleans)
http://www.lsumc.edu/

Tulane University Medical Center (New Orleans)

http://www1.omi.tulane.edu/

Maine

University of New England College of Osteopathic Medicine (Biddeford)*

http://www.aacom.org/unecom.htm

Maryland

Johns Hopkins University School of Medicine (Baltimore)

http://infonet.welch.jhu.edu/som/

http://www.med.jhu.edu/admissions/

Uniformed Services University, Health Sciences School of Medicine (Bethesda)

http://www.usuhs.mil/medschool/index.html

University of Maryland School of Medicine (Baltimore)

http://som1.umaryland.edu/

Massachusetts

Boston University Medical Campus, School of Medicine

http://www.bumc.bu.edu/

Harvard Medical School (Boston)

http://www.hms.harvard.edu/

Tufts University School of Medicine (Boston)

http://www.tufts.edu/med/

University of Massachusetts Medical School (Worcester)
http://www.ummed.edu/

Michigan

Michigan State University College of Human Medicine (East Lansing)
http://www.chm.msu.edu/

University of Michigan Medical School (Ann Arbor)
http://www.med.umich.edu/medschool/

Wayne State University School of Medicine (Detroit)
http://www.med.wayne.edu/

Minnesota

Mayo Medical School (Rochester)
http://www.mayo.edu/mms/MMS_Home_Page.html

University of Minnesota at Duluth, School of Medicine
http://www.d.umn.edu/medweb/

University of Minnesota Medical School (Minneapolis)
http://www.med.umn.edu/

Mississippi

The University of Mississippi Medical Center (Jackson)
http://umc.edu/medicine/

Missouri

Saint Louis University School of Medicine*
http://www.slu.edu/colleges/med/

University of Missouri, Columbia, School of Medicine
http://www.hsc.missouri.edu/~medicine/

University of Missouri, Kansas City, School of Medicine
http://research.med.umkc.edu/

Washington University St. Louis School of Medicine
http://medinfo.wustl.edu/

Nebraska

Creighton University School of Medicine (Omaha)
http://medicine.creighton.edu/

University of Nebraska College of Medicine (Omaha)
http://www.unmc.edu/

Nevada

University of Nevada, Reno, Medical School and Biosciences
http://www.unr.edu/med

New Hampshire

Dartmouth Medical School (Hanover)
http://www.dartmouth.edu/dms/

New Jersey

New Jersey Medical School (Newark)
http://www.umdnj.edu/njmsweb

Robert Wood Johnson Medical School (Piscataway)
http://www2.umdnj.edu/rwjpweb/

New York

Albany Medical College (Albany)
http://www.amc.edu/Academic/index.htm

Albert Einstein College of Medicine of Yeshiva University (Bronx)
http://www.aecom.yu.edu/

Columbia University College of Physicians and Surgeons (New York)
http://cpmcnet.columbia.edu/dept/ps/

Weill Medical College of Cornell University (New York)
http://www.med.cornell.edu/

Mount Sinai School of Medicine (New York)
http://www.mssm.edu/

New York Medical College (Valhalla)
http://www.nymc.edu/

City University of New York Medical School (New York)
http://med.cuny.edu/

New York University School of Medicine (New York)
http://www.med.nyu.edu/som/index.html

State University of New York at Stony Brook, School of Medicine
http://www.informatics.sunysb.edu/som/

State University of New York, Health Science Center at Brooklyn, College of Medicine
http://www.hscbklyn.edu/COM/

State University of New York, Health Science Center at Syracuse
http://www.hscsyr.edu/

University of Buffalo School of Medicine and Biomedical Sciences
http://www.smbs.buffalo.edu/

University of Rochester School of Medicine and Dentistry
http://www.urmc.rochester.edu/SMD/

North Carolina

Bowman Gray School of Medicine at Wake Forest University (Winston-Salem)
http://isnet.is.wfu.edu/

Duke University School of Medicine (Durham)
http://www2.mc.duke.edu/depts/som/

East Carolina University School of Medicine (Greenville)
http://www.med.ecu.edu/DEPTMENU.HTM

University of North Carolina at Chapel Hill, School of Medicine
http://www.med.unc.edu/welcome.htm

North Dakota

University of North Dakota School of Medicine & Health Sciences (Grand Forks)

http://www.med.und.nodak.edu/

Ohio

Case Western Reserve University School of Medicine (Cleveland)

http://mediswww.meds.cwru.edu/

Medical College of Ohio, School of Medicine (Toledo)

http://www.mco.edu/smed/smedmain.html

Northeastern Ohio Universities College of Medicine (Rootstown)

http://www.neoucom.edu/

Ohio State University College of Medicine (Columbus)

http://www.med.ohio-state.edu/

University of Cincinnati College of Medicine

http://www.med.uc.edu/htdocs/medicine/uccom.htm

Wright State University School of Medicine (Dayton)

http://www.med.wright.edu/

Oklahoma

University of Oklahoma College of Medicine (Oklahoma City)

http://www.medicine.ouhsc.edu/

Oregon

Oregon Health Sciences University (Portland)
http://www.ohsu.edu/

Pennsylvania

MCP Hahnemann University, School of Medicine (Philadelphia)
http://www.auhs.edu/medschool/medschl.html

Pennsylvania State University College of Medicine (Hershey)
http://www.collmed.psu.edu/hmc/colmed.htm

Temple University School of Medicine (Philadelphia)
http://www.temple.edu/medschool/

Thomas Jefferson University, Jefferson Medical College (Philadelphia)
http://jeffline.tju.edu/CWIS/JMC/jmc.html

University of Pennsylvania School of Medicine (Philadelphia)
http://www.med.upenn.edu/

University of Pittsburgh School of Medicine
http://www.dean-med.pitt.edu/

Rhode Island

Brown University Division of Biology and Medicine (Providence)
http://biomed.brown.edu/Medicine.html

South Carolina

Medical University of South Carolina, College of Medicine (Charleston)
http://www2.musc.edu/medicine.html

University of South Carolina School of Medicine (Columbia)
http://www.med.sc.edu/

South Dakota

University of South Dakota School of Medicine (Vermillion)
http://www.usd.edu/med/

Tennessee

East Tennessee State University, James H. Quillen College of Medicine (Johnson City)
http://qcom.etsu.edu

Meharry Medical College (Nashville)
http://web.fie.com/htbin/Molis/MolisSummary?FICE=003506

University of Tennessee Memphis, College of Medicine
http://www.utmem.edu/medicine/

Vanderbilt University School of Medicine (Nashville)
http://www.mc.vanderbilt.edu/medschool/

Texas

Baylor College of Medicine (Houston)
http://www.bcm.tmc.edu/

College of Medicine at Texas A&M University (College Station)
http://tamushsc.tamu.edu/COM/COMmain.html

Texas Tech University Health Sciences Center, School of Medicine (El Paso, Lubbock & Odessa)
http://www.ttuhsc.edu/pages/med.htm

University of Texas Health Science Center at San Antonio Medical School
http://www.uthscsa.edu/som/som_main.htm

University of Texas Medical Branch at Galveston
http://www.utmb.edu/

University of Texas at Houston Health Science Center, Medical School
http://www.med.uth.tmc.edu/

University of Texas Southwestern Medical School at Dallas
http://www.swmed.edu/home_pages/publish/sms_catalog/1smscat.html

Utah

University of Utah School of Medicine (Salt Lake City)
http://www.med.utah.edu/som/

Vermont

The University of Vermont College of Medicine (Burlington)
http://www.med.uvm.edu/

Virginia

Eastern Virginia Medical School (Norfolk)
http://www.evms.edu/

School of Medicine, Medical College of Virginia/Virginia Commonwealth University (Richmond)
http://www.medschool.vcu.edu/

University of Virginia Health Sciences Center, School of Medicine (Charlottesville)
http://www.med.virginia.edu/schools/medschl.html

Washington

University of Washington School of Medicine (Seattle)
http://www.washington.edu/medical/som/index.html

West Virginia

Marshall University School of Medicine (Huntington)
http://musom.marshall.edu/

West Virginia University Robert C. Byrd Health Sciences Center School of Medicine (Morgantown)
http://www.hsc.wvu.edu/som/

Wisconsin

Medical College of Wisconsin (Milwaukee)
http://www.mcw.edu/

The University of Wisconsin Medical School (Madison)
http://www.medsch.wisc.edu/index.html

Canadian Medical Schools

Alberta

University of Alberta Faculty of Medicine and Oral Health Sciences (Edmonton)
http://www.med.ualberta.ca/

University of Calgary Faculty of Medicine (Calgary)
http://www.ucalgary.ca/UofC/faculties/Medicine/

British Columbia

The University of British Columbia Faculty of Medicine (Vancouver)
http://www.med.ubc.ca/

Manitoba

University of Manitoba Faculty of Medicine (Winnepeg)
http://www.umanitoba.ca/medicine/home.html

Newfoundland

Memorial University of Newfoundland Faculty of Medicine (St. John's)
http://www.med.mun.ca/med/

Nova Scotia

Dalhousie University Medical School (Halifax)
http://www.mcms.dal.ca/index.html

Ontario

McMaster University Faculty of Health Sciences (Hamilton)
http://www-fhs.mcmaster.ca/

Queen's University School of Medicine (Kingston)
http://meds-ss10.meds.queensu.ca/medicine/

University of Ottawa Faculty of Medicine
http://www.uottawa.ca/academic/med/

University of Toronto Faculty of Medicine
http://utl1.library.utoronto.ca/www/medicine/index.htm

University of Western Ontario Faculty of Medicine (London)
http://www.med.uwo.ca/

Quebec

McGill University Faculty of Medicine (Montreal)
http://www.med.mcgill.ca/

Universite Laval Faculty of Medicine (Ste-Foy)
http://www.fmed.ulaval.ca/

University of Montreal Faculty of Medicine (Montreal)
http://medes3.med.umontreal.ca/

University of Sherbrooke Faculty of Medicine (Sherbrooke)
http://www.usherb.ca/Programmes/fmed.htm

Saskatchewan

University of Saskatchewan College of Medicine (Saskatoon)
http://www.usask.ca/medicine/index.html

Medical Schools: Lists

Accredited Medical Schools of the U.S. and Canada

http://www.aamc.org/meded/medschls/

Compiled by the Association of American Medical Colleges.

Medical Schools

http://www.collegenet.com/geograph/medical.html

Lists medical schools with addresses, enrollment, tuition and, when available, Internet links.

Peterson's Guide to Medical Schools

http://www.petersons.com/medical/

Provides list of schools offering allopathic and osteopathic medical degrees, as well as MCAT test preparation.

Tore B. Sjoboden's Medical School Links!

http://www.anat.dote.hu/~tore/medfak/

Links to international and U.S. schools of medicine.

United States and Canada Medical Schools

http://www.mc.vanderbilt.edu/~aubrey/medstu/medical_schools.html

Vanderbilt University List of U.S. and Canadian Medical Schools

http://www.mc.vanderbilt.edu/~aubrey/medstu/medical_schools.html

A list of the online U.S. and Canada medical schools that have an entry in the *Directory of American Medical Education*, Association of American Medical Colleges, 1994-1995, 41st Edition.

U.S. News & World Report Online, Medical Schools Ranking

http://www.usnews.com/usnews/edu/beyond/gradrank/med/gdmedt1.htm

List of American medical schools that can be sorted by rank, tuition cost, average MCAT score, and other indicators.

Yahoo's List of Medical Schools

http://dir.yahoo.com/Health/Medicine/Education/Medical_Schools/

Links to U.S. and international medical school websites.

General Medical Education Information

American Medical College Application Service
http://www.aamc.org/stuapps/admiss/amcas/start.htm
Centralized application processing service for applicants to participating medical schools.

American Medical Student Association
http://www.amsa.org/
Membership organization with services and resources for both medical and pre-med students. Site features information on committees and interest groups, resources, legislative affairs, news and *The New Physician* magazine.

The Interactive Medical Student Lounge
http://www.medstudents.net/
Lots of resources for medical and pre-medical students, including information about med school application and financial aid, a message service, links to medical websites, and other features.

The Mature Medical Student
http://falcon.cc.ukans.edu:80/~cwpowell/
One individual's story of attending medical school at an older age.

The Medical Education Page
http://www.scomm.net:80/~greg/med-ed/
Site for medical and pre-medical school students developed by a second-year medical student. Provides links to medical schools, news sources, frequently asked questions (FAQs), ftp sites and medical indexes.

The Medical Education Software Homepage
http://www.webcom.com/~wooming/mededuc.html
Site features reviews of medical education software.

Monster Healthcare
http://www.medsearch.com/
Online job postings for those in search of, or recruiting for health care positions. Searches can be personalized by clicking on "My Monster."

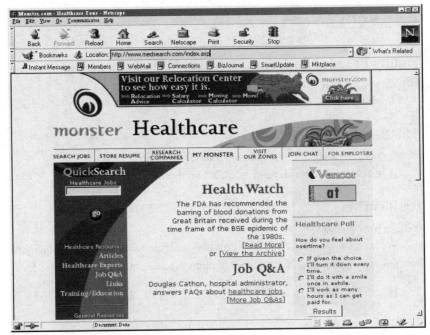

Monster Healthcare. *http://www.medsearch.com/index.asp*

Miscellaneous Medical Education Page

http://www.fcm.missouri.edu/medical/mismed.htm

Valuable links to discussion groups, indexes, tools, and more for medical school and pre-medical school students.

The Princeton Review Online: Medicine

http://www.review.com/medical/find/med_schools_search.html

Princeton Review Online's medical school search engine. Enter your specific criteria and receive statistics and a description of schools which may fit your profile.

WWW Med School Lists

http://premed.edu/medschls.html

Helpful information and support for pre-medical school students.

Residency

Family Practice Residency Program Web Guide
http://www.geocities.com/CapeCanaveral/Lab/1775/fp.htm

An online guide to family practice residency programs in the United States.

The Residency Page
http://www.webcom.com/~wooming/residenc.html

A list of medical residencies available on the web. Select specialty.

ResidentNet
http://www.residentnet.com/

Website for surgical residents. Provides information on surgical techniques, board review tips, career and fellowship opportunities, and links to other sites.

MEN'S HEALTH

Circumcision

Circumcision Information and Resource Pages
http://www.cirp.org/

Technical, medical and patient material on circumcision, including the American Academy of Pediatrics' Policy Statement on circumcision.

Circumcision Issues
http://www.eskimo.com/%7egburlin/circ.html

Links to information on the different types of male circumcision practiced around the world.

Doctors Opposing Circumcision
http://faculty.washington.edu/gcd/DOC/

Homepage for a physician organization that opposes routine natal circumcision. Provides information and links.

Mothers Against Circumcision
http://www.mothersagainstcirc.org/index.html

Searchable site with information on circumcision.

Cosmetic Surgery

Cosmetic Surgery for Men
http://www.phudson.com/male.html

This page provides information on the different types of cosmetic surgeries for men. It is part of "E-sthetics Cosmetic Plastic Surgery" site, which is authored by Patrick Hudson, MD, a board-certified plastic surgeon.

Fathering

Fathering Magazine
http://www.fathermag.com/

This online monthly magazine has articles on various aspects of being a father.

Fertility & Infertility
See also: Sexual & Reproductive Health - Fertility.

How to Enhance Your Fertility
http://www.coolware.com/health/medical_reporter/malefertility.html

Advice for men on how to enhance their fertility and have a healthier baby.

Male Factor Infertility
http://www.ivf.com/male.html

Site maintained by the Atlanta Reproductive Health Center provides information on male infertility and in-vitro fertilization.

Fitness & Health

Duke University's Healthy Devil On-Line: Men's Health
http://h-devil-www.mc.duke.edu/h-devil/men/men.htm

Topics covered include erectile dysfunction, premature ejaculation, testicular self-examination, and urinary tract infections.

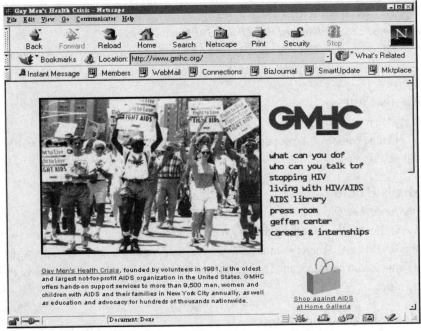

Gay Men's Health Crisis. http://www.gmhc.org/

Gay Men's Health Crisis

http://www.gmhc.org

Homepage for famous AIDS advocacy and support group. Provides information on how to live with HIV, as well as ways in which people can fight AIDS through volunteering, advocacy and contributions.

Healthtouch: Men's Health

http://www.healthtouch.com/level1/leaflets/120307/120307.htm

Includes information for men on heart disease, cholesterol, kidney and urologic health, sexually transmitted diseases, and prostate problems.

A Man's Life

http://www.manslife.com/

Health and fitness articles for men, along with other columns and news geared to men.

Medic: Men's Health Issues
http://medic.med.uth.tmc.edu/ptnt/00000391.htm
Information on diet and exercise for a healthy heart, prostate cancer screening and benign prostatic hyperplasia.

Men's Fitness
http://www.mensfitness.com/
Online edition of the popular magazine which covers fitness, nutrition, health and sex for men.

Men's Health
http://menshealth.com/mens_index.html
Online version of the popular magazine for men. Website includes departments such as Personal Trainer with information on fitness and exercise, Eat This with information on nutrition, and Executive Suite with information on getting ahead at the office.

Men's Health Consulting
http://www.menshealth.org/
Website for consulting firm that helps health organizations set up effective men's health programs. The site offers information about its services, and a sample of the firm's HEALTH *MEN*TOR, a questionnaire to help men assess their diet, physical health, sexual health and attitudes.

Not For Men Only: The Male Health Center Internet Education Site
http://www.malehealthcenter.com/
Information for men on exercise, erections, and guidelines regarding regular physical examinations.

Tulane University: Men's Health Links
http://www.tulane.edu/~health/text/mens_health.htm
Links to other sites on the Internet devoted to men's physical and mental health.

Urologic and Male Genital Diseases
http://www.mic.ki.se/Diseases/c12.html
Information from the Karolinska Institute Library on male urologic diseases. Includes links to articles and ability to search MEDLINE.

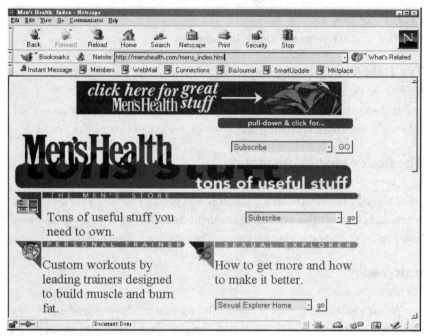

Men's Health *http://menshealth.com/mens_index.html*

Gynecomastia

Gynecomastia
http://www.surgery.uiowa.edu/surgery/plastic/gyneco.html

Information on this condition, in which men develop enlarged breasts. Site designed by the University of Iowa Plastic Surgery Department.

Gynecomastia - Correction of Enlarged Male Breasts
http://www.plasticsurgery.org/surgery/gyne.htm

Information about breast reduction surgery to correct gynecomastia in men. Site produced by the Plastic Surgery Information Service, American Society of Plastic & Reconstructive Surgeons and Plastic Surgery Education Foundation.

Hair Loss

See also: Skin & Connective Tissue/Dermatology - Hair Loss.

The Bald Man's Home Page

http://www.thebaldman.com/

Includes the Bald Man's Live Hair Chat Room, The Baldman's Forum ("ask a doctor"), research and articles, horror stories, jokes and commercial products.

The Bosley Medical Institute

http://www.bosley.com/home.html

This site allows you to click on the baldness pattern similar to your own to find out about hair restoration options. Learn about the history of coping with hair loss, how to choose the best option for you, and how to find a good doctor.

Hair Today

http://www.hairtoday.com/

A hair loss and treatment resource offering new articles and product reviews each month. The site's "Ask An Expert" section gives answers to questions on surgery, nutrition and hair systems.

The Hairloss Information Center

http://hairloss.com/

Includes free evaluation, pamphlets, and consumer information about hair loss.

Regrowth!

http://www.regrowth.com/

Hair loss headlines, frequently asked questions (FAQs), discussion group and mailing list.

Impotence

Impotence Information Center

http://www.medic-drug.com/impotence/impotence.html

Site provides comprehensive information on impotence and FDA-approved treatments. Information is a public service of Medic Home Health Care, a JCAHO-accredited health care provider.

Impotence: It's Reversible

http://www.cei.net/~impotenc/

Basic but reassuring information on impotence, how to treat it, and where to get more information.

Impotence Resource Site

http://www.impotence.org/

This site, for both patients and medical professionals, provides information and basic facts on the causes and treatment of impotence. A women's perspective is offered and participation in an online survey is invited.

Successfully Treating Impotence

http://www2.impotent.com/

Online guide to impotence and its treatments. Features links to related sites, information for health care professionals, and information for users of *Caverject*, an impotence treatment.

Penile Surgery

Penile Lengthening and Enlargement Surgery Center for Men

http://www.2020tech.com/mensurg/

Site produced by the Surgery Center for Men in Beverly Hills. Provides information about penile enlargement surgery, before-and-after photos, and frequently asked questions (FAQs).

Penis Enlargement Surgery

http://www.SURGEON.org/penis.htm

Information about and referrals to penile lengthening and augmentation treatments. Site includes size statistics and art gallery.

The Reed Centre for Ambulatory Urological Surgery

http://www.penisdoctor.com/

Includes information about penile enlargement, penile prosthetic implants, vasectomy, vasectomy reversal, circumcision, male breast reduction, and Peyronie's disease.

Prostate Cancer

American Cancer Society's Prostate Cancer Resource Center
http://www3.cancer.org/cancerinfo/res_home.asp?ct=36

Includes the "Man to Man Prostate Cancer Education and Support Program" which offers group education, one-on-one visitation and telephone support, a quarterly newsletter and free patient education information.

Brady Urological Institute Approach to Prostate Cancer
http://prostate.urol.jhu.edu/prostate/prostate.html

Information on prostate cancer, prevention, diagnosis and treatment.

CaP CURE
http://www.capcure.org/

Website for the Association for the Cure of Cancer of the Prostate. Find information about prostate cancer, how to live with it, and ongoing research.

Male Cancer
http://www.allhealth.com/mens/cancers/

Find information on prostate cancer, penile cancer and testicular cancer, including current news articles which change daily. Part of the allHealth.com site.

OncoLink Information on Prostate Cancer
http://oncolink.upenn.edu/disease/prostate/

Provides general information, symptom management advice, answers to frequently asked questions, recommendations for prostate cancer screening and diagnostics, and information about risk factors and prevention.

Prostate Cancer Help Zone
http://www.prostate-cancer.com/

Information about prostate cancer treatment options, stages, recovery, support groups and a glossary of terms. In addition, professional resources and information are provided. The page was developed by Shering Oncology/Biotech as a service for prostate cancer survivors, their families, friends and health care providers.

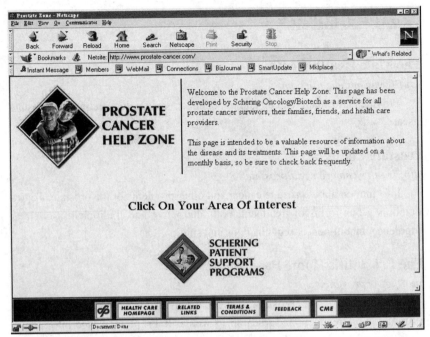

Prostate Cancer Help Zone. *http://www.prostate-cancer.com/*

Prostate Cancer InfoLink

http://www.comed.com/Prostate/index.html

Site provides a lot of information as well as support for men with prostate cancer.

"Real Men Cook" to Fight Prostate Cancer

http://www.cinenet.net/~prostate/awareness/

Site for a nonprofit educational and support organization whose goal is to fight prostate cancer and promote early detection. Since 1990 the group has contributed more than $500,000 to education. Find information here about the organization, prostate cancer, prevention guidelines and further links.

University of Michigan Prostate Cancer Program

http://www.cancer.med.umich.edu/prostcan/

A resource for prostate cancer information. Features pertinent articles from medical journals, information on clinical trials, treatment options and links to other resources.

Prostate Health

The Male Health Centres
http://www.malehealth.com/

Provides information about and treatment of erectile dysfunction and prostate disease.

Prostate Pointers
http://rattler.cameron.edu/prostate/

Information about prostate cancer and other problems of the prostate. Topics include various forms of treatment, both alternative and traditional, as well as impotence, incontinence, organizations and studies.

The Prostatitis Home Page
http://www.prostate.org/

Homepage for the Prostatitis Foundation. Provides clinical and patient information on treatment and research, as well as links, pointers, and information about a prostate e-mail list.

Testicular Cancer

Men: Examining Your Testicles May Save Your Life
http://www.coolware.com/health/medical_reporter/testicles.html

In addition to telling how to perform a testicular self exam, this site describes the symptoms of testicular cancer and the risk factors.

Testicular Cancer
http://www.noah.cuny.edu/cancer/ushc/testic.html
http://www.noah.cuny.edu/cancer/nci/cancernet/201121.html

Two NOAH (New York Online Access to Healthcare) sites provide information about testicular cancer, including testicular self examination.

Testicular Cancer Resource Center
http://www.acor.org/diseases/TC/

Information about testicular cancer and self-examination, as well as a list of questions to ask your doctor.

Testicular Self-Exam

http://h-devil-www.mc.duke.edu/h-devil/men/tse.htm

Provides information on how to perform a testicular self exam and the warning signs of cancer.

Vasectomy

All About Vasectomy

http://www.plannedparenthood.org/BIRTH-CONTROL/allaboutvas.htm

Provides information about what a vasectomy is and how it works. Page is authored by Planned Parenthood.

The Patient's Guide to Vasectomy Reversal

http://cait.cpmc.columbia.edu/dept/urology/vasr0000.html

Informative page gives men information on vasectomy reversal surgery and what to expect. Written by Harry Fisch, M.D., director of the Male Reproductive Center and a member of the Department of Urology at Columbia-Presbyterian Medical Center in New York.

MENTAL HEALTH

Anxiety

Anxiety Disorders Association of America

http://www.adaa.org/

This organization promotes the prevention and cure of anxiety disorders, and seeks to enhance the lives of those who have such disorders. The site provides information and resources for both lay people and health care professionals.

Attacking Anxiety

http://www.sover.net/~schwcof/

Free booklets and newsletters on anxiety and post-traumatic stress disorder.

Center for Anxiety and Stress Treatment

http://www.stressrelease.com/

Resources to help people overcome anxiety and stress, including books and audio tapes, an anxiety symptom checklist, advice about panic attacks, and a list of stress busters.

Managing Your Anxiety

http://www.vh.org/Patients/IHB/FamilyPractice/AFP/December/DecFour.html

Site developed by the Children's Hospital of Iowa provides advice on managing anxiety. Defines anxiety, lists its symptoms, offers suggestions on how to control and reduce it, and provides addresses and phone numbers of support groups.

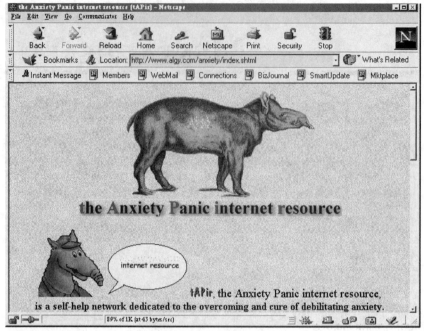

tAPir, the Anxiety Panic Internet Resource. *http://www.algy.com/anxiety/index.shtml*

Meditation/Relaxation Exercises

http://members.tripod.com/~Aquamoon/medit.html

A variety of relaxation exercises that can be accessed online or printed out.

National Panic/Anxiety Disorder Newsletter

http://www.NPADNews.com/

Newsletter for sufferers of panic attacks and anxiety disorders.

Online Screening for Anxiety (OSA)

http://www.med.nyu.edu/Psych/screens/anx.html

A 10-question test to determine if you have an anxiety problem.

Stress Education Center

http://www.dstress.com/

Articles and other publications about stress and stress management; links, seminar registration, and products such as audio tapes.

tAPir: The Anxiety Panic Internet Resource
http://www.algy.com/anxiety/index.shtml

A self-help network helping people overcome debilitating and disruptive anxiety, fears and phobias. The site offers information about treatment, online support groups, and links to other Web resources.

Treatment of Panic Disorder
http://text.nlm.nih.gov/nih/cdc/www/85txt.html

A conference statement from the National Institutes of Health on the treatment of panic disorders.

Children
See also: Children's Health/Pediatrics.

American Academy of Child and Adolescent Psychiatry
http://www.aacap.org/web/aacap/

This site includes fact sheets to help children and their families and is available in English, Spanish and French. Discusses issues such as adoption, bedwetting, abuse, divorce, TV violence, grief, medications, and suicide. Also covers the Academy's activities and publications, legislative and clinical updates, practice guidelines and research.

Suicide by Teens
http://www.he.net/~bwtc/library/suicteen.html

Information on the incidence and causes of teen suicide.

Symptoms of Depressed Children
http://www.mentalhealth.com/mag1/p5h-dp06.html

Information from the Harvard Medical School Mental Health Letter regarding the diagnosis of depression in children.

Violence on Television: What Children Learn and What Parents Can Do
http://www.apa.org/pubinfo/violence.html

The American Psychological Association states the findings of several studies on the effect violent television programming has on children, and steps parents can take to mitigate that effect.

Counseling/Therapy

See also: Psychiatry/Psychology, later in this chapter.

Marriage Builders

http://www.marriagebuilders.com/

Learn ways to overcome marital conflicts and restore love from psychologist and author Dr. Willard Harley, Jr., Ph.D.

Depression

See also: Pregnancy & Childbirth - Postpartum Depression.

Clinical Depression Screening Test

http://sandbox.xerox.com/pair/cw/testing.html

A test to help the visitor determine if he or someone he knows is suffering from clinical depression. The site also provides information on depression and treatment.

Depression and Mental Health Sources on the Internet

http://stripe.Colorado.EDU/~judy/depression/

Links to organizations' sites, personal homepages, newsgroups and mailing lists related to depression. Also features a list of the best and worst things to say to someone who is depressed.

Depression FAQ

http://avocado.pc.helsinki.fi/~janne/asdfaq/index.html

Provides information on depression, as well as its causes, treatment and relation to substance abuse.

Depression. . . When the Sadness Just Won't Stop

http://www.blarg.net/~charlatn/Depression.html

Information about depression and treatment, as well as links to other Web resources pertaining to depression in children, suicide, and mental health.

Dr. Ivan's Depression Central

http://www.psycom.net/depression.central.html

Clearinghouse for information on depression and other mood disorders, divided helpfully by topic. Includes an area with a large introduction to depression, especially how it is defined, how it is treated and FAQS. Links.

Internet Depression Resources List
http://www.execpc.com/%7Ecorbeau/
Site provides information about depression, manic depression, panic attacks, suicide and treatment options.

Melatonin and Seasonal Affective Disorder
http://hometown.aol.com/mindbend2/index.htm
This site includes research, information and links to other sites about melatonin and its effects on seasonal affective disorder (SAD).

Online Depression Screening Test
http://www.med.nyu.edu/Psych/screens/depres.html
Use this test to check if you're depressed, or access other psychiatric screening tests. Site hosted by the New York University Department of Psychiatry.

Serotonin: The Neurotransmitter for the 90's
http://www.fairlite.com/ocd/articles/ser90.shtml
Technical research paper written by Ronald F. Borne, Ph.D., University of Mississippi, School of Pharmacy.

Wing of Madness: A Depression Guide
http://www.wingofmadness.com/index.htm
Discusses clinical depression and its effect on children, teenagers and women. Features links, articles, and recent news on the subject.

Emotional Support
See also: Self Help and Support Groups, later in this chapter.

Emotional Support on the Internet
http://www.faqs.org/faqs/support/emotional/resources-list/
Bi-monthly posting of different resources with addresses and instructions on how to reach them or post a listing. Everything from newsgroups addressing abuse issues to listservers relating to gay parenting. Links to suicide prevention and intervention counseling.

False Memory Syndrome

Evaluate False Memory Foundation Material with Respect and Caution
http://www.northcoast.com/~dka/caution.htm
> Advises people to treat false memory claims with caution.

False Memory Syndrome Foundation
http://advicom.net/~fitz/fmsf/
> Describes false memory syndrome, the purpose and activities of the Foundation, and offers a mailing list for updates.

Grief and Bereavement
See also: Death & Dying - Grief and Bereavement; Pregnancy - Miscarraiges.

Grief Resources
http://www.cp-tel.net/pamnorth/grief.htm
> A good list of Web resources for people suffering from loss and grief.

GROWW: Grief Recovery
http://www.groww.com/gr.htm
> Chat room for people who are experiencing loss.

Living With Grief When a Loved One is Dying
http://www.caregivertips.com/
> When a loved one is dying, it is often difficult to consider one's own needs and wants. This site offers some useful tips for survivors prior to the actual loss of a loved one, such as advice on how to be with someone who is dying, family morale, and notes of encouragement.

A Place to Honor Grief
http://www.webhealing.com/honor.html
> Website where people can honor a person in their lives who has died by writing about their own grief and healing, which in turn will help others cope with similar feelings.

SANDS(Vic)

http://www.sandsvic.org.au/

A support group for parents who have experienced miscarriage, stillbirth, or neonatal death.

Homelessness and Mental Illness

Community Access Information Resource Network

http://www.cairn.org/

A nonprofit agency that provides housing, funding and advocacy for people with psychiatric disabilities.

Mental Illness and Homelessness

http://nch.ari.net/mental.html

Fact sheets on mental health issues related to homelessness and other information. From the National Coalition for the Homeless.

Mental Health

The Center for Mental Health Services

http://www.mentalhealth.org/

Billed as a knowledge exchange network, this site provides information on prevention, treatment and rehabilitation services for mental illness. Also features a School Violence Prevention initiative.

Dr. Bob's Mental Health Links

http://uhs.bsd.uchicago.edu/~bhsiung/mental.html

Also known as "Dr. Bob's Virtual En-psych-lopedia," this site contains many Web links concerning mental health, and a limitless number of related organizations, academic sites and publications.

Drugs for Treating Mental Health

http://pharminfo.com/disease/mental/

Lists mental diseases and their medications. Also provides drug information.

Internet Mental Health
http://www.mentalhealth.com/

An encyclopedia of mental health information. Look up disorders and medications, and find links to magazines, software demos, and other mental health sites.

The Madness Group
http://www.peoplewho.org/Madness/

Electronic forumof advocacy and support for people who experience mood swings, fear, voices and visions. People can exchange their strategies for dealing with these things, as well as for dealing with and changing the mental health system.

Mental Health Infosource
http://www.mhsource.com/

Search engine for mental health issues on the internet. Also includes regular columns, chat rooms, mail lists, and links to patient advocacy groups, information on different mental disorders, and a professional directory.

Mental Health Net
http://mentalhelp.net/

Very sophisticated site has thousands of mental health resources covering abuse, anxiety, bipolar disorder, depression, eating disorders, personality disorders, schizophrenia, and more. Features a weekly updated "In The News" section, as well as professional resources in psychology, psychiatry and social work. Search engine provided. Offers full-service e-mail.

National Institute of Mental Health
http://www.nimh.nih.gov/

Offers public information on specific mental disorders, educational programs on depression and panic disorder, as well as information for scientists on grants and research activities, news and events.

Self-Injury: You are Not the Only One
http://www.palace.net/~llama/psych/injury.html

Site helps people who intentionally hurt themselves to understand what they are doing psychologically and to get help.

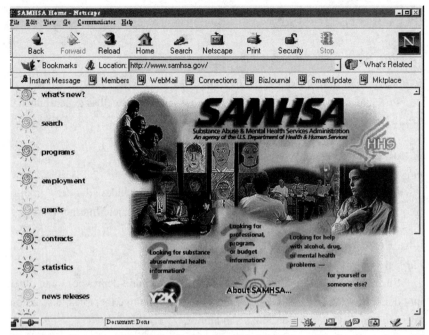

Substance Abuse and Mental Health Services Administration. *http://www.samhsa.gov/*

The Shyness Home Page

http://www.shyness.com/

This site, which is sponsored by the Shyness Institute in Portola Valley, California, provides Internet resources for people suffering from severe shyness.

Specifica

http://www.realtime.net/~mmjw/

Find links to other websites offering help and information on a variety mental health problems.

Substance Abuse and Mental Health Services Administration

http://www.samhsa.gov/

SAMHSA is an agency of the Department of Health and Human Services. Its site provides information on substance abuse and mental health, as well as lists of substance abuse treatment centers and mental health providers.

Mood Disorders

Bipolar Planet
http://www.tcnj.edu/~ellisles/BipolarPlanet/

Provides a link to free online help for those in crisis as well as general mental health links.

Moodswing.Org
http://moodswing.org/

Online resources for people with bipolar disorder. Includes advocacy groups, frequently asked questions (FAQs), books, support groups, and Internet links.

The Pendulum Pages
http://www.pendulum.org/

Site offers information and support for bipolar (manic-depression) and other mood disorders. Articles, books, support groups, alternative therapies, discussion area, mailing list, medication, links and humor.

Obsessive-Compulsive Disorder

O.C.D. Resource Center
http://www.ocdresource.com/ocdresource.nsf

Introduction to the causes, symptoms and treatment of obsessive-compulsive disorder (OCD); OCD resources.

O.C.D. Web Server
http://www.fairlite.com/ocd/

Contains a bulletin board, abstracts, articles, information on medications, and links to mental health sites related to obsessive-compulsive disorder. Includes advice on how to deal with OCD, personal accounts, and web links.

Obsessive-Compulsive Anonymous
http://members.aol.com/west24th/index.html

A fellowship of people who remain anonymous in order to share their personal stories, and to help others recover from obsessive-compulsive disorder (OCD).

Obsessive-Compulsive Disorder

http://www.psyc.memphis.edu/students/abramowitz/ocd.htm

A general description of OCD and a bibliography for those seeking self-help and for health care professionals.

Obsessive-Compulsive Foundation

http://www.ocfoundation.org/

Information on what obsessive-compulsive disorder is and how it's treated in both adults and children. Site also features an OCD screening test, and a list of online resources.

Organizations

National Mental Health Association

http://www.nmha.org/

The NMHA is a citizen volunteer advocacy organization dedicated to improving the mental health of all. This site has news about NMHA activities, its advocacy efforts (including public policy and legislative alerts), and community outreach and prevention issues. Jumplist includes a good description of helpful websites to visit. Direct e-mail links to the President, Vice President, Senate, House of Representatives, and First Lady.

PsychNET

http://www.apa.org/

The American Psychological Association page includes information for the general public, psychologists, and students interested in a career in mental health care.

World Federation of Mental Health

http://www.wfmh.com/

An international nonprofit advocacy organization founded in 1948 to advance the prevention of mental and emotional disorders, the proper treatment and care of those with such disorders, and the promotion of mental health. The Federation achieves its goals through public education programs such as World Mental Health Day, research through collaborating centers at major universities, consultation to the United Nations and other agencies.

Personality Disorders

Astraea's Multiple Personality Resources and Controversies
http://www.asarian.org/~astraea/household/

A website for people with multiple personalities to communicate with each other and share their experiences of how they are treated.

Avoidant Personality Disorder
http://www.mentalhealth.com/dis/p20-pe08.html

Tells what the disorder is, treatment, research, and provides an online diagnosis.

Borderline Personality Disorder Information
http://www.stanford.edu/~corelli/borderline.html

Describes borderline personality disorder, its symptoms, etiology, and treatment.

BPD Central
http://www.BPDCentral.com/

Provides information on borderline personality disorder (BPD) and how a person can care for themself if they have it, including therapists and programs that can help, as well as online resources and books. Features a helpful list of indicators to help a person determine if they are in a relationship with someone who has BPD.

BPD Experiences
http://members.aol.com/BPDCentral/bpdexp.html

People with BPD explain what it's like to struggle with the disorder, and provide suggestions on positive ways others can interact with them.

Essential Information on Trauma and Dissociation
http://www.mcs.net:80/~kathyw/trauma.html

Information about dissociative identity disorder (DID) and its effects on children who've suffered traumatic events. Site has links to many related pages, both personal and professional, including the SIDRAN Foundation, and the International Society for the Study of Dissociation.

International Society for the Study of Dissociation
http://www.issd.org/

Nonprofit professional organization that promotes research and training in the identification and treatment of dissociative disorders. The site provides professional and public education.

Laura's Home Page
http://huizen.dds.nl/%7Elaura_d/

Personal account of a person who has learned to overcome her borderline personality disorder, and ideas about BPD.

Multiple Personality Disorder and Dissociation Resources
http://www.vuw.ac.nz/~anita/dissociation.html

A list of resources (including books and Web links) concerning MPD and dissociative disorders.

Online Screening for Personality Disorders
http://www.med.nyu.edu/Psych/screens/pds.html

Twenty questions to determine if you have a personality disorder.

Paranoid Conditions: A Guide for Families
http://www.mentalhealth.com/book/p42-gpar.html

Web page advertising book on paranoid conditions. Lists table of contents, and ordering information.

SIDRAN Foundation
http://www.sidran.org/

A national nonprofit group devoted to education, advocacy and research for early recognition and treatment of trauma-related stress in children, and the treatment of adults suffering from trauma-generated disorders.

The Spectrum of Dissociative Disorders: An Overview of Diagnosis and Treatment
http://www.voiceofwomen.com/centerarticle.html

Information about the various dissociative disorders, and their treatment. Written by Joan A. Turkus, M.D. Includes references.

Psychiatry/Psychology

Abnormal Psychology Project
http://www.chs.chico.k12.ca.us/Staff/kohencla.htm

Students in Mr. Kohen's psychology class studied various mental illnesses, and used the WWW to collect information. They have compiled their sources here at this site. Topics covered include addictive behaviors, anorexia, autism, dissociative disorders, depression, obsessions and compulsion, personality disorders and schizophrenia, among others.

The American Psychoanalytic Association
http://apsa.org/

Professional organization of psychoanalysts. Offers information describing psychoanalysis, and information for members about organization activities, meetings and programs. Literature search, newsletter, journal information and access are provided, along with list of additional related links.

International Journal of Psychiatry in Medicine
http://www.dartmouth.edu/~ijpm/about.html

This journal, which seeks to advance psychosocial and biological theory, methods and treatment as they apply to primary care, contains articles on mental disorders, physician-patient interactions; educational programs; biomedical etiologies of mental symptoms, geriatrics, and, health services. The website includes abstracts, editorials, and instructions to authors.

The Keirsey Temperament Sorter II
http://www.keirsey.com/cgi-bin/keirsey/newkts.cgi

Take an online personality test that sorts results according to the Myers-Briggs method. Identifies four personality types: artisan, idealist, guardian, and rational.

Medscape Psychiatry
http://www.medscape.com/Home/Topics/psychiatry/psychiatry.html

Current news, journal articles, treatment information and links related to mental illness and psychiatry.

Psych Central

http://psychcentral.com/

Maintained by Dr. John Grohol, Psych Central provides online resources for mental health information. Features newsgroups, mailing lists, websites, books, articles, surveys, and checklists, as well as a suicide helpline.

Psych Web

http://www.psychwww.com/

Psychology-related information for students and teachers of psychology. Includes a browsable web version of Freud's *The Interpretation of Dreams*, as well as other books, brochures and articles; links to commercial sites, journals, discussion groups; and a psychology quiz.

Psychiatric Society for Informatics

http://www.psych.med.umich.edu/

Promotes the use of information technology in psychiatry. Website provides information about the organization and its activities.

Psychiatry Information for the General Public

http://www.med.nyu.edu/Psych/public.html

Access several online screening tests for depression, anxiety, sexual disorders, attention deficit disorder and personality disorders. Links to websites offering treatment information, advocacy groups, and search engines.

PsycINFO

http://www.apa.org/psycinfo/

PsycINFO is a part of the American Psychological Association that creates products to help researchers locate psychological literature relevant to their research topics. These products include *Psychological Abstracts* and the PsychINFO Database, which can be accessed here.

Psychology in Daily Life

http://www.apa.org/pubinfo/

Information about current mental health topics such as health insurance parity, and mental health patients' bill of rights. Site also features a Help Center where visitors can get assistance and advice for their problem.

Shoshanna's Psychiatric Survivor's Guide
http://www.harborside.com/home/e/equinox/

According to this site, it's OK to be mentally ill, but mental health professionals would have you believe otherwise in order to control people and situations which the mental health profession cannot comprehend. To make its point, the site lists famous people who have been diagnosed with mental illness.

Psychoanalysis

The American Psychoanalytic Foundation
http://www.cyberpsych.org/apf/index.htm

This no-nonsense site describes the objectives and programs of the APF, provides links to organizations and publications on the Internet, and offers a listing of all its members as well as a literature search engine.

The Brill Library of the New York Psychoanalytic Institute
http://plaza.interport.net/nypsan/

Also known as "Freudnet," this site describes the program and activities of the Institute, as well as provides access to its library, which contains more than 40,000 books, articles and reprints dealing with psychoanalysis and related fields. Also contains the Freud Archives, a collection of Internet resources related to Sigmund Freud's life and works.

Sigmund Freud - Father of Psychoanalysis
http://www.austria-info.at/personen/freud/index.html

Includes a brief biography of Freud, a description of the significance of his work and some of the influence he had on contemporary theory. Site is maintained by the Austrian National Tourist Office.

Schizophrenia

Schizophrenia
http://www.psy.med.rug.nl/0012/

Site devoted to information about schizophrenia developed by the Department of Psychiatry at the University of Groningen.

Schizophrenia Digest

http://www.vaxxine.com/schizophrenia/

Site contains information and news about schizophrenia, as well as books, videos, seminars and workshops.

Schizophrenia Pages

http://www.mentalhealth.com/dis/p20-ps01.html

Internet Mental Health's schizophrenia pages features both American and European descriptions, online diagnosis, and treatment resources.

Schizophrenia: Questions and Answers

http://www.psy.med.rug.nl/0031/

Frequently asked questions are answered, such as "What is it?" and "How is it treated?" Offers subscription to *Schizophrenia Bulletin*.

Schizophrenia Update : The Email Newsletter

http://www.schizophrenia.com/help/NewsL2.html

Weekly e-mail on schizophrenia includes news, updates on research, success stories, and reviews of other websites.

schizophrenia.com

http://www.schizophrenia.com/

A nonprofit information, support and education center which offers basic information about the disease such as its causes, diagnosis and medications, as well as in-depth information for families, friends and patients diagnosed with it. Site features discussion and chat areas, and a search of 200 top psychology websites.

VA-Yale Schizophrenia Biological Research Center

http://www.yale.edu/vayale/

Website for the Center, which is located at the Connecticut Veteran's Administration Health Center and is part of Yale University's School of Medicine.

Self-Help and Support Groups

National Mental Health Consumer's Self-Help Clearinghouse
http://www.mhselfhelp.org/index2.html

A technical assistance center established in 1986 and funded by a grant from the Federal Center for Mental Health Services. Helps mental health consumers to plan, provide, and evaluate mental health and community support services. Valuable information on how to start a self-help group.

Self-Help and Psychology Magazine
http://www.shpm.com/

Offers numerous "zones" to learn about self-help and psychology issues. Written by mental health professionals for the discussion of general psychology as applied to everyday life. Articles, news, reviews, books, professional resources and links.

Starting a New Online Support Group
http://www.grohol.com/howto.htm

This site is a friendly and informative "how-to" about starting a new online support group. It provides examples and a step-by-step guide.

Suicide

The Samaritans
http://mentalhelp.net/samaritans/

The Samaritans is a volunteer group that offers confidential emotional support to suicidal and despairing individuals via e-mail, phone, personal visit and letter.

San Francisco Suicide Prevention
http://www.sfsuicide.org/

A volunteer service offering telephone intervention to people in crisis. Contact them by phone or e-mail.

Suicide Awareness/Voices of Education

http://www.save.org/

Informative site discussing the link between depression and suicide. Includes questions and answers, common misconceptions, symptoms of depression, suicide danger signals, how to help friends or yourself, and a list of recommended books.

Suicide - FAQ

http://www.lib.ox.ac.uk/internet/news/faq/archive/suicide.info.html

Frequently asked questions about suicide, from Oxford University Libraries. In addition to questions and answers, the site has links to other suicide prevention resources on the Web.

Trauma

Nate's Traumatology Page

http://dolphin.upenn.edu/~prentice/trauma.html

Traumatology is the study of the effects of traumatic events on individuals, groups and society. This site provides information on ongoing research and links to other relevant sites.

Post Traumatic Stress Resources Web Page

http://www.long-beach.va.gov/ptsd/stress.html

Information and links on post traumatic stress syndrome occurring from any cause. Includes links for veterans of different military conflicts.

Warning Signs of Trauma-Related Stress

http://www.apa.org/practice/ptsd.html

Helpful information, including symptoms to watch out for.

MUSCLES & MUSCULOSKELETAL DISORDERS

Covered in this chapter: *Arthritis; Back/Spinal Problems; Chronic Fatigue Syndrome; Fibromyalgia; Knees; Musculoskeletal Diseases; Repetitive Strain Injuries; Rheumatology; Syringomyelia.*

Related chapters: *Bones/Orthopedics; Chiropractics; Neuromuscular Disorders.*

Arthritis

Ah! (Arthritis Help)
http://rheuma.bham.ac.uk/primer.html

Primer on rheumatic diseases for those with no prior knowledge. Discusses inflammatory arthritis, back pain, sciatica, connective tissue disease and children's arthritis.

Animal Arthritis
http://www.altvetmed.com/arthriti.html

A discussion of the effects of arthritis on dogs and cats, and holistic and complimentary treatment for it.

Arthritis Foundation
http://www.arthritis.org/

A great deal of information and links relating to arthritis. Includes advocacy and support organizations, public information and fact sheets, news and research updates as well as access to the medical journal *Arthritis Today*, and a listing of treatment centers.

Arthritis Information Center
http://www.arthritisinformation.net/

General information on arthritis and joint pain.

Arthritis Today
http://www.arthritis.org/at/

Magazine for people who have arthritis, published by the Arthritis Foundation. Subscribe here at the site, or check the archives.

ArthritisLink
http://easyweb.easynet.co.uk/~pgardiner/index.htm

A UK site with information about the different types of arthritis and arthritis drugs. Links to the Irish Society of Rheumatology and other arthritis-related sites.

Coping with Arthritis
http://www.fda.gov/fdac/features/296_art.html

An article that originally appeared in *FDA Consumer* that covers the common types of arthritis and ways in which people can deal with them.

Doctor's Guide to Arthritis Information and Resources
http://www.pslgroup.com/ARTHRITIS.HTM

Medical news and drug information, discussion groups and newsgroups.

Elfstrom's Arthritis and Rheumatology Resources
http://www.sunnybrook.utoronto.ca:8080/~elfstrom/arthritis/index.html

Articles and reference material for patient self-education. The articles are written by David Elfstrom, a person with chronic inflammatory arthritis, and cover such topics as how to talk to your doctor, arthritis medications and ulcers, and whether knuckle-cracking causes arthritis.

Intramural Clinical Studies
http://www.nih.gov/niams/clinical/

A current listing of clinical studies being conducted by the National Institute of Arthritis, Musculoskeletal and Skin Diseases, a branch of the NIH. Diseases being studied include rheumatoid arthritis, synovitis and lupus glomerulonephritis.

Multipurpose Arthritis and Musculoskeletal Disease Center
http://hacuna.ucsd.edu/ra/

Hosted by the University of California, San Diego, this page has information for researchers studying the genetic epidemiology of arthritis. It offers programs to help analyze genetic data, and a list of other arthritis-related resources.

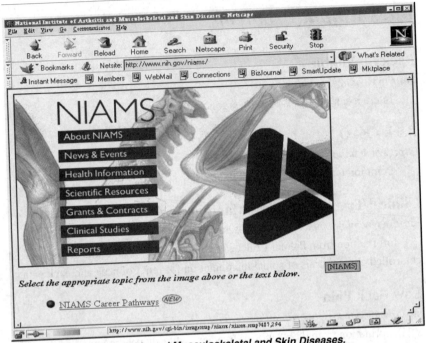

National Institute of Arthritis and Musculoskeletal and Skin Diseases.
http://www.nih.gov/niams/

National Institute of Arthritis and Musculoskeletal and Skin Diseases

http://www.nih.gov/niams/

This site describes the research of this NIH branch, and offers fact sheets, brochures, reports and other information about the many forms of arthritis and diseases of the musculoskeletal system and the skin.

Thumb Arthritis

http://www.handsurgery.com/arthritis.html

Information about arthritis of the thumb, and treatment including surgery for severe cases, from the Southeastern Hand Center in Florida.

Understanding Osteoarthritis & Rheumatoid Arthritis

http://www.myna.com/~jbrodie/arth.htm

Information on how to obtain two educational videos.

Back/Spinal Problems

Back Be Nimble

http://www.backbenimble.com/

Internet sales of back-friendly ergonomic devices.

Back - FAQ

http://www.impaccusa.com/frameset.html

Common questions about back pain.

Clinical Trials of Cervical Manipulation

http://www.mbnet.mb.ca/~jwiens/research.txt

Information from Palmer College of Chiropractic about results of randomized controlled clinical trials of spinal manipulation for relief of neck and back pain.

Low Back Pain

http://www.aaos.org/wordhtml/pat_educ/lowback.htm

Information from the American Academy of Orthopaedic Surgeons. Provides answers on why low back pain is so common, its causes, treatment options, when surgery is needed, and prevention.

Patient's Guide to Low Back Pain

http://www.sechrest.com/mmg/back/backpain.html

Information on the anatomy of the back, symptoms of lower back problems, and treatment options.

Scoliosis

http://www.rad.washington.edu/mskbook/scoliosis.html

Information for doctors on how to diagnose scoliosis.

Spinal Cord Injury Links

http://www.medsupport.org/scinav.htm

Information and links related to spinal cord injuries, published by MedSupport FSF (Friends Supporting Friends), an organization that provides education and assistance to persons with disabilities and their caregivers.

Spine & Peripheral Nerve Surgery Center

http://neurosurgery.mgh.harvard.edu/spine-hp.htm

Information about spinal surgery from Massachusetts General Hospital and Harvard Medical School. Also includes links to information about treatment of spinal tumors, sciatica and low back pain.

Spine Surgery

http://www.spine-surgery.com/

Includes articles, information and online consultation about spine surgery.

Texas Back Institute

http://www.texasback.com/

Site claims that the TBI is the largest spine specialty clinic in the United States. Get advice on when to see a doctor, treatment options, and what to do if you're injured on the job.

Chronic Fatigue Syndrome

Also known as Chronic Fatigue & Immune Dysfunction Syndrome (CFIDS) and Myalgic Encephalomyelitis (ME).

American Association for Chronic Fatigue Syndrome

http://www.aacfs.org/

Nonprofit organization of research scientists, physicians, licensed medical healthcare professionals and other individuals and institutions interested in promoting the exchange of ideas for chronic fatigue syndrome (CFS) research and patient care. Offers periodic reviews of current clinical, research and treatment ideas on CFS for the benefit of CFS patients and others, as well as newsletter, journal, position papers, member news, links to other CFS sites and a selected bibliography.

Ask NOAH: Chronic Fatigue Syndrome

http://www.noah.cuny.edu/wellconn/chronicftge.html

Common questions and answers about chronic fatigue syndrome and related conditions. Includes causes, tests, treatment and recent literature.

CFS News & Information

http://www.cfs.inform.dk/

Information on chronic fatigue syndrome (CFS), and a discussion of the controversy around asserting the legitimacy of this disorder. Major topics include news, research, hypotheses of causes, CFS and exercise, treatment, fibromyalgia and related conditions.

Chronic Fatigue Syndrome

http://chronicfatigue.about.com/

Site offers advocacy, treatment, diagnosis, mailing list, information for doctors, and much more. Includes feature articles, support groups and many links.

Chronic Fatigue Syndrome

http://www.ncf.carleton.ca:80/freenet/rootdir/menus/social.services/cfseir/CFSE IR.HP.html

Links to electronic resources, newsletters, government agencies and articles related to chronic fatigue syndrome.

Chronic Fatigue Syndrome/Myalgic Encephalomyelitis

http://www.cais.com/cfs-news/

News, information, resources, discussion groups and links about CFS/ME.

Chronic Fatigue Syndrome - One Man's Recovery

http://www.cfs-recovery.org/

Personal story and information on chronic fatigue syndrome and candida related complex, and its connection with aspartame.

Chronic Fatigue Syndrome Page

http://www.geocities.com/HotSprings/Spa/4526/

Patient survey, and information on this syndrome which is characterized by profound exhaustion.

From Fatigued to Fantastic

http://www.endfatigue.com/Book/chapter1.html

Information on CFS and selections from a book discussing chronic fatigue syndrome, related fatigue disorders, and their possible causes; a newsletter which includes summaries of research, reviews and a questions and answers sections; links and more.

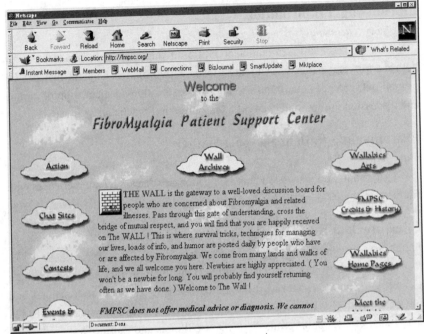

Fibromyalgia Patient Support Center, *http://fmpsc.org/*

My Chronic Fatigue & Immune Dysfunction Syndrome Page

http://www.geocities.com/HotSprings/1683/index.html

Major topics include general information, research, advocacy, associations, children and adolescents with CFIDS, related illnesses and more.

New Concepts in Cause and Treatment of CFIDS

http://www2.rpa.net/~lrandall/see1.html

Outline and transcription of a lecture which discusses pathological causes and therapy.

Fibromyalgia

See also: Pain & Pain Management.

Canberra Fibromyalgia and Chronic Fatigue Syndrome Page

http://www.spirit.net.au/~masmith/

Information from Australia about fibromyalgia and CFS, and their treatments.

Fibromyalgia Information
http://www.cais.com/cfs-news/fibro.htm

This page contains information about fibromyalgia and pain management for both doctors and patients, including a patient information handout that can be printed out. Provides many links to relevant associations, patient support groups and discussion groups, and even offers resources in French and Spanish.

Fibromyalgia Patient Support Center
http://fmpsc.org/

Chat rooms and discussion board for patients to discuss their experiences with fibromyalgia.

Fibromyalgia Resources
http://www.hsc.missouri.edu/~fibro/index.html

Maintained by the Missouri Arthritis Rehabilitation Research and Training Center, this site offers frequently asked questions (FAQs) for both patients and physicians and a list of resources including associations and newsletters in the US and Canada, and support groups in Missouri, Illinois and California.

Joy's World's Best Sites for Fibromyalgia Survivors
http://home.earthlink.net/~fotojoy/index.html

This page, which is maintained by Joy, a fibromyalgia survivor, provides information on fibromyalgia, suggestions on what to do if you have just been diagnosed, and links to other helpful sites.

A Physician's Guide to Fibromyalgia Syndrome
http://www.hsc.missouri.edu/fibro/fm-md.html

Basic information on the disease, its etiology, diagnosis and treatment.

Knees

Common Knee Injuries
http://sportsmedicine.about.com/msubkneeinjuries.htm?pid=2789&cob=home

Information about various types of knee injuries and treatments.

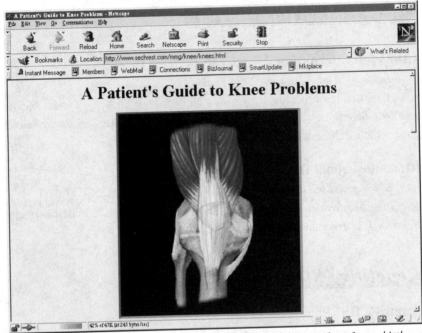

A Patient's Guide to Knee Problems, http://www.sechrest.com/mmg/knee/knees.html

The Knee Sources
http://www.orthop.washington.edu/knee/

Provided by the Washington Department of Orthopedics, this site gives information about the sources of knee pain, and exercises that can be performed to strengthen the knee and alleviate pain.

A Patient's Guide to Artificial Knee Replacement
http://www.sechrest.com/mmg/tkr/index.html

Information about knee replacement surgery and recovery.

A Patient's Guide to Knee Problems
http://www.sechrest.com/mmg/knee/knees.html

A general guide to various knee problems, including ACL tears, torn meniscus, kneecap problems and bursitis.

Musculoskeletal Diseases

CliniWeb International: Musculoskeletal Diseases
http://www.ohsu.edu/cliniweb/C5/C5.html

Here, find resources and information on bone and cartilage diseases; fascitis and foot deformities; hand, jaw, joint and muscular diseases; musculoskeletal abnormalities; rheumatic disease; and tennis elbow.

Musculoskeletal Diseases
http://www.mic.ki.se/Diseases/c5.html

This site provides a huge number of links to information on musculoskeletal diseases. It is maintained by Sweden's Karolinska Institute.

Repetitive Strain Injuries

Amara's RSI Page
http://www.amara.com/aboutme/rsi.html

Information about repetitive strain injuries, especially those caused by using computers, treatment and prevention.

Carpal Tunnel Syndrome Page
http://www.netaxs.com/%7Eiris/cts/welcome.html

Information about carpal tunnel syndrome, including its link to using a computer keyboard and solutions. Links to related CTS and ergonomic sites.

Chicago Legal Net: Carpal Tunnel Syndrome
http://www.chicagolegalnet.com/carpal.htm

Information about receiving worker's compensation for carpal tunnel syndrome.

Computer-Related Repetitive Strain Injury
http://engr-www.unl.edu/ee/eeshop/rsi.html

Site describes computer-related repetitive strain injuries and how to prevent them, since prevention is easier than treatment. It also offers books and links to related Internet sites, and information about products to reduce repetitive strain.

Repetitive Strain Injuries: The Hidden Cost of Computing

http://webreference.com/rsi.html

Information on RSI, its causes, symptoms, prevention and treatment.

Repetitive Strain Injury Recovery Page

http://home.clara.net/ruegg/index.htm

Information on recognizing signs of RSI, how to treat it and how to avoid it. Also features links to other related sites.

Repetitive Stress Injuries

http://planet-hawaii.com/~billpeay/TECHT08.html

A seven-part series on repetitive stress injuries with links to other related pages.

RSI Network Newsletters

http://www.ctdrn.org/rsinet.html

Subscription publication provides articles, news and product information of interest to those interested in repetitive strain injuries. Access archives at site.

Typing Injury FAQ

http://www.tifaq.org/

Educational site providing a variety of information about repetitive stress injuries, particularly typing.

Rheumatology

See also: Arthritis, earlier in this chapter.

American College of Rheumatology

http://www.rheumatology.org/

Site for organization composed of physicians, health professionals and scientists who are educators, researchers, and advocates of the care of people with arthritis and rheumatic and musculoskeletal diseases. Provides information on membership, education, publications, research and patient information.

Syringomyelia

Syringomyelia: Do You Have These Symptoms?
http://www.syringo.org/

Page can be viewed in either English or Spanish, and provides information on symptoms of syringomyelia (which include back pain, headache, weakness, shoulder and/or leg pain, and numbness in the hands) and causes. Links to related websites for patients.

Syringomyelia Fact Sheet
http://www.ninds.nih.gov/patients/disorder/syringo/syringfs.htm

Syringomyelia occurs when a cyst forms on the spinal cord, eventually destroying the center of the spinal cord and resulting in pain, weakness, and stiffness. Find out about the different forms of the disease, its diagnosis, treatment, and current research.

NEUROLOGICAL DISORDERS

Epilepsy

Alliance for Epilepsy Research
http://www.epilepsyresearch.org/research.htm
List of links and information on epilepsy from various sources.

Andrew Patrick's Epilepsy Resources
http://debra.dgbt.doc.ca/~andrew/epilepsy/resources.html
List of links to medical centers, associations, individual web pages, and related epilepsy resources.

Anti-Epileptic Medications
http://www.epipro.com/meds.html
Information on the drugs often provided to control epileptic seizures. Includes side effects and drug interactions, and descriptions of what happens if dosage is too small or too big.

CyberSpasm
http://www.hps.com/tomftp/cyberspasm/
Home of the Epilepsy Web Ring. Links, famous "flappers," members directory, archives and more.

Epilepsy and Brain Mapping Program

http://www.epipro.com/

Describes the program, provides treatment and research information, and answers to frequently asked questions.

Epilepsy Discussion Board

http://debra.dgbt.doc.ca/cgi-bin/epilepsy-board.cgi

Post or respond to an inquiry.

The Epilepsy Foundation of America

http://www.efa.org/indexf.htm

Includes epilepsy information, research, advocacy and news features. Also includes links, a page for kids with epilepsy, and an online journal.

Epilepsy in Young Children

http://www.geocities.com/HotSprings/1000/

This site is intended as a support platform for parents and other caregivers of children with epilepsy. The main portion consists of stories of individual children contributed by the parents (or other caregivers) of these children. Each story includes an e-mail address of the parents, so that visitors can get in touch with them if they wish. You can search for stories by child's name, age, diagnosis, or treatment. There is also an e-mail group at this site.

Epilepsy International

http://epilepsy-international.com/english/

Includes information on epilepsy history, medical resources, bulletin board, drugs, and women and epilepsy. In addition, find a professional center, links and a reference section.

Epilepsy Links

http://www-hsl.mcmaster.ca/tomflem/epilep.html

Frequently asked questions, articles and organizations.

Epilepsy Resource Center

http://members.aol.com/healwell/epilepsy.htm

Epilepsy books, medical news, online resources, chat rooms, web rings and links.

Epilepsy Resources

http://www.geocities.com/Wellesley/9641/epilepsy.html

Includes personal experiences of living with epilepsy.

Frequently Asked Questions

http://137.172.248.46/frequent.htm

Basic information on epilepsy, names of people with epilepsy, types of seizures, causes and triggers, diagnosis, coping and more information.

Important Issues in Epilepsy

http://epilepsy-international.com/english/issues/issmain.html

Summary papers on diverse subjects important in the care and day-to-day function of individuals with epilepsy. Includes diet, legal aspects, drug monitoring, and vagal nerve stimulation.

Ketogenic Diet

http://www.stanford.edu/group/ketodiet/ketobinder.html

Information on the high fat/low sugar and low carbohydrate diet that has been used to help control seizures in children with intractable epilepsy. Guidelines for checking if diet is appropriate and, if so, how to follow it.

Medinex Epilepsy Discussion Board

http://www.medinex.com/epilepsy.shtml

In addition to access to the discussion board, this site offers links to support groups and epilepsy information sites.

Seizure Types

http://epilepsyontario.org/faqs/seizures/index.html

There are over forty types of seizures.

Washington University Comprehensive Epilepsy Program

http://www.neuro.wustl.edu/epilepsy/

Find information about epilepsy medications and surgery. Connect with epilepsy Internet sites, publications, support groups and services, and epilepsy discussion groups.

Your TBI, ABI and Epilepsy Home Away from Home
http://www.canddwilson.com/tbi/tbiepil.shtml

Lots of resources and links to traumatic brain injury, acquired brain injury, and epilepsy, as well as poems, quotations and stories that display the every day experiences of those with epilepsy and brain injury.

General Resources

Central Nervous System Diseases
http://www.mic.ki.se/Diseases/c10.228.html

Large list of links to articles and websites, courtesy of the Karolinska Institute of Sweden.

Frequently Asked Questions about Neurological Problems
http://www.neus.ccf.org/patients/faq.html

Questions cover various neurological diseases.

Gateway to Neurology at Massachusetts General Hospital
http://132.183.145.103

Online patient and caregiver services which include bulletin boards and chat rooms, information about the neurology department, links and more.

Neurological Disorders
http://faculty.washington.edu/chudler/disorders.html

Internet resources on Alzheimer's, epilepsy, neuro-immunology, pediatric neurology, aphasia, Huntington's, neuro-otology, phobias, Bell's Palsy, Parkinson's and more.

Neurological/Psychiatric
http://www.vh.org/Patients/IHB/OrgSys/NeuroPsych.html

Patient information from the Virtual Hospital.

Neurology Online
http://www.neurology.org/

Official journal of the American Academy of Neurology. You must be an AAN member and journal subscriber to obtain full text of articles. Visitors can view table of contents and abstracts.

NeuroNet
http://www.neuronet.org/

Online resource center for the neurology profession. It is organized under four diseases: Dementia, Acute Stroke, Epilepsy and Multiple Sclerosis; and access is limited to physicians only. Pre-registration is required.

Neuropsychology Central
http://www.neuropsychologycentral.com/

This site describes the field of neuropsychology, which is the investigation of brain and behavior.

Neurosciences on the Internet
http://www.neuroguide.com/

"A searchable and browsable index of neuroscience resources available on the Internet. Includes neurobiology, neurology, neurosurgery, psychiatry, psychology, cognitive science sites and information on human neurological diseases."

Oliver Sack's Home Page
http://www.oliversacks.com/

Oliver Sacks is an author and neurologist. Site describes his books and presents excerpts, interviews, lectures, and links.

Yahoo! Neurological Diseases
http://dir.yahoo.com/Health/Diseases_and_Conditions/Neurological_Diseases/

Directory of sites on different neurological disorders.

Guillain-Barre Syndrome

Acute Immune Polyneuropathies (Guillain-Barre) Syndrome
http://www.neuro.wustl.edu/neuromuscular/antibody/gbs.htm

Classification of neuropathies and GBS-like syndromes. Guillain-Barre involves the development of progressive muscle weakness and respiratory paralysis associated with absent reflexes, usually after an infection.

Guillain-Barre Association

http://www.ozemail.com.au/~guillain/

Information about the Association and the disease. Site provides links, case histories, and separate guides for patients, for laypeople and for professionals.

Guillain-Barre Syndrome Fact Sheet

http://www.ninds.nih.gov/patients/disorder/guillain/guillain.htm

General GBS information from the National Institutes of Health, National Institute of Neurological Disorders and Stroke.

Guillain-Barre Syndrome Menu

http://neuro-www.mgh.harvard.edu/forum/GuillainBarreSyndromeMenu.html

Web forum for discussion of this disease.

Guillain-Barre Syndrome

http://www.mayohealth.org/mayo/9708/htm/guillain.htm

Information from the Mayo Clinic.

Guillain-Barre Syndrome Support Group of the U.K.

http://www.gbs.org.uk/

The information found at this site will be helpful, no matter where you live.

Huntington's Disease

Caring for People with Huntington's Disease

http://www.kumc.edu/hospital/huntingtons/

Information sheet for patients, family members, friends and the general public. Huntington's Disease (HD) is an inherited, degenerative neuropsychiatric disorder. Lots of links.

Communication Strategies for those with Huntington's Disease

http://www.kumc.edu/hospital/huntingtons/communication.html

Principles and strategies for enhancing communication with a HD patient.

Facing Huntington's Disease: A Handbook for Families and Friends

http://neuro-chief-e.mgh.harvard.edu/mcmenemy/facinghd.html

Online booklet discusses medical facts, genetic facts, diagnosis, coping, disease progression, and further sources of help.

Genome Map

http://www.ncbi.nlm.nih.gov/cgi-bin/SCIENCE96/nph-gene?HD

The HD gene maps to chromosome 4. This site considers the genetic description of the disease, and offers links to gene, protein and mRNA sequencing data.

Huntington Disease

http://www3.ncbi.nlm.nih.gov:80/htbin-post/Omim/dispmim?143100

Clinical information about HD.

Huntington's Disease

http://www.interlog.com/~rlaycock/2nd.html

News, information and links.

Huntington's Disease Fact Sheet

http://www.kumc.edu/instruction/medicine/neurology/hd.html

Describes this neurodegenerative disorder that affects motor, mood and cognition.

Huntington's Disease Information on the Internet

http://www.telerama.com/~mccarren/

Links to selected Huntington sites.

Huntington's Disease Lighthouse

http://table.jps.net/~wuf/

Tips on understanding Huntington's disease. Includes research news, legislative issues, personal care discussion, and a healthy skepticism of drugs.

Huntington's Disease Menu

http://neuro-www.mgh.harvard.edu/forum/HuntingtonsDiseaseMenu.html

Discussion and web forum.

Huntington's Disease Society of America

http://www.hdsa.org/

Support, research, information and grants.

Huntington's Links

http://www.geocities.com/Pentagon/Base/1284/

Check out the articles and resources, or read a diary of a Huntington's patient.

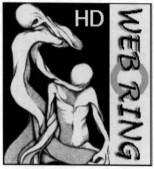

Huntington's Web Ring

http://www.hackers.demon.co.uk/webring.html

Information on how to join the web ring, and how to visit its member sites.

Teens and Huntington's Disease

http://www3.pei.sympatico.ca/stephen.hurst/
TEENHD.HTM

Support group for teens around the world who are affected in any way by Huntington's disease.

Huntington's Web Ring.
http://www.hackers.demon.co.uk/

Multiple Sclerosis

Drug Infonet's Multiple Sclerosis Sites

http://www.druginfonet.com/ms.htm

Links to several multiple sclerosis (MS) sites on the web.

International Multiple Sclerosis Support Foundation

http://209.132.43.204/

MS resources, arranged by topic. As well as "the usual," topics include: glossary, humor, newsletter, nutrition, recipes, theories, and an area for teens.

Jooly's Joint

http://www.mswebpals.org/realind.htm

Group which shares personal experiences with multiple sclerosis and seeks to give and receive support; for people with multiple sclerosis and their families.

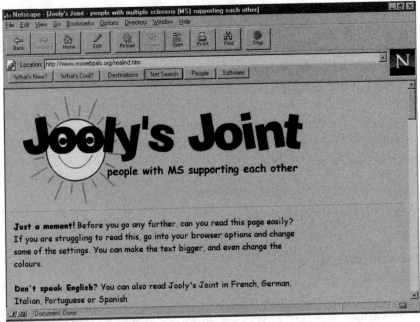

Jooly's Joint. *http://www.mswebpals.org/realind.htm*

MS Direct Discussion Forum
http://dean.sporleder.aquila.com/

Post a new message, search the archives, or respond to an article already posted.

MS Crossroads
http://www.helsinki.fi/~ahalko/ms.html

Many links to MS information sites, personal pages, research, treatment and helpful software.

Multiple Sclerosis
http://www-medlib.med.utah.edu/kw/ms

An introduction to MS for medical students and physicians in training. The site provides a guide to the disease and includes a patient video.

Multiple Sclerosis Foundation
http://www.icanect.net/msf/

Information about the services offered by the Foundation, frequently asked questions (FAQs), and a newsletter.

National Multiple Sclerosis Society

http://www.nmss.org/

MS information, resources, links, and information about the Society.

The World of Multiple Sclerosis

http://www.ifmss.org.uk/

Directory of national MS societies, a description of the disease, and answers to frequently asked questions. You can also find a list of publications, a section for professionals, resources and support.

Neurofibromatosis

Neurofibromatosis, Inc.

http://www.nfinc.org/

Neurofibromatosis (NF) is a genetic disorder of the nervous system that causes tumors to form on the nerves anywhere in the body, at any time. Site provides NF information (effects, references, misconceptions), resources, a bulletin board, links and support.

Neurofibromatosis Online Service

http://nf.org/

Neurofibromatosis tumors may affect bones and skin, and sometimes lead to mental disability. This site provides information for patients, their families and health care professionals about the disease, its diagnosis and genetic management. Also provided are counseling and support groups, literature references and online resources.

Neurofibromatosis - von Recklinghausen's Disease - Acoustic Neuroma

http://neurosurgery.mgh.harvard.edu/NFR/

General information on neurofibromatosis and related disorders. Also includes links to related sites and photographs which demonstrate the visible aspects of the disease.

Organizations

American Academy of Neurology

http://www.aan.com/

Information about neurology and disorders of the brain and nervous system, organization resources and membership, meetings and research efforts.

Mind Online

http://www.mindonline.com/

Homepage of the Michigan Institute of Neurological Disorders.

National Institute of Neurological Disorders and Stroke

http://www.ninds.nih.gov/

News and neurological health information, including guides to stroke, epilepsy and Parkinson Disease; general interest information on neurological conditions and publications available from the NINDS; clinical alerts and advisories.

Society for Neuroscience

http://www.sfn.org/

Includes several neuroscience-related journals and meeting information.

Parkinson's Disease

Awakenings

http://www.parkinsonsdisease.com/

This is an open forum for all with an interest in Parkinson's disease (PD). Information is divided into three main categories, which include living with PD, guidance for primary care doctors, and information and news for specialists. It aims to improve understanding and management of the condition.

Even More Links

http://neuro-chief-e.mgh.harvard.edu/parkinsonsweb/Main/Other/More2.html

Links to Parkinson's disease websites.

Exercises for the Parkinson Patient
http://www.cnsonline.org/www/archive/parkins/park-03.txt

Describes ten basic exercises which, if performed daily, can help the Parkinson's patient maintain muscle power and tone, and help to prevent deformities of the limbs and spine.

National Parkinson Foundation, Inc.
http://www.parkinson.org/

The Foundation is devoted to finding the cause and cure for Parkinson's, educating professionals about the early warning signs for the disease, educating patients and their loved ones, providing diagnostic and therapeutic services, and improving the quality of life for those who suffer from this disease. Site offers Parkinson facts, news, events, patient/caregiver resources, clinical studies and a library.

Parkinson's Disease Message Board
http://www.healthboards.com/parkinsons-disease/

Search the boards, or post your own message.

Parkinson's List Information
http://neuro-chief-e.mgh.harvard.edu/parkinsonsweb/Main/Other/listserv.html

Read for instructions on how to search the Parkinson archives.

Parkinson's News from the Front Line
http://www.cloudnet.com/~mandms/

"Webpaper" for the Parkinson's community. Invites visitors to send in their own stories and articles.

The Parkinson's Web
http://pdweb.mgh.harvard.edu/

Information about Parkinson's disease, how to cope with it, where to find support, recent research updates and publications, surgical procedures, advocacy efforts and links.

Research News on Parkinson's Disease
http://www.nhgri.nih.gov/DIR/LGDR/PARK2/

From the National Human Genome Research Institute.

Pediatric Neurology

Child Neurology Home Page
http://www.waisman.wisc.edu/child-neuro/index.html
> Information for parents and professionals.

Child Neurology Society
http://www1.umn.edu/cns/index.htm
> Professional association of pediatric neurologists.

Neurological Disorders in Children
http://www.bethisraelny.org/inn/
> Individual disorders and general information.

Rett Syndrome

International Rett Syndrome Association
http://www.rettsyndrome.org/
> Members of this organization include parents, relatives, physicians, therapists, researchers and friends, all interested in providing a better future for girls with Rett Syndrome. Site offers advice on communicating and educating patients, links and support groups, a directory of fundraising events, and information on research grants.

Living with Rett Syndrome
http://hometown.aol.com/Rsmother/livingrs.html
> Site tells a personal story of living with Rett's, as well as medical issues, "Rettchicks" stories, parents' stories, treatment and therapy, communication aids, online magazine about Rett's, assistive technology and much more.

Our Rett Syndrome Page
http://www.bundlings.com/irsg.htm
> Rett syndrome is a neurological disorder effecting girls. One of the first symptoms is decreased muscle tone, but it has behavioral and developmental symptoms as well. Site offers recommended readings and videos, advice for families on getting support, parent tips, a personal story, and other resources.

Rett Syndrome Links
http://www.execpc.com/~tamratam/rettlinks.html

Long list of associations, informational sites, mail lists and personal stories.

The Rett Syndrome Study Web
http://www.studyweb.com/med/rettsyn.htm

Suggests valuable sites from which one can learn about Rett's.

Tourette Syndrome

The Facts about Tourette Syndrome
http://members.tripod.com/~tourette13/

Basic information, links, and connection to newsgroup and Tourette mailing list. To subscribe, send e-mail to *majordomo@igc.apc.org*, and put "subscribe sunrise-tourette" (without the quotes) in the body, and nothing else.

Famous People with Tourette Syndrome
http://neuro-www2.mgh.harvard.edu/tsa/AboutTS/famouspeople.html

Biographical and historical information on well-known people who have or have had Tourette syndrome, which is characterized by spectrum of motor and/or vocal tics and associated symptoms.

Guide to the Diagnosis and Treatment of Tourette Syndrome
http://www.mentalhealth.com/book/p40-gtor.html

This online booklet is intended to provide information to physicians, psychologists, nurses, and other professionals. Friends and family members will also find it helpful, however.

A Neurologist's Notebook
http://neuro-www2.mgh.harvard.edu/TSA/AboutTS/notebook.html

Chapter from Oliver Sacks' book, *The Anthropologist from Mars*, which features a chapter on a Canadian surgeon and amateur pilot with TS.

The Nova Scotia Tourette Syndrome Site
http://www.chebucto.ns.ca/Health/Tourette/TS.html

Includes frequently asked questions, articles, mailing lists, and Internet links.

Tourette Syndrome Association, Inc.
http://tsa.mgh.harvard.edu/
What Tourette's is (and isn't), medical and scientific information, publications and activities. There is also a page entitled, "Just for Laughs."

Tourette Syndrome Fact Sheet
http://www.ninds.nih.gov/patients/disorder/tourette/tourette.htm
Answers to frequently asked questions and information from the National Institute of Neurological Disorders and Stroke.

Tourette Syndrome Primer
http://www.chadd.org/tsprime.htm
Good overview on the disorder, discussion of genetics, and list of books and organizations that can offer more information or personal stories.

Tourette Syndrome: Virtual Hospital
http://www.vh.org/Patients/IHB/Psych/Tourette/TouretteSyndrome.html
Handout from the University of Iowa's Virtual Hospital includes links to articles on Tourette's, motor and vocal tics, associated symptoms, attention deficit/hyperactivity disorder, and other related problems.

Tuberous Sclerosis

Global Tuberous Sclerosis Information Link
http://members.aol.com/gtsil/ts/index.htm
Tuberous sclerosis is a genetic disorder that causes benign tumors on various organs, including the brain, kidneys, heart, skin and lungs. This website includes a newsletter, news room, lots of links, a book list and more.

Lisa's Tuberous Sclerosis Site
http://www.title14.com/ts/
Lisa's personal story, experience with laser surgery, CT scans, chat site, and links.

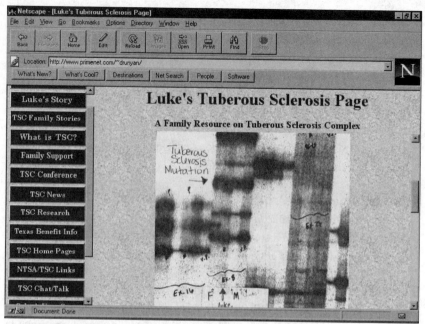

Indicates chromosome mutation for Tuberous Sclerosis, as displayed at Lukes Tuberous Sclerosis Page. http://www.primenet.com/~drunyan/

Luke's Tuberous Sclerosis Page

http://www.primenet.com/~drunyan/

Family support site. Provides an explanation of the disease, family stories, tuberous sclerosis complex (TSC) news, research and links.

National Tuberous Sclerosis Association

http://www.ntsa.org/

The National Tuberous Sclerosis Association (NTSA) is the only national organization solely devoted to serving individuals with TS and their families.

NEUROMUSCULAR DISORDERS

Amyotrophic Lateral Sclerosis

ALS Association
http://www.ALSA.org/

Amyotrophic lateral sclerosis (a.k.a. ALS or Lou Gehrig's disease) is a fairly common disorder of the nervous system. Life expectancy upon diagnosis is usually two to four years, but many with this disease live much longer. The ALS Association encourages, funds and monitors research for a cure, supports patients and families, and educates the general public and government representatives about this disease.

ALS Network
http://alsnetwork.en.com/index.html

This site offers a great deal to those affected by amyotrophic lateral sclerosis. It tracks individual treatment programs and progress, serves as a support for PALS (people with ALS) and their families and caregivers, and demonstrates "there is life beyond ALS" with its suggestions regarding adaptive technology and more. Find exercises that prevent stiffness and pain, ways to minimize the risk of falling, nutritional recommendations, new medications and treatments to fight the disease.

ALS Survival Guide
http://www.lougehrigsdisease.net/

Provides basic information, news, legal/financial aid, advocacy, vital statistics, treatment information, adaptive technology, and many more resources and information on ALS.

Ask NOAH About Amyotrophic Lateral Sclerosis
http://www.noah.cuny.edu/neuro/neuropg.html#ALS

Site offers fact sheets, care and treatment, special considerations, and information resources for consumers.

Drug Trials
http://www.bcm.tmc.edu/neurol/struct/als/als8.html

Information on drugs for ALS that have been shown to improve survival or slow disease progression.

Charcot-Marie-Tooth

Charcot-Marie-Tooth
http://disability.ucdavis.edu/Clearinghouse/Virtual_Library/Disease_Database/ Charcot-Marie-Tooth_Disease_Links.html

List of links to organizations and information about this disease, which is a slowly progressive, neuromuscular disorder which can affect the feet, legs, hands, arms, spine, vocal cords, breathing and other areas of the body.

Charcot-Marie-Tooth Association
http://www.charcot-marie-tooth.org/

This organization is devoted to educating the public, supporting patients and promoting a cure to Charcot-Marie-Tooth disease (CMT). Site offers medical alerts, publications (newsletter and fact sheets), a discussion forum, and a list of resources.

CMT International
http://www.cmtint.org/

Website for a world-wide organization run by and for people who have Charcot-Marie-Tooth disease. The organization publishes a newsletter and a variety of pamphlets. Site offers a list of drugs to avoid, as well as a list of physicians, and information on scholarships.

General Resources

European Neuromuscular Centre

http://enmc.spc.ox.ac.uk/

Provides information on the diagnosis and epidemiology of neuromuscular diseases.

Human Muscle Gene Map

http://www.bio.unipd.it/~telethon/Diet/Hmgm/main_map.html

"A comprehensive, high resolution genomic transcript map of human skeletal muscle."

Muscle Power

http://www.disabilitynet.co.uk/groups/musclepower/

National organization of people with neuromuscular impairments.

MuscleNET

http://telethon.bio.unipd.it/

MuscleNET provides information on neuromuscular disorders, cardiomyopathies and the recent advances of the scientific research on these subjects. It also contains a study companion in muscle biology, and many links.

Neuromuscular Conditions Information

http://www.kumc.edu/gec/support/neuromus.html

Lots of links to websites.

Neuromuscular Disease Center

http://www.neuro.wustl.edu/neuromuscular/

Information on neuromuscular disorders, neuromuscular evaluation, autoantibody testing, patient information, links to related sites and additional references.

Neuromuscular Disease Database

http://disability.ucdavis.edu/Clearinghouse/Virtual_Library/

Includes information about amyotrophic lateral sclerosis, muscular dystrophy, polio, spinal muscular atrophy, Charcot-Marie-Tooth syndrome, and dozens of other neuromuscular diseases.

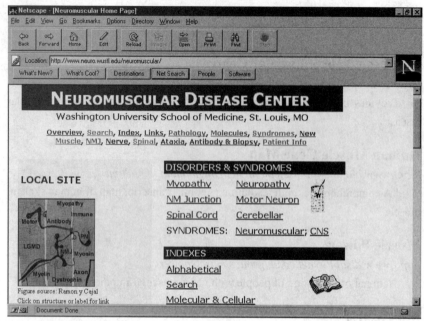

Neuromuscular Disease Center. http://www.neuro.wustl.edu/neuromuscular/

Neuromuscular Diseases

http://www.mic.ki.se/Diseases/c10.668.html

Long list of links to neuromuscular diseases, organized by disease.

Neuromuscular Diseases in the MDA Program

http://www.mdausa.org/disease/

Find out the disease characteristics, usual age of onset, progression and inheritance type, and a comprehensive list of web materials on forty different neuromuscular diseases.

Neuromuscular Disorders Links

http://hsl.mcmaster.ca/tomflem/neuromus.html

Link to sites about some of the most common neuromuscular disorders.

Muscular Dystrophy

Ask NOAH about: Muscular Dystrophy
http://www.noah.cuny.edu/neuro/musdys.html
Covers disease basics, genetics, diagnosis, care and treatment, and resources.

Congenital Myotonic Dystrophy
http://www.myotonicdystrophy.com/
Site provides a great deal of information on this form of muscular dystrophy, including medical, genetic and social information, research, personality and psychological effects, speech, research, treatment and personal stories. There is also a discussion forum, e-mail group, and list of activities and games children with this disorder like to do.

Fact Sheet: Myotonic Muscular Dystrophy
http://www.mda.org.au/specific/mdamyt.html
Information on this form of muscular dystrophy that tends to affect adults.

Genetics Primer
http://www.muscular-dystrophy.org/information/Research/genetics.html
Good, laymen's explanation of genetics and how chromosomal abnormalities can cause havoc; in this case, by causing muscular dystrophy.

Glossary of Terms
http://www.muscular-dystrophy.org/information/glossary.html
Definitions of terms encountered in the discussion of muscular dystrophy.

The Haynes Family's Duchenne Muscular Dystrophy Home Page
http://www.geocities.com/CapeCanaveral/8676/
Information about Duchenne muscular dystrophy (DMD) and one family's experience.

Leiden Muscular Dystrophy Pages
http://www.dmd.nl/
Discusses the disease including the genes and proteins involved, and provides diagnostic databases, research and diagnostic news.

Muscular Dystrophy Association of Australia
http://www.mda.org.au/

General and specific muscular dystrophy information, research and links to Ryan's Café, a site to help people with MD get in touch with each other and discuss problems related to MD.

Muscular Dystrophy Association - USA
http://www.mdausa.org/

You can watch a "replay" of the most recent MDA telethon, hosted by Jerry Lewis. Also contains information on the neuromuscular diseases, clinics and services, research, publications, and ways to help.

Muscular Dystrophy by Giovanni Naso
http://www.rtmol.stt.it/users/gnaso/muscdyst.html

A parent of a child with muscular dystrophy shares the information he has collected on this disease, including laboratory studies, treatment options, pyschological and scoiological considerations, and more.

Muscular Dystrophy Message Board
http://www.healthboards.com/muscular-dystrophy/

Post your own message, respond to another's, or browse through exchanges others have had.

Myotonic Dystrophy: An Information Booklet for Individuals and Families
http://www.vtmednet.org/~m145037/vhgi_mem/myodys/myodys_head.htm

Also known as Dystrophia Myotonica (DM), this disease consists of muscle weakness and myotonia (inability of muscles to relax after use) which gets more severe over time.

Parent Project: Muscular Dystrophy Research
http://www.parentdmd.org/

The Parent Project seeks to expedite treatment and cure of Duchenne and Becker muscular dystrophy by funding education and research.

A Parent's Muscular Dystrophy Page

http://users.neworld.net/woliver/md.html

Page discusses one of the most common types of muscular dystrophy, Duchenne's. This is an inherited neuromuscular disorder characterized by rapid progression of muscle degeneration.

Myasthenia Gravis

Life with Myasthenia

http://pages.prodigy.com/lifewithmg/

The goal of this site is to connect those with myasthenia gravis with information, and with each other. It offers a list of organizations, e-mail support groups, publications, personal experiences, daily living hints and much more. Myasthenia gravis is a chronic autoimmune disease that causes weakness in the voluntary muscles, and can lead to paralysis.

Myasthenia Gravis Links

http://pages.prodigy.net/stanley.way/myasthenia/

Organizations, clinical information, life style and individual stories, support groups and more.

Myasthenia Gravis Survival Guide

http://www.med.unc.edu//wrkunits/2depts/neurolog/mgfa/mgf-surv.htm

This is a guide to allow the myasthenic patient to learn about the disease and the health care system so that he or she can participate in important discussions with caregivers and make informed decisions about available treatment options.

NURSING

Discussion Groups

Legal Nurse Discussion Group
http://firms.findlaw.com/lncforum/

A forum for medical/legal professionals to discuss relevant issues pertaining to their discipline. Although it is not free, there are advantages to joining.

NURSENET
http://www.ualberta.ca/~jrnorris/nursenet/nn.html

Collections of different discussions on nursing topics.

Nurses World Message Board
http://www.nursesworld.com/boards.htm

There are two boards here, one exclusively for employment issues and the other for discussion of general nursing issues.

Psychiatric-Nursing Discussion List
http://www.mailbase.ac.uk/lists/psychiatric-nursing/

How to join, browse or search archives, contribute and respond.

Rural Nursing Discussion List
http://www.texastown.com/rural_nursing/

Topics of interest often include educational backgrounds needed for rural nursing, incentives for employment of nurses in rural areas, special concerns of patients specific to the rural residents, and many others.

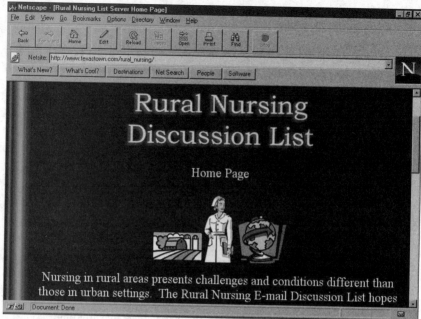

Rural Nursing E-mail Discussion List. *http://www.texastown.com/rural_nursing/*

Education

Continuing and Distance Education for Nurses and Health Care Professionals

http://www.cde.psu.edu/Nursing/

Upcoming and recent programs offered by the Penn State School of Nursing.

NURSEONE

http://www.nurseone.com/

This site provides online continuing education courses aimed to improve or refresh the knowledge base of interested nurses. These courses are available for free through the Internet to anyone equipped to read URL documents. Testing and CEU certification is available via online e-mail, and fees are paid after completion.

Nursing Education

http://www.nursingeducation.net/

Emergency nursing, medsurg nursing, continuing education, test questions and more.

Nursing Education of America

http://www.nursingeducation.org/index2.html

Nonprofit organization that offers a wide selection of continuing education courses for nurses, ranging from general interest to mental health, critical care and more.

Nursing Matters

http://www.nursingmatters.com/

"Nationally accredited to provide continuing education at your convenience." Course catalog available for browsing.

Online and Other CEUs

http://www.nursingnet.org/ceu.htm

List of online courses and seminars for the nursing professions.

Virtual Nursing College

http://www.langara.bc.ca/vnc/

"The VNC is a virtual learning and teaching environment that is dedicated to the education and professional development of nurses everywhere." It contains free MEDLINE searches, lab and diagnostic tests, pharmacology and drug resources, nursing informatics, nursing research, nursing terminology and more.

Emergency Care

Emergency Nurses Association

http://www.ena.org/enainfo/member.html

National organization for emergency nurses. Membership includes journal, newsletter, and voting rights, as well as information on meetings and continuing education.

Emergency Nursing World

http://enw.org/

Great practical information for emergency nurses. Includes clinical articles, research applied to clinical practice, associations and journals, and many other tools.

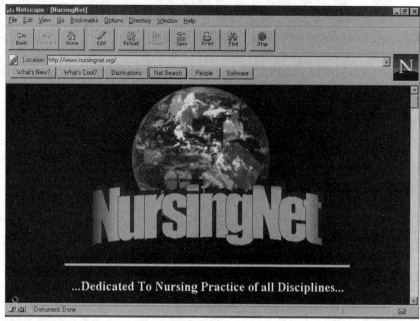

NursingNet. http://www.nursingnet.org/

General Resources

Cyber-Nurse
http://www.cyber-nurse.com/
Chat rooms and educational material.

CyberNurse
http://www.cybernurse.com/
Created by nursing professionals to serve their peers, this page includes valuable nursing resources and interactive links.

Hardin Meta Directory - Nursing
http://www.lib.uiowa.edu/hardin/md/nurs.html
Collection of sites that contain many links to nursing information.

Nursing and Health Care Resources on the Net
http://www.shef.ac.uk/~nhcon/
Global resources for nurses and other health care professionals. Organized by region, organization, therapy, and specialty.

Nursing and Health Professionals Internet Directory

http://www.slackinc.com/allied/allnet.htm

Major categories include general sites, anaesthesia, associations, education, eldercare, employment, EMS, nutrition, and publications.

Nursing World

http://www.nursingworld.org/

All about the American Nurses Association, an affiliation of associations and organizations that represents the nation's Registered Nurses. Topics include back issues of *The American Nurse*, continuing education, classified ads, e-mail lists, and special programs which focus on ethics and human rights, ethnic/racial minority fellowship, and international nursing. Site contains a news area, reading room, and a reference room, as well as resources for safety and health, nursing standards and more.

NursingCenter.com

http://www.NursingCenter.com/

Electronic educational, research and practice resources for nurses. Includes a long list of journal links, continuing education material, forum discussions, a career center, and a list of nursing organizations.

NursingNet

http://www.nursingnet.org/

This site's goal is to educate the public about the nursing profession, and to serve as a forum for medical professionals and students to find and distribute information on nursing and medicine. Site features nursing images, the NursingNet mentoring program, Nurseweek, a number of chat rooms and discussion forums, as well as sections that provide nurse practitioners references, emergency nursing and EMS links, pharmaceutical information, and career opportunities.

Resources for Nurses and Families

http://pegasus.cc.ucf.edu/~wink/

Resources are arranged by topic, and include: academic organizations, clinical practice, general health and government information, hospitals and medical center links, print and online journals, general nursing and health, specialty nursing, nursing informatics, nursing tutorials, nursing and health care listservs, and more.

Thomas Moll's Cool Nursing Site of the Week

http://www.odyssee.net/~fnord/nurselink.html

Links to the last month's picks of "cool nursing sites," and archives of all past choices.

The "Virtual" Nursing Center

http://www-sci.lib.uci.edu/HSG/Nursing.html

A practicing nurse or nursing student, and indeed anyone interested in nursing, would be hard pressed to find an aspect of the profession that is not covered at this site. The "Virtual" Nursing Center offers medical references (dictionaries and glossaries for a range of specialties), and material on metabolic pathways and genetic databases, online continuing eduction, nursing journal links, medical literature and patent searches, hospital and health care statistics and links, nursing courses and tutorials on a wide array of topics, clinical tutorials, nursing protocols and procedures, various interactive cases, laboratory diagnostic tools and clinical calculators, as well as nursing school and nursing association links.

Virtual Nurse Link Resources

http://virtualnurse.com/Link/pages/

Over 5000 links at this site. Provides description, and viewer ratings.

WholeNurse

http://www.wholenurse.com/

Index of thousands of nursing-related sites. Categories include: alternative health, diseases and illnesses, drug resources, education, employment, government, informational sites, legal and ethics, leisure, managed care, medical sites, medical specialties, mental health, patient education, job resources, references and wellness information.

History

The History of Nursing

http://gnv.fdt.net/~dforest/hxindex.htm

Perspectives of nursing his/herstory.

Night Shift

Night Shift Survival Tips

http://enw.org/NightShift.htm

There are advantages and disadvantages of working the night shift, and here are some suggestions for making it easier.

Nurse-Midwifery

See also: Pregnancy & Childbirth - Midwifery.

American College of Nurse-Midwives

http://www.acnm.org/

Professional education, find a nurse-midwife, midwifery education and more. A certified nurse-midwife (CNM) is a registered nurse who is educated in both nursing and midwifery.

Internet Midwifery Resources

http://www-personal.umich.edu/~dswalker/internet.html

List of sites on nursing, midwifery, and nurse-midwifery programs around the country.

Journal of Midwifery and Women's Health

http://www.elsevier.nl:80/inca/publications/store/ 5/0/5/7/7/4/

Formerly the Journal of Nurse-Wifery.

Midwifery Today

http://www.midwiferytoday.com/

Information on this quarterly magazine.

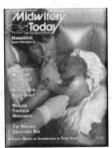

Midwifery Today.
http://www.midwifery today.com/

National Association of Neonatal Nurses

http://www.nann.org/

Supports and promotes neonatal nursing via providing a unified voice, advocacy efforts, and public education.

Online Birth Center: Midwifery, Pregnancy, Birth and Breastfeeding

http://www.efn.org/~djz/birth/birthindex.html

Links for nurse-midwives, including career information, newsgroups, organizations, alternative and general health resources.

Nurse Practitioners

American College of Nurse Practitioners

http://www.nurse.org/acnp/

National nonprofit organization that serves as a voice for nurse practitioners (NPs) and NP associates.

NP Central

http://www.nurse.net/np/

Information for and about nurse practitioners.

Nurse Practitioner Resources

http://nurseweb.ucsf.edu/www/arwwebpg.htm

Sites of interest and of use to nurse practitioner students.

The Virtual PNP

http://home.earthlink.net/~emgoodman/virtualpnp.htm

This site serves pediatric nurse practitioners, offering case studies, clinical insights, professional and NP links, and resources for employment and education.

Nursing Humor

Emergency Nursing Humor

http://enw.org/Humor.htm

Lots of humor for this crowd that thrives in a high-stress environment.

Home Health Humor

http://www.whidbey.com/ihn/humor.html

Funny, true stories from home health personnel.

Journal of Nursing Jocularity

http://www.jocularity.com/

There's a lot of material at this site designed to bring a smile.

Weird Nursing Tales

http://users.twave.net/texican/

Doctor jokes and unusual nursing stories.

Too Live Nurse

http://www.vgernet.net/toolive/toolive2.html

Educational and humorous music for health care professionals. Too Live Nurse has performed around the country, and they have even been featured on the nationally-syndicated "Doctor Demento Show."

Nursing Theory

Complexity and Chaos in Nursing

http://www.scsu.ctstateu.edu/scsu/chaos-nursing/index.html

Although this journal does not seem to be around anymore, interesting articles from past issues are still located here. The rather heady goal was to consider topics such as "chaos theory and complexity theory derivations from the natural sciences and the social sciences, annotated bibliographies, research findings, applications of theory to practice and the analyses of individual concepts within the paradigms."

Introduction to Nursing Theory

http://jan.ucc.nau.edu/~erw/nur301/theory/ntheory/index.html

This site accompanies a course taught at Northern Arizona University, but provides lots of information for anyone interested in nursing theories.

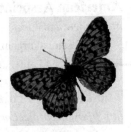

Nursing Science Resource Site

http://www.users.arn.net/~patoland/list.html

Links to and description of sites that provide "timely resources about nursing theory and research."

Nursing Science Resource Site.
http://www.users.arn.net/~patoland/list.html

The Nursing Theory Page
http://www.ualberta.ca/~jrnorris/nt/theory.html

This collection of links to references about nursing theories is a colloborative effort by an international group. There are links to a number of theory sites, information on nursing models around the world, and more. A thoughtful site for all interested in caregiving.

Resource Bibliography in Cross-Cultural Nursing
http://weber.u.washington.edu/~ethnomed/theory2.htm

Resources are arranged alphabetically, by author.

Self-Care Deficit Nursing Theory
http://www.hsc.missouri.edu/~son/scdnt/scdnt.html

Discussion and dissemination of information about this theory of nursing advanced by Dorothea Orem.

Organizations

American Association of Colleges of Nursing
http://www.aacn.nche.edu/

As this site mentions, nursing is the nation's largest health care profession. The AACN acts as a voice for nursing programs around the nation, and their site offers curriculum standards, the latest statistics, legislative advocacy, books reports and position statments, member programs and career opportunities.

American Association of Critical-Care Nurses
http://www.aacn.org/

Professional organization of critical care nurses provides lots of resources for its members and others.

The Florence Project, Inc.
http://florenceproject.org/

This site is maintained by an advocacy organization that is comprised of nurses who believe that health care should not be motivated by economic gain. "An equal-access and high quality health care system is a human right, not a privilege."

NIH Clinical Center Nursing Department

http://www.cc.nih.gov/nursing/

Find employment opportunities, nursing department staff resources, an alphabetical index of nursing policies, standards of practice, nursing and health related websites.

Publications

Journal of Neonatal Nursing

http://www.bizjet.com/jnn/

This journal is published six times each year and contains information for any professional involved in the care of pre-term babies. Access the Internet edition at this site (guests are permitted), learn how to subscribe, and join in discussion forums.

Journals and Publications

http://www.nursingnet.org/journals.htm

Links to a number of nursing journals and publications.

Nursing Journals

http://dir.yahoo.com/Health/Nursing/News_and_Media/Journals/

List of and links to journals that serve the nursing profession.

Online Nursing Journals

http://www.ajn.org/journals/

Table of contents, abstracts, and full-text nursing articles from Lippincott's large library of nursing journals are available here.

Research

Canadian Nurse Researcher Database

http://NurseResearcher.com/

Offers an interactive database for nurse researchers.

Midwest Nursing Research Society

http://www.mnrs.org/

Information about nursing research, funding sources, publications, program meetings, and about the Society.

National Institute of Nursing Research

http://www.nih.gov/ninr/

This organization is part of the National Institutes of Health, and it supports research in promoting the care of individuals. Find out about the research programs, legislative activities, conferences and publications of this organization. Site contains research, news, events, fact sheets, frequently asked questions (FAQs) and further resources about nursing research.

Southern Nursing Research Society

http://www.snrs.org/

Members have access to the *Southern Online Journal of Nursing Research*, a newsletter, abstracts, news and discussion groups. There are also opportunities for networking, and funding and training programs. Site describes the benefits of joining and tells you how to become a member.

Take a Break

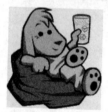

NurseLounge.com.
http://www.nurse lounge.com/

The Break Room

http://www.nursesworld.com/break.htm

Check out this site to help you get "centered."

NurseLounge.com

http://www.nurselounge.com/

This site invites nurses to take a break: "If you are looking for some diversions from the rigors of every day, how about venting in the Discussion Forum, or browse some cool and useful places on the web[?]" As well as diversions, you will also find a lot of helpful nursing information at this site.

ORGANIZATIONS

Academic Orthopaedic Society
http://www.a-o-s.org/

Academy for Eating Disorders
http://www.acadeatdis.org/

Academy of General Dentistry
http:/www.agd.org/

The Acoustic Neuroma Association Home Page
http://neurosurgery.mgh.harvard.edu/ana/

ACT-UP New York
http://www.actupny.org/

Addiction Research Foundation
http://www.arf.org/

Administration for Children and Families
http://www.acf.dhhs.gov/

Administration on Aging
http://www.aoa.dhhs.gov/

Adult Children of Alcoholics World Service Organizations
http://www.adultchildren.org/

Agency for Health Care Policy and Research
http://www.ahcpr.gov/

Agency for Toxic Substances and Disease Registry
http://www.atsdr.cdc.gov/

AIDS Action
http://www.aidsaction.org/

Al-Anon and Alateen
http://www.Al-Anon-Alateen.org/

Alcoholics Anonymous World Services
http://www.alcoholics-anonymous.org/

Alliance for Epilepsy Research
http://www.epilepsyresearch.org/research.htm

Alliance for Technology Access
http://www.ataaccess.org/

Alliance of Genetic Support Groups
http://www.geneticalliance.org/

ALS Association
http://www.ALSA.org/

Alzheimer's Association
http://www.alz.org/

American Academy of Allergy, Asthma and Immunology
http://www.aaaai.org/

American Academy of Child and Adolescent Psychiatry
http://www.aacap.org/web/aacap/

American Academy of Dermatology
http://www.aad.org/

American Academy of Family Physicians
http://www.aafp.org/

American Academy of Hospice and Palliative Medicine
http://www.aahpm.org/

American Academy of Medical Acupuncture
http://www.medicalacupuncture.org/

American Academy of Neurology
http://www.aan.com/

American Academy of Orthopaedic Surgeons
http://www.aaos.org/

American Academy of Osteopathy
http://www.aao.medguide.net/

American Academy of Otolaryngology, Head and Neck Surgery
http://www.entnet.org/

American Academy of Pain Management
http://www.aapainmanage.org/index.html

American Academy of Pediatric Dentistry
http://www.aapd.org/

American Academy of Pediatrics
http://www.aap.org/

American Academy of Pharmaceutical Physicians
http://www.aapp.org/

American Anorexia Bulimia Association
http://www.aabainc.org/

American Association for Chronic Fatigue Syndrome
http://www.aacfs.org/

American Association for the Study of Liver Disease
http://hepar-sfgh.ucsf.edu/

American Association for the Surgery of Trauma
http://www.aast.org/

American Association of Blood Banks
http://www.aabb.org/

American Association of Colleges of Nursing
http://www.aacn.nche.edu/

American Association of Colleges of Osteopathic Medicine
http://www.aacom.org/

American Association of Critical-Care Nurses
http://www.aacn.org/

American Association of Clinical Endocrinologists
http://www.aace.com/

American Association of Colleges of Osteopathic Medicine
http://www.aacom.org/

American Association of Dental Schools
http://www.aads.jhu.edu/

American Association of Diabetes Educators
http://www.aadenet.org/

American Association of Immunologists
http://www.scienceXchange.com/aai/

American Association of Kidney Patients
http://www.aakp.org/aakpteam.html

American Association of Naturopathic Physicians
http://www.naturopathic.org/

American Association of Pediatric Dentistry
http://aapd.org

American Association of Poison Control Centers
http://www.aapcc.org/

American Association of Respiratory Care
http://www.aarc.org/

American Association of Retired Persons
http://aarp.org/

American Association of Tissue Banks
http://www.aatb.org/

American Association on Mental Retardation
http://www.aamr.org/

American Board of Family Practice
http://www.abfp.org/

The American Cancer Society
http://www.cancer.org/

American Chiropractic Association
http://www.amerchiro.org/

American College of Cardiology
http://www.acc.org/

American College of Gastroenterology
http://www.acg.gi.org/

American College of Healthcare Executives
http://www.ache.org/

American College of Legal Medicine
http://www.aclm.org/

American College of Medical Practice Executives
http://www.mgma.com/acmpe/index.html

American College of Nurse-Midwives
http://www.acnm.org/

American College of Physicians
http://www.acponline.org/

American College of Rheumatology
http://www.rheumatology.org/

American College of Surgeons
http://www.facs.org/

American Council for Headache Education
http://www.achenet.org/index.html

American Council of Exercise
http://www.acefitness.org/

American Council of the Blind
http://www.acb.org/

American Council on Science and Health
http://www.acsh.org/medical/index.html

American Dental Association Online
http://www.ada.org/

American Diabetes Foundation
http://www.diabetes.org/

American Dietetic Association
http://www.eatright.org/

American Environmental Health Foundation
http://www.aehf.com/

American Foundation for AIDS Research
http://www.amfar.org/

The American Foundation for the Blind
http://www.igc.apc.org/afb/

American Foundation of Thyroid Patients
http://www.thyroidfoundation.org/

American Gastroenterological Association
http://www.gastro.org/

American Heart Association
http://www.americanheart.org/

American Holistic Health Association
http://ahha.org/

American Hospital Association
http://www.aha.org/

American Hyperlexia Association Home Page
http://www.hyperlexia.org/

American Institute for Cancer Research
http://www.aicr.org/

American Institute of Ultrasound in Medicine
http://www.aium.org/

American Liver Foundation
http://sadieo.ucsf.edu/alf/alffinal/homepagealf.html

American Lung Association
http://www.lungusa.org/

American Lyme Disease Foundation, Inc.
www.ALDF.com/

American Macular Degeneration Foundation
http://www.macular.org/

American Medical Association
http://www.ama-assn.org/

The American Medical Women's Association
http://www.amwa-doc.org/

American Meditation Institute
http://www.americanmeditation.org/

American Nephrology Nurses Association
http://anna.inurse.com/

The American Optometric Association
http://www.aoanet.org/

American Pain Foundation
http://www.painfoundation.org/

American Pain Society
http://www.ampainsoc.org/

American Pediatric Surgical Association
http://ped-surg.org/

American Physical Therapy Association: Geriatrics Section
http://geriatricspt.org/

American Porphyria Foundation
http://www.enterprise.net/apf/

The American Psychoanalytic Association
http://apsa.org/index.htm

The American Psychoanalytic Foundation
http://www.cyberpsych.org/apf/index.html

The American Psychological Association
http://www.apa.org/

American Public Health Association
http://www.apha.org/

American Red Cross
http://www.redcross.org/

American Sleep Disorder Association
http://www.asda.org/

American Social Health Association
http://www.ashastd.org/

American Society for Aesthetic Plastic Surgery
http://surgery.org/

American Society for Gastrointestinal Endoscopy
http://www.asge.org/

American Society for Nutritional Sciencies
http://www.faseb.org/asns/

American Society of Addiction Medicine
http://www.asam.org/

American Society of Anesthesiologists
http://www.asahq.org/

American Society of Cataract and Refractive Surgery-American Society of Ophthalmic Administrators
http://www.ascrs.org/

American Society of Clinical Pathologists
http://www.ascp.org/

American Society of Dermatology
http://www.asd.org/

American Society of Health-System Pharmacists
http://www.ashp.org/a

American Society of Hematology
http://www.hematology.org/

American Society of Hypertension
http://www.ash-us.org/

American Society of Law, Medicine & Ethics
http://www.aslme.org/

American Society of Transplant Physicians
http://www.a-s-t.org/index.htm

American Society of Transplantation
http://www.a-s-t.org/

The American Speech-Language Association
http://www.asha.org/

American Spinal Injury Association
http://www.asia-spinalinjury.org/

American Stroke Association
http://americanheart.org/Stroke/index.html

American Sudden Infant Death Syndrome Institute
http://www.sids.org/

American Thoracic Society
http://www.thoracic.org/

American Tinnitus Association
http://www.teleport.com/~ata/

The Arc of the United States
http://TheArc.org/welcome.html

The Association for the Study of Dreams
http://www.ASDreams.org/

Association of American Medical Colleges
http://www.aamc.org/

Association of Emergency Physicians
http://www.aep.org/index.html

Association of Schools of Public Health
http://www.asph.org/

Association of State and Territorial Health Officials
http://www.astho.org/about.html

Association of Women Surgeons
http://www.womensurgeons.org/

Asthma and Allergy Foundation of America
http://www.aafa.org/

Autism Society of America
http://www.autism-society.org/asa_home.html

The Bone Marrow Foundation
http://www.bonemarrow.org/

The Brain Tumor Society
http://www.tbts.org/

Bureau of Alcohol, Tobacco and Firearms
http://www.atf.treas.gov/

Canadian Organization for Rare Disorders
http://www.bulli.com/~cord/

CARE
http://www.care.org/

Center for Aging
http://garnet.berkeley.edu/~aging/

Center for Human Simulation
http://www.uchsc.edu/sm/chs/

Center for Reproductive Law and Policy
http://www.crlp.org/

Center on Budget and Policy Priorities
http://cbpp.org/

Center for International Health Information
http://www.cihi.com/

Centers for Disease Control and Prevention
http://www.cdc.gov/

Centre for the Epidemiology of Infectious Diseases
http://www.ceid.ac.uk/

Charcot-Marie-Tooth Association
http://www.charcot-marie-tooth.org/

Child Neurology Society
http://www1.umn.edu/cns/index.htm

Children's Liver Alliance (CLA)
http://www.livertx.org/viewer.html

Children's Organ Transplant Association
http://www.cota.org/

Choice in Dying
http://www.choices.org/

The Coalition for Medicare Choices
http://www.medicarechoices.org/

Cocaine Anonymous World Services
http://www.ca.org/

College of American Pathologists
http://www.cap.org/

Council for Affordable Health Insurance
http://www.cahi.org/

The Council for Responsible Genetics
http://www.gene-watch.org/

Crohn's and Colitis Foundation of America
http://www.ccfa.org/

Cystic Fibrosis Foundation
http://www.cff.org/

Dermatology Foundation
http://www.dermfnd.org/

Diabetes Action Research and Education Foundation
http://www.daref.org/

Diabetes Education and Research Center
http://www.libertynet.org/~diabetes/

The Drug Policy Foundation
http://www.dpf.org/

Ehlers-Danlos National Foundation
http://www.ednf.org/

Emergency Nurses Association
http://www.ena.org/enainfo/member.html

The Endocrine Society
http://www.endo-society.org/

Endometriosis Association
http://www.ivf.com/endoassn.html

The Epilepsy Foundation of America
http://www.efa.org/

The Family AIDS Network
http://www.familyaidsnet.org/

Family Violence Prevention Fund
http://www.igc.org/fund/

Federal Emergency Management Agency
http://www.fema.gov/

FRAXA Research Foundation
http://www.FRAXA.org/

The Glaucoma Foundation
http://www.glaucoma-foundation.org/info/

Glaucoma Research Foundation
http://www.glaucoma.org/

Guillain-Barre Association
http://www.ozemail.com.au/~guillain/

Health Care Financing Administration
http://www.hcfa.gov/

Health Care Liability Alliance
http://www.hcla.org/

The Health Consumer Alliance
http://healthconsumer.org/

Healthcare Financial Management Association
http://www.hfma.org/

Helicobacter Foundation
http://www.helico.com/

The Hemlock Society
http://www.hemlock.org//

Hepatitis C Foundation
http://www.hepcfoundation.org/

Hepatitis Research Foundation
http://www.hepatitis.ca/

Hereditary Disease Foundation
http://www.hdfoundation.org/

History of Sciency Society
http://depts.washington.edu/hssexec/

Holistic Dental Association
http://simwell.com/hda/

Hospice Foundation of America
http://www.hospicefoundation.org/

Huntington's Disease Society of America
http://www.hdsa.org/

Hydrocephalus Association
http://neurosurgery.mgh.harvard.edu/ha/

Immunization Action Coalition
http://www.immunize.org/

Institute for Child Health Policy
http://mchnet.ichp.ufl.edu/

Institute of Food Technologists
http://www.ift.org/

Institute of Medicine
http://www4.nas.edu/IOM/IOMHome.nsf

Institutes for the Achievement of Human Potential
http://www.iahp.org/

International Albinism Center
http://lenti.med.umn.edu:90/iac/

International Association of Physicians in AIDS Care
http://www.iapac.org/

International Chiropractors Association
http://www.chiropractic.org/

International Committee of the Red Cross
http://www.icrc.org/

International Diabetes Foundation
http://www.idf.org/

International Diabetic Athletes Association
http://www.diabetes-exercise.org/

International Dyslexia Association
http://www.interdys.org/

International Food Information Council
http://ificinfo.health.org/

International Harm Reduction Association
http://www.ihra.org.uk/default.htm

International Myeloma Foundation
http://myeloma.org/

International Plastic, Reconstructive and Aesthetic Surgery
http://www.ipras.org/

International Rett Syndrome Association
http://www.rettsyndrome.org/

International Society for Computer Aided Surgery
http://www.iscas.org/

International Society for Heart & Lung Transplantation
http://www.ishlt.org/

International Society for Infectious Diseases
http://www.isid.org/

International Society of Abortion Doctors
http://alpha.nedernet.nl/~ngva/isadindex.htm

International Society of Refractive Surgery
http://www.isrs.com/

Internet Dermatology Society
http://www.telemedicine.org/ids.htm

Interstitial Cystitis Association
http://www.ichelp.com/

Joint Commission on Accreditation of Healthcare Organizations
http://www.jcaho.org/

Joint Council of Asthma, Allergy and Immunology
http://www.jcaai.org/

The Juvenile Diabetes Foundation
http://www.jdf.org/index.html

Kidney Cancer Association
http://www.nkca.org/index.stm

Kidney Dialysis Foundation
http://www.kdf.org.sg/

Leukemia Society of America
http://www.leukemia.org/

Life Extension Society
http://www.clark.net/pub/kfl/les/les.html

Lupus Foundation of America
http://www.lupus.org/

Lyme Disease Foundation, Inc.
http://www.lyme.org/index2.html

Lymphoma Research Foundation
http://www.lymphoma.org/

Make-a-Wish Foundation
http://www.wish.org/

Maternal and Child Health Bureau
http://www.mchb.hrsa.gov/

Medical Group Management Association
http://www.mgma.com/

Medical Protection Society
http://www.mps.org.uk/medical/

Medical Research Council of Canada
http://www.mrc.gc.ca/

Melanoma Research Foundation
http://www.melanoma.org/

Midwest Nursing Research Society
http://www.mnrs.org/

Minority Health Professionals Foundation
http://www.minorityhealth.org/

Mothers' Voices United to End AIDS
http://www.mvoices.org/

The Multiple Myeloma Research Foundation
http://www.multiplemyeloma.org/

Multiple Sclerosis Foundation
http://www.icanect.net/msf/

Muscular Dystrophy Association of Australia
http://www.mda.org.au/

Muscular Dystrophy Association - USA
http://www.mdausa.org/

Narcotics Anonymous World Services
http://na.org/index.htm

National Academy of Sciences/National Academy of Engineering/Institute of Medicine/National Research Council
http://www.nas.edu/

National Adrenal Disease Foundation
http://www.medhelp.org/nadf/

National AIDS Fund
http://www.aidsfund.org/

National Arthritis Foundation
http://www.arthritis.org/

National Association for Children of Alcoholics
http://www.health.org/nacoa/

National Association for Chiropractic Medicine
http://www.chiromed.org/

National Association for Public Health Statistics and Information Systems
http://www.naphsis.org/

National Association of Developmental Councils
http://www.igc.apc.org/NADDC/

National Association of Nurse Practitioners
http://www.nurse.org/acnp/

The National Association of Women's Health Professionals
http://www.nawhp.org/

National Association to Advance Fat Acceptance
http://www.naafa.org/

National Ataxia Foundation
http://www.nwwin.com/houston/mall-a/ataxia.htm

National Black Child Development Institute
http://www.nbcdi.org/

The National Cancer Institute
http://www.nci.nih.gov/

National Center for Complementary and Alternative Medicine
http://nccam.nih.gov/

National Center for Food Safety and Technology
http://www.iit.edu/~ncfs/

National Center for Health Statistics
http://www.cdc.gov/nchswww/default.htm

National Center for Infectious Diseases
http://www.cdc.gov/ncidod/

National Center for Injury Prevention and Control
http://www.cdc.gov/ncipc/ncipchm.htm

National Center on Elder Abuse
http://www.gwjapan.com/NCEA/

National Coalition for Cancer Research
http://www.cancercoalition.org/index.html

National Coalition for the Homeless
http://nch.ari.net/

National Coalition on Health Care
http://www.americashealth.org/

National College of Naturopathic Medicine
http://www.ncnm.edu/

National Committee for Quality Assurance
http://www.ncqa.org/

National Enuresis Society
http://www.peds.umn.edu/Centers/NES/

National Eye Institute
http://www.nei.nih.gov/

The National Federation of the Blind
http://www.nfb.org/default.htm

National Foundation for Infectious Diseases
http://www.nfid.org/

National Foundation for the Treatment of Pain
http://www.paincare.org/

National Foundation for Transplantation
http://transplants.org/

National Health Care for the Homeless Council
http://www.nhchc.org/

National Health Information Center
http://nhic-nt.health.org/

National Heart, Lung and Blood Institute
http://www.nhlbi.nih.gov/index.htm

National Hemophilia Foundation
http://www.hemophilia.org/

National Hospice Organization
http://www.nho.org/

National Incontentia Pigmenti Foundation
http://medhlp.netusa.net/www/nipf.htm

National Institute of Allergy and Infectious Diseases
http://www.niaid.nih.gov/

National Institute of Arthritis and Musculoskeletal and Skin Diseases
http://www.nih.gov/niams/

National Institute of Child Health and Human Development
http://www.nichd.nih.gov/

National Institute of Deafness and Other Communication Diseases
http://www.nih.gov/nidcd/

National Institute of Dental and Craniofacial Research
http://www.nidr.nih.gov/

National Institute of Diabetes and Digestive and Kidney Diseases
http://www.niddk.nih.gov/

National Institute of Environmental Health Sciences
http://www.niehs.nih.gov/

National Institute of General Medical Sciences
http://www.nih.gov/nigms/

National Institute of Mental Health
http://www.nimh.nih.gov/

National Institute of Neurological Disorders and Stroke
http://www.ninds.nih.gov/

National Institute of Nursing Research
http://www.nih.gov/ninr/

National Institute of Transplantation
http://www.transplantation.com/

National Institute on Aging
http://www.nih.gov/nia/

National Institute on Alcohol Abuse and Alcoholism
http://www.niaaa.nih.gov/

National Institute on Drug Abuse
http://www.nida.nih.gov/

National Institutes of Health
http://www.nih.gov/

National Jewish Medical and Research Center
http://www.njc.org/

National Kidney Foundation
http://www.kidney.org/

National Lymphedema Network
http://www.lymphnet.org/

National Marrow Donor Program
http://www.marrow.org/

National Mental Health Association
http://www.nmha.org/

National Multiple Sclerosis Society
http://www.mnss.org/

The National Organization for Rare Disorders, Inc.
http://www.rarediseases.org/

National Organization for Women
http://www.now.org/

National Osteoporosis Foundation
http://www.nof.org/

National Ovarian Cancer Coalition
http://www.ovarian.org/

National Parkinson Foundation, Inc.
http://www.parkinson.org/

National Psoriasis Foundation
http://www.psoriasis.org/

National Public Health Information Coalition
http://nphic.org/

National Rural Health Association
http://www.nrharural.org/

The National Science Foundation
http://www.nsf.gov/

The National Sleep Foundation
http://www.sleepfoundation.org/

National Stroke Association
http://www.stroke.org/

National Transplant Assistance Fund
http://www.transplantfund.org/

National Tuberous Sclerosis Association
http://www.ntsa.org/

National Vitiligo Foundation
http://www.nvfi.org/

National Women's Health Resource Center
http://www.healthywomen.org/

Nicotine Anonymous
http://www.nicotine-anonymous.org/

North American Syringe Exchange Network
http://www.nasen.org/NASEN_II/index.html

Obsessive-Compulsive Foundation
http://www.ocfoundation.org/

Occupational Safety and Health Administration
http://www.osha.gov/

Office of Women's Health
http://www.4woman.org/owh/index.htm

Overeaters Anonymous
http://www.overeatersanonymous.org/

PanAmerican Health Organization
http://www.paho.org/

PBC (Primary Biliary Cirrhosis) Foundation
http://www.nhtech.demon.co.uk/pbc/index.html

Physicians Committee for Responsible Medicine
http://www.pcrm.org/

Physicians for a National Health Program
http://www.pnhp.org/

Planned Parenthood Federation of America
http://www.plannedparenthood.org/

Public Health Foundation
http://www.phf.org/

Radiological Society of North America
http://www.rsna.org/

RAND Health
http://www.rand.org/organization/health

Rape Abuse & Incest National Network
http://www.rainn.org/

Safe Works AIDS Project
http://safeworks.org/

Scleroderma Foundation
http://www.scleroderma.com/

Sidran Foundation
http://www.sidran.org

Sjogren's Syndrome Foundation
http://www.sjogrens.com/

Society for Clinical Trials
http://www.sctweb.org/

Society for Endocrinology
http://www.endocrinology.org/

Society for Investigative Dermatology
http://www.sidnet.org/index.htm

Society for Neuroscience
http://www.sfn.org/

Society of Cardiovascular and Interventional Radiology
http://www.scvir.org/

Society of Critical Care Medicine
http://www.sccm.org/

Society of Environmental Toxicology and Chemistry
http://www.setac.org/

Southern Nursing Research Society
http://www.snrs.org/

Special Olympics International
http://www.specialolympics.org/

The Spina Bifida Association of America
http://www.sbaa.org/

Thyroid Foundation of Canada
http://home.ican.net/~thyroid/Canada.html

Tourette Syndrome Association, Inc.
http://tsa.mgh.harvard.edu/

The Transplantation Society
http://www.unos.org/frame_Default.asp

UNICEF
http://www.unicef.org/

United Cerebral Palsy Association
http://www.ucpa.org/

United Network for Organ Sharing
http://www.unos.org/

U.S. Department of Health and Human Services
http://www.os.dhhs.gov/

U.S. Environmental Protection Agency
http://www.epa.gov/

U.S. National Library of Medicine
http://www.nlm.nih.gov/

U.S. Nuclear Regulatory Commission
http://www.nrc.gov/

U.S. Public Health Service
http://phs.os.dhhs.gov/phs/phs.html

The Vascular Disease Foundation
http://www.vdf.org/

Veterans Health Administration
http://www.va.gov/health/index.htm

WHO Division of Emergency and Humanitarian Action
http://www.who.int/eha/

Women for Sobriety Inc.
http://www.womenforsobriety.org/

The World Association for Disaster and Emergency Medicine
http://www.pitt.edu/HOME/GHNet/wadem/wadem.html

World Federation of Hemophilia
http://www.wfh.org/

World Federation of Mental Health
http://www.wfmh.com/

World Health Organization
http://www.who.int/

World Organization of Family Doctors
http://www.wonca.org/

Xeroderma Pigmentosum Society, Inc.
http://www.xps.org/

OSTEOPATHY

Access AOA

http://www.am-osteo-assn.org/
Resources and information for the general public and professionals about osteopathy, from the American Osteopathic Association.

American Academy of Osteopathy

http://www.aao.medguide.net/
Offers courses, publications (e.g., online journal, newsletter, yearbooks and reprints of original works), information about the Academy and the profession.

American Association of Colleges of Osteopathic Medicine

http://www.aacom.org/
Informative and professional site.

Cranial Osteopathy Page

http://vzone.virgin.net/big.phil/index1.htm
Site promotes cranial osteopathy, which it explains as "a very gentle, yet extremely powerful, system of osteopathic medicine which uses the patient's 'Cranial Rhythm'. . . for evaluation and treatment."

The D.O. Difference

http://www.gvh-svh.org/dodiffer.html
Good description of the principles of osteopathic medicine.

Gregory's Osteopathic Links

http://www.osteopathic.com/gregory/
Comprehensive list of Internet resources. Categories include: Important Starting Points for Pre-Med Students, Recent Osteopathic Developments, Medical Schools, Hospitals and Medical Centers, Physicians on the Internet, Medical Associations, Online Publications, Medical Student Home Pages, and Miscellaneous Links.

How I Found Osteopathic Medicine

http://www.geocities.com/HotSprings/Villa/2617/osteo.htm

Personal statement from a doctor of osteopathic medicine.

Osteopathic Medical Web Ring

http://www.osteopathicmedicine.org/

Information on how to become a part of the Osteopathic Web Ring, which boasts over 110 members.

Osteopathic Medicine International WWW Resource Website

http://www.rscom.com/osteo/

This site offers a very good definition of osteopathy, as "a system of health care. . . based on the theory that the body is capable of making its own remedies against disease and other toxic conditions." Site provides information on the founder of osteopathy, Andrew Taylor Still, links to osteopathy sites around the world, an Internet journal, and more.

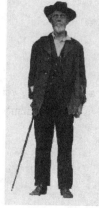

Osteopathic.Com

http://www.osteopathic.com/

Learn about osteopathic medicine and locate a practitioner in your area. If you are a student, chat with colleagues or receive advice from those more experienced. Physicians may access career resources, or they may promote their own services.

Still Alive

http://www.rscom.com/osteo/journal/intro.htm

Journal about the science and art of osteopathic manipulative medicine and naturopathic medicine.

Still Alive. http:// www.rscom.com/osteo/ journal/intro.htm

What is a D.O.?

http://dale.hsc.unt.edu:80/~brent/whatisado.html

Explains what a Osteopathic Physician (D.O.) is, and how one differs from a Allopathic Physician (M.D.)

PAIN & PAIN MANAGEMENT

Alternative Treatments

Magnet Therapy

http://www.ivanhoe.com/docs/backissues/magnettherapy.html

Information on how magnets and magnetic fields help to treat pain.

Cancer Pain

Cancer Pain

http://www.medsch.wisc.edu/WHOcancerpain/

Publication from the World Health Organization to help support international efforts to alleviate needless suffering from cancer pain.

Pain Management for the Cancer Patient

http://pharmacy.drake.edu/faculty/A_Blash/
PHA191-327/thcpati/cancer_pain/UNTITLED/
home.htm

Briefly deescribes pharmacologic methods (narcotic and non-narcotic) and alternative therapies (e.g., radiation and surgery, neurosurgery, neurostimulation and behavioral) for the treatment of cancer pain.

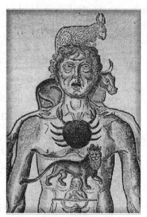

Pain Management for the Cancer Patient. *http://pharm acy.drake.edu/faculty/A_Blash /PHA191-327/thcpati/cancer_ pain/UNTITLED/home.htm*

Talaria: The Hypermedia Assistant for Cancer Pain Management

http://www.stat.washington.edu/TALARIA/TALARIA.html

Site for health care providers covering pain management in cancer patients. It provides tools, such as a calculator for converting drug dosages and a multimedia instructional video, a library of technical references, and links to web resources.

Chronic Pain

American Chronic Pain Association

http://www.theacpa.org/

Provides support and information for people with chronic pain.

Chronic Pain: Hope through Research

http://www.nih.gov/health/chip/ninds/cronpain/

This online booklet published by the National Institutes of Health offers great information about chronic pain, methods of management, research and where to go for help.

InfoMIN Chronic Pain

http://www2.rpa.net/~lrandall/

Frequently updated information on chronic pain and links to other resources, including the Merck Manual online.

North American Chronic Pain Association of Canada

http://www3.sympatico.ca/nacpac/

Self-help organization for people with chronic pain. On the site, find a list of Canadian support groups and links to pain information.

Talkway Chronic Pain Support Group

http://decaf.talkway.com/cgi-bin/cgi?request=enter&group=alt.support.
chronic-pain

News and discussion group for chronic pain. Discover suggestions and opinions from other pain sufferers.

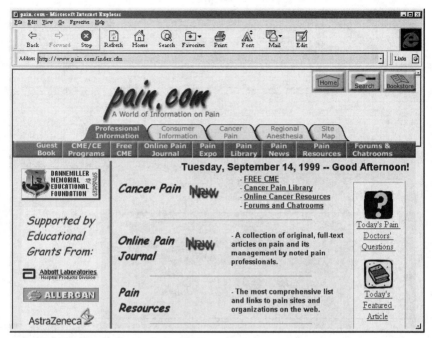

pain.com *http://www.pain.com/index.cfm*

General Pain

Doctor's Guide to Pain Management Information & Resources
http://www.Pslgroup.com/PAINMGT.htm

This site offers medical news and alerts, discussion groups, new developments, pain management information and many helpful related websites.

Pain Management Online
http://www.painmngt.com/

Information on a variety of pain topics and links to various sites.

Pain Resources for Patients and Their Families
http://weber.u.washington.edu/~crc/CRCpage/patients.html

Extensive resource. Features hundreds of links to a variety of pain and health resources for both health care providers and pain sufferers.

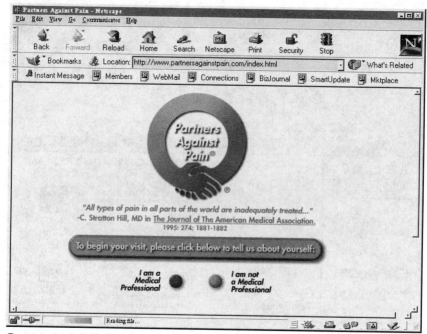

Partners Against Pain. *http://www.partnersagainstpain.com/index.html*

Pain.com

http://www.pain.com/index.cfm

Helpful site for both pain sufferers and doctors, hosted by the Dannemiller Foundation and sponsored by several pharmaceutical companies. It features daily news and articles, an online pain journal, a section devoted to cancer pain, an "ask the doctor" forum, and a list of other pain resources on the Web. The site also helps people around the country find local pain clinics. Includes expert interviews on cancer pain, headache pain, back pain and interventional pain therapies. For professionals, the site offers free continuing medical education courses, a virtual library and professional links.

Partners Against Pain

http://www.partnersagainstpain.com/index.html

This site provides information and advice about caring for people in pain. It is divided into resources for both medical professionals and non-professionals, and includes news, books, pain control guides, support groups, and suggestions for controlling side-effects. Medical professionals can obtain continuing education credits, patient education materials, and information on prescribing medications.

Headaches & Migraines

American Council for Headache Education (ACHE)
http://www.achenet.org/index.html

A nonprofit physician-patient partnership whose goal is to advance headache prevention and treatment. Site offers information, helps visitors find a headache doctor, provides discussion forums and a migraine disability assessment survey.

Glaxol Wellcome's Migraine Resource Center
http://www.migrainehelp.com/

Site provides a lot of information about migraines, including diagnosis, suggestions on how to cope, news, support and related links. Also offers information on the pharmaceutical company's migraine drug Imitrex, and a free trial offer.

Migraine Association of Canada
http://www.migraine.ca/

Information about the association and its programs. Features a section just for kids, and offers a migraine-friendly cookbook.

Migraine FAQs
http://www.meldrum.demon.co.uk/migraine/

Frequently asked questions concerning migraines and their prevention and treatment.

The Migraine Information Site
http://www.niagara.com/migraine/

Links and information for migraine sufferers.

Migraine: The Non-Pharmaceutical Medical Magazine
http://www.etonhall.com/mig1.htm

Explains migraines and advocates treatment by electrostimulation.

Ronda's Migraine Page.com
http://www.migrainepage.com

Site has many helpful features, including an online journal for migraine sufferers to post their personal experiences, a log-in discussion forum, and links to critiqued resources for support and medication information.

Organizations

American Pain Foundation
http://www.painfoundation.org/
   Provides information, education and advocacy for people suffering from pain who are not getting adequate pain relief.

American Pain Society
http://www.ampainsoc.org/
   Educational and scientific organization dedicated to helping people in pain. Members include health care workers who research and treat pain, and advocate for patients in pain.

American Society for Pain Relief, Research and Education
http://www.cris.com/~jgupta/ASPRRE.htm
   Nonprofit society of both physicians and non-physicians that seeks to improve the status of pain management throughout the world. Site lists steps to improve pain management, and provides useful links.

National Foundation for the Treatment of Pain
http://www.paincare.org/
   This nonprofit organization provides support for patients who are suffering from intractable pain, their families, friends and the physicians who treat them.Site presents perspectives on pain management, pain treatment advocacy news, lots of information on migraines, a helpline, and a number of medical, legal, psychiatric and research links.

Pain Study

The Institute for the Study and Treatment of Pain
http://www.istop.org/
   A nonprofit organization dedicated to the study and treatment of soft-tissue pain, especially using intramuscular stimulation.

International Association for the Study of Pain

http://www.halcyon.com/iasp/

International organization of medical professionals dedicated to pain research and improving patient care. Site offers information about IASP, continuing education opportunities, public information and pain resources.

Palliative Care

Palliative Care for Children

http://www.wwdc.com/death/iwg/children.html

International Work Group's statement on the treatment of terminally ill children and the needs of a dying child.

University of Ottowa Institute of Palliative Care

http://www.ochin.on.ca/pallcare/

University-based institute for research, education and administration of palliative care. Palliative care focuses on the needs of the patient and the family when cure for a life-threatening illness, such as cancer or AIDS, is no longer available. This site provides information for the terminally ill and their caregivers to help make the patient's final days more comfortable, and to help patients and their families move toward this reality with comfort, reassurance and strength.

Surgical Pain

Pain Control After Surgery: A Patient's Guide

http://pain.roxane.com/library/AHCPR/apmp1.html

Online brochure offers information on how to help control pain after surgery.

Postoperative Pain Management

http://www.usyd.edu.au/su/anaes/VAT/Pain.html

Comments and information on postoperative pain, prepared by the Virtual Anaesthesia Textbook. Note: "Unrelieved pain after surgery is often unhealthy; fortunately, it is preventable or controllable in an overwhelming majority of cases. Pain control may have a further benefit of improving clinical outcome by reducing the incidence of postoperative complications."

PATHOLOGY

Blood/Hematology

Hematopathology Index

http://www-medlib.med.utah.edu/WebPath/HEMEHTML/HEMEIDX.html

Seventy-five images of blood samples showing standard peripheral blood and marrow findings, RBC and bone marrow disorders, leukemias,lymph nodes and Non-Hodgkin's lymphomas, myeloma, Hodgkin's and splenic issues.

Histology Lesson: Blood

http://www.mc.vanderbilt.edu/histo/blood/

Find out everything you ever wanted to know about blood, including the difference between and function of erythrocytes, platelets, and leukocytes.

Cancer/Oncology

Cancer Cytopathology Online

http://www.canceronline.wiley.com/cchome.html

This full-text, web version of *CANCER CYTOPATHOLOGY*, a section of the journal *CANCER*, offers access to current issues. Articles focus on: analytic cytopathology, fine-needle aspiration, gynecologic and nongynecologic cytopathology, immunocytochemistry and molecular diagnostics.

Pathology Simplified

http://www.erinet.com/fnadoc/path.htm

Good information for patients about lung cancer, breast cancer, and Pap smears. Includes photo archives and hotlinks.

Tumor Board

http://www.tumorboard.com/

This site calls itself the world's largest source of copyright-free digital pathology images. Browse through the image library, comment on a case or contribute your own image to the database.

Cardiovascular

Cardiovascular Index

http://www.dml.georgetown.edu/webpath/CVHTML/CVIDX.html

Over 100 images of the heart, healthy and diseased.

Society for Cardiovascular Pathology

http://pathology.jhu.edu/scvp/

Find out about membership, meetings, publications, educational materials, and other cardiovascular-related sites.

HIV/AIDS

AIDS Pathology

http://www-medlib.med.utah.edu/WebPath/TUTORIAL/AIDS/AIDS.html

The textbook includes a general discussion of the pathophysiology of HIV infection, organ system pathology of AIDS, and descriptions of the opportunistic infections and neoplasms associated with AIDS, and a general discussion of issues, including safety and education, related to the AIDS epidemic.

Pathology and Treatment

http://www.thebody.com/encyclo/pathology_overview.html

Overview of discussion from the *Encyclopedia of AIDS*.

Kidneys/Nephrology

1999 Atlas of Renal Pathology
http://ajkd.wbsaunders.com/atlas/
From the National Kidney Foundation.

Renal Pathology Tutorial
http://www.gamewood.net/rnet/renalpath/tutorial.htm
Demonstrates normal kidney cellular structure, and some of the diseases that cause the nephrotic syndrome.

Liver/Hepatology

Atlas of Liver Pathology
http://www.vh.org/Providers/Textbooks/LiverPathology/Text/AtlasLiver Pathology.html
Index of a multimedia textbook on liver pathology by Frank A. Mitros, M.D., of the University of Iowa College of Medicine. Access text, tables and images.

Review of the Pathology of the Liver
http://www.meddean.luc.edu/lumen/MedEd/orfpath/pthcntnt.htm
Shows normal liver histology images, general pathology, and liver samples demonstrating cirrhosis, viral hepatitis, other viruses, infections, parasitic infestation, toxic and drug hepatitis. Accompanied with brief explanatory text.

Organizations

American Society of Clinical Pathologists
http://www.ascp.org/
Information on the organization's membership requirements, programs and publications. Members can search for a job.

American Society of Cytopathology

http://www.cytopathology.org/

Find out about membership, scientific meetings, the Society's position papers and training programs. Features a list of ASC-accredited laboratories, public education information and related websites.

College of American Pathologists

http://www.cap.org/

Site provides meeting and membership information, pathology information for students and others, news, online resources for professionals, educational material, public interest and advocacy efforts.

Links to Pathology Organizations

http://www.wramc.amedd.army.mil/departments/Pathology/org.htm

Links to general pathology organizations, anatomic/surgical pathology organizations, clinical pathology organizations, both national and international.

Pathology Resources

American Journal of Pathology

http://www.amjpathol.org/

Search for articles, select an issue from the archives, view the current month's table of contents, and subscribe.

Emory University Department of Pathology & Laboratory Medicine

http://www.cc.emory.edu/PATHOLOGY/

Details on Emory's pathology program and collaborative research efforts.

Hardin MD Pathology & Laboratory Medicine

http://www.lib.uiowa.edu/hardin/md/path.html

An extensive list of pathology-related sites, including many university pathology departments.

HistoWeb

http://www.kumc.edu/instruction/medicine/anatomy/histoweb/

A great learning tool for students and physicians. Covers cell structure, over a dozen different body systems and organs, histopathology and more.

Internet Resources for Pathology and Laboratory Medicine

http://www.pathology.med.umich.edu/pathresourceak/path_resources.html

Provides a listing of pathology departments that can be found on the web, listservers and databases, journals, commercial and regulatory links, positions available/wanted, as well as sub-specialty (e.g., neuropathology, gynecologic pathology, veterinary pathology, etc.) resources.

PathIT Pathology Online

http://www.pathit.com/

Includes images and text on anatomic, clinical, veterinary, forensic and quantitative pathology, as well as morphometrics (the measurement of forms or structures of organisms) and pathology informatics.

Pathology Sites and Resources

http://www.people.cornell.edu/pages/wef2/path2.html

Long list of pathology resources includes case studies, professional organizations, academic departments and more.

Pathology on the Web

http://www.anapath.necker.fr/APWEngl/APWEB/APweb

Internet resources, both general and specialized.

Pathology Services Inc. Newsletters

http://www.pathsrv.com/psi/newsltrs.html

Includes *Pathology Review* (Vols. 1-7) and *Oral Pathology Review* (1992-1997) newsletters.

Pathology to Go!

http://www.wramc.amedd.army.mil/departments/Pathology/links.htm

Walter Reed Army Medical Center Pathology links page to educational, organizational and hospital pathology websites.

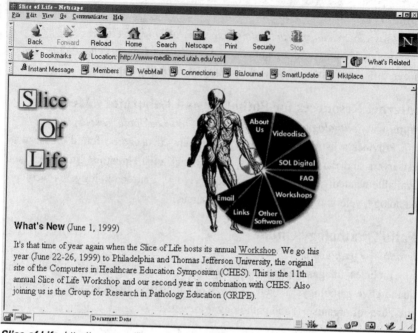

Slice of Life *http://www-medlib.med.utah.edu/sol/*

Pathwise

http://pathwise.com/

Pathology translation service for consumers, so that they can understand their diagnostic pathology reports.

Slice of Life

http://www-medlib.med.utah.edu/sol/

A nonprofit project based at the University of Utah in Salt Lake City which develops educational multimedia videodisks called Slice of Life. Each one contains more than 12,000 images of the body from the departments of pathology, radiology, neurology, and anatomy, and the Utah state medical examiner's office.

The Urbana Atlas of Pathology

http://www.med.uiuc.edu/PathAtlasf/titlepage.html

A six volume atlas that includes cardiovascular, endocrine, pulmonary, renal and general pathology. Extensive images in *.gif and *.jpg format.

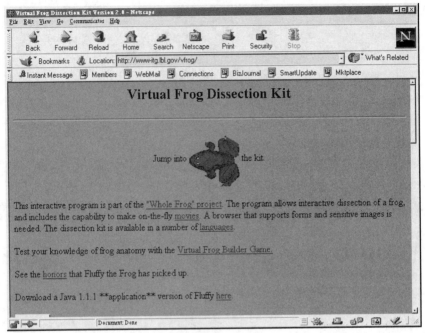

Virtual Frog Dissection. http://www-itg.lbl.gov/vfrog/

Virtual Frog Dissection Kit

http://www-itg.lbl.gov/vfrog/

Dissect a frog without getting your hands messy or smelling chloroform! This program allows you to dissect a frog on the computer, then test your knowledge of frog anatomy with the Virtual Frog Builder Game. For those who prefer live frogs, sample then order the "Sounds of North American Frogs" CD from the Smithsonian Library.

WebPath: The Internet Pathology Laboratory for Medical Education

http://www-medlib.med.utah.edu/WebPath/webpath.html

Electronic laboratory of over 1900 images with text and tutorials demonstrating gross and microscopic pathologic findings associated with human disease states.

PREGNANCY & CHILDBIRTH

Birth & Birthing Alternatives

Birthplan.com
http://birthplan.com/

Guides expectant couples in creating a birth plan; i.e., a list of preferences for their birth experience. View a sample plan.

Birth Psychology
http://www.birthpsychology.com/

Explore the mental and emotional dimensions of pregnancy and birth, as experienced by both mother and child. Information has been obtained from journal articles, personal stories and news.

Childbirth.org
http://www.childbirth.org/

"Birth is a natural process, not a medical procedure." This site helps women to understand all aspects and options of pregnancy and childbirth, and to select the best care. It has many educational and informative links and features, including first-hand birthing stories, and a customizable list of things new parents will need.

Homebirth
http://www.home-birth.org/

Information about home birth, and stories from women who chose to have their babies at home. Provides links to other websites related to birthing and midwifery.

Home Birth, Water Birth

http://home.i1.net/~abbie/birthpics.html

A personal story with pictures of a home water birth.

Multiple Birth Resources

http://expectingmultiples.com/

Program offering class instruction and a video series to educate and help parents achieve a healthy multiple birth.

Perineal Massage

http://www.childbirth.org/articles/massage.html

Tells how to perform perineal massage, a technique that can reduce the risk of tearing or the need for episiotomy.

The Safety of Home Birth: The Farm Midwives Study

http://www.thefarm.org/charities/mid.html

Text of a study which appeared in the *American Journal of Public Health* regarding the safety of home births. It was conducted by the Farm Midwives, a pro-vegetarian group in rural Tennessee. The study found that lay midwife-attended home births were as safe as conventional hospital births for non high-risk women.

Waterbirth Website

http://www.wenet.net/~karil/index.html

Learn about this method of birthing, which is supposed to be more gentle and empowering to both mother and baby. A video documentary and list of water-birthing centers are available to order.

Birth Defects

Neonatal Diseases and Abnormalities

http://www.mic.ki.se/Diseases/c16.html

This extensive collection of links assembled by the Karolinska Institute includes organizations, indexes and research facilities dealing with genetic, neonatal and developmental disorders, from jaundice and fetal alcohol syndrome, to cystic fibrosis and Down syndrome.

Preventing Birth Defects and Developmental Disabilities

http://www.cdc.gov/nceh/pubcatns/1994/cdc/brosures/surv-epi.htm#surv-epi

A brochure from the Centers for Disease Control and Prevention. It provides online surveillance and epidemiology data, as well as links to related sites.

Wide Smiles: Cleft Lip and Palate Resources

http://www.widesmiles.org/

Website for a group that offers support and information to parents of children born with cleft lips and palates.

Breastfeeding

Breastfeeding and Working

http://motherstuff.com/html/breastfd-work.html

Links to other sites offering information and support to women who continue to breastfeed when they go back to work.

Breastfeeding.com

http://www.breastfeeding.com/

Provides information, support, humor, news, advocacy, and supplies to help women with breastfeeding. Includes video clips that illustrate proper technique, and a question-and-answer section.

FAQ about Breastfeeding

http://www.lalecheleague.org/FAQ/FAQMain.html

Quick answers to the most frequently asked questions about La Leche League, breastfeeding, pumping and weaning.

La Leche League

http://www.lalecheleague.org/

This award-winning website for the famous breastfeeding advocacy group provides information about the organization and its meetings, helps visitors find local groups and lactation consultants, and offers catalogues and books.

Lactation Expert
http://www.parentsplace.com/expert/lactation

Having trouble breastfeeding, or just have questions? Get expert advice from a lactation consultant.

The Nursing Corner
http://ww.snugglebaby.com/nursing_corner.html

Although most people think breastfeeding should come easily, it sometimes doesn't. This site provides stories that show that even if things don't start off exactly as planned, if you have the right support and information you can usually "work things out" and go on to have a beautiful and rewarding nursing relationship.

Cesarean Section

Cesarean Childbirth
http://mentalhelp.net/factsfam/cbirth.htm

General information on cesarean sections in frequently asked question (FAQ) format.

Cesarean Section Homepage
http://www.childbirth.org/section/section.html

This site provides a long list of informative articles and web links about C-sections and pregnancy.

CSection.Com
http://www.csection.com

This website gives the rate of cesarean sections (C-sections) performed at specific hospitals. It calculates the rate for each hospital in a state as a percentage of all inpatient births reported to the state, adjusting for a number of known risk factors.

International Cesarean Awareness Network Homepage
http://www.childbirth.org/section/ICAN.html

Information sheets on C-sections, how to prevent unnecessary ones, and vaginal birth after C-section.

Understanding Cesarean Birth

http://www.noah.cuny.edu/pregnancy/march_of_dimes/birth/csection.html

Site addresses basic questions about C-sections, including indications for and benefits, risks and effects of this procedure.

Midwifery

See also: Nursing - Nurse-Midwifery.

American College of Nurse-Midwives

http://www.acnm.org/

The ACNM promotes nurse-midwifery through research, education, practice and advocacy. Visit this website to get information about becoming a nurse-midwife; to learn more about what they do; to find a nurse-midwife if you are expecting; or to help with lobbying/legislative efforts.

Marilyn's Midwifery Page

http://www.midwifery2000.com/

Information about midwifery, and links to other related websites.

Midwifery Today

http://www.midwiferytoday.com/

Access to this quarterly magazine with information on midwife services.

Miscarriages

For Those Who Have Had Miscarriages

http://www.ivf.com/misc.html

This guide from IVF.Com is for parents who have recently experienced the death of a child through miscarriage, stillbirth or other perinatal loss. It contains compassionate facts and words of comfort.

Frequently Asked Questions about Miscarriage

http://brook006.mc.duke.edu/mc/miscarriage.html

Questions and information are grouped into the following general areas: words of support, causes and technical information, bleeding during pregnancy, molar pregnancy, how long to wait before trying again, and other resources.

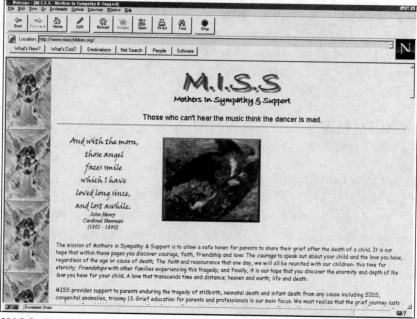

M.I.S.S.: Mothers in Sympathy and Support. http://www.misschildren.org/

Hygeia

http://www.connix.com/~hygeia/

Register at this site to communicate with others about the loss of a pregnancy or child.

Infertility & Miscarriage Research Summaries

http://www.chem-tox.com/infertility/

Provides summaries and references to some important research articles discussing miscarriage and infertility, particularly as relates to environmental causes.

M.I.S.S.: Mothers in Sympathy and Support

http://www.misschildren.org/

A place for parents to share their grief after the death of a child.

SANDS (Vic)

http://www.sandsvic.org.au/

A support group for parents who have experienced miscarriage, stillbirth, or neonatal death. Includes resource and support links, a dedication wall, and a chat room, as well as a section especially for fathers.

Neonatology

See also: Children's Health/Pediatrics - Neonatology.

Fetal.Com

http://www.fetal.com/

Information for physicians and parents regarding prenatal diagnosis, amniocentesis, ultrasound, maternal-serum screening and other diagnostic tests used in the evaluation of an unborn child.

The Journal of Neonatal Nursing

http://www.bizjet.com/jnn/default.html

Internet edition includes full text of articles for subscribers, or summaries for visitors.

Neonatology on the Web

http://www.neonatology.org/

A long list of resources with brief descriptions of each site's contents. Includes career information, clinical information, teaching files and more. Geared to professionals.

Neonatology Web Pages

http://www.neonatology.org/neo.links.web.html

Links to homepages of many academic and hospital neonatology programs.

NICU Resident's Guidebook

http://www.med.jhu.edu/peds/neonatology/neo/ResidentGuidebook/
ResidentGuidebook.htm

From Johns Hopkins University; updated yearly.

Patient Information on Neonatology

http://www.vh.org/Patients/IHB/Peds/Neonatal/Neonatal.html

Includes a list of recommended sites for parents of premature babies, or parents of babies with other problems.

Premature & Newborn

http://www.pediatrics.org/cgi/collection/premature_and_newborn

Citations, abstracts and full text for selected articles appearing in the journal *PEDIATRICS*.

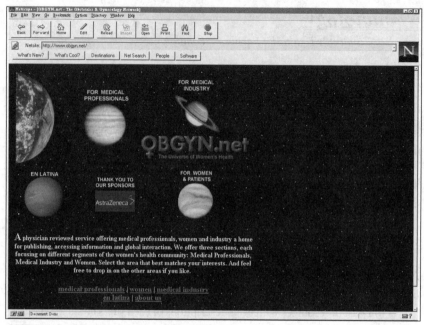

OBGYN.net. *http://www.obgyn.net/*

Vysis

http://www.vysis.com/hm_crc_hm.asp

Offers consumer information on prenatal testing.

Obstetrics & Gynecology

The American College of Obstetricians and Gynecologists

http://www.acog.com/

Information for the public includes patient education, a doctor search, legislative news, and more. Information for health professionals includes course listings, meeting and membership facts, technical help, and access to the *Journal of Ob-Gyn.*

Dr. Pranikoff's Ob/Gyn Web Library

http://www.uc.edu/~pranikjd/

Includes the obstetrics web library and the gynecologic web library, with many links grouped by topic.

Gynaecology, Obstetrics and Paediatrics

http://www.sciencekomm.at/journals/medicine/gyna.html

Gynecology and obstetric medical journal links.

Links of Interest to Obstetrics & Gynecology

http://www.museum.state.il.us/isas/oblink.html

Includes academic departments, e-mail lists, databases, journals and more.

MedWebPlus: Obstetrics

http://www.medwebplus.com/subject/Obstetrics.html

Links to obstetrics sites on the web. Various subsets include: academic departments, manuals, practice guidelines, societies and more.

OB/Gyn Net

http://www.obgyn.net/

This is "a physician reviewed service." Information is divided into three sections: for medical professionals, women and patients, and the medical industry. Site available in Spanish and Portuguese.

Postpartum Depression

Depression After Delivery (DAD)

http://www.behavenet.com/dadinc/

Information about postpartum depression (PPD), including who is affected, what causes it, treatment methods, and how to distinguish between "baby blues" and PPD, which is more serious.

The Marce' Society

http://www.cam.net.uk/home/marce.uk/

International society for psychological disorders after childbirth based in London. Society aims to raise awareness of these disorders, and encourage discussion and research. Site provides information, a newsletter and postpartum depression assistance through links to support organizations.

Postpartum Depression

http://www.chss.iup.edu/postpartum/

Offering social support, information and research.

Postpartum Depression Support and Education
http://infotrail.com/dad/dad.html

Homepage for the Cleveland, Ohio chapter of Depression After Delivery (DAD). Group offers support and education to women experiencing postpartum depression.

Postpartum Education for Parents (PEP)
http://www.sbpep.org/

PEP was founded in 1977 by a group of mothers to offer support to each other after the births of their children. This nonprofit organization is staffed by trained parent volunteers, and it offers information and support for postpartum distress, as well as for parenting skills and raising "spirited" (i.e., difficult) children. Site contains many links to other posppartum support sites, as well as to helpful general parenting sites.

Westcoast Motherhood Adjustment Services
http://www.geocities.com/Heartland/1805/

Based in Vancouver, British Columbia, this nonprofit organization's website provides information about "baby blues," postpartum depression, postpartum anxiety, postpartum obsessive compulsive disorder, and postpartum psychosis.

Pregnancy

BabyTime
http://www.clicked.com/babytime/

"Everything you need... to help you have a well-informed pregnancy." Information, support and product links.

Fitness for Two
http://www.noah.cuny.edu/pregnancy/
march_of_dimes/pre_preg.plan/
fit42is.html

This public health information sheet discusses the benefits of exercise during pregnancy, as well as safety issues, sports, and postpartum exercising.

The Miracle of Life

http://www.dibbs.net/~tragates/
Tracey.htm
   A graphic journey from egg to infant, with descriptive text.

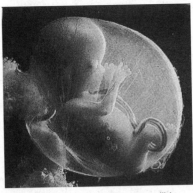

MotherStuff

http://www.motherstuff.com/
   Links and brief descriptions to Internet resources on pregnancy as well as birthing, parenting, mothering, miscarriage, premature babies, breastfeeding and midwifery. Calls itself "a meta-index of mother-knowledge."

The Miracle of Life. http://www.dibbs. net/~tragates/Tracey.htm

Plus-Size Pregnancy Website

http://www.vireday.com/plus/
   Discusses the special concerns of large women who are preparing for pregnancy, who are pregnant, or who have recently given birth. Links to helpful sites.

A Positive Pregnancy

http://members.aol.com/NancyRoman/Preg2.html
   Read many different women's pregancy stories.

Pregnancy

http://www.parentsplace.com/pregnancy
   Site offers a pregnancy calendar, due date calculator, baby name finder, newsletter and information on nutrition, tests, complications, loss and breastfeeding.

Pregnancy and Fitness

http://lifematters.com/medicalinfo.html
   Guidelines for exercise during pregnancy.

Pregnancy and Labor Corner

http://www.parenthoodweb.com/parent_cfmfiles/pregnancy_labor.cfm
   Extensive resource includes information on natural labor techniques, midwives, childbirth classes, comfort while pregnant, medications and hundreds of other issues. Polls, discussion groups and an ovulation calculator are also offered.

Pregnancy Calculator

http://www.magma.ca/~rgiffen/PregnancyCalculator.html

Calculate due date or current gestational age.

The Pregnancy Institute

http://www.preginst.com/

Site for this nonprofit organization that studies normal pregnancies.

Pregnancy Links

http://www.childbirth.org/articles/preglinks.html

Main topics include pregnancy basics, complications, emotions, exercise, frequently asked questions, labor, lifestyle, signs, symptoms, testing, and pregnancy week-by-week.

Pregnancy Signs

http://www.ausoft.com/pregnancy/

Signs and symptoms of pregnancy, time of appearance, and other possible reasons they might appear.

Storknet

http://www.storknet.org/

Online pregnancy community that includes chat room, message boards, pregnancy and parenting journals, and more.

Things Which Might Complicate Pregnancy

http://www.motherstuff.com/html/pregnant-things.htm

E.g., asthma, diabetes, lupus, anemia and other conditions.

Premature Birth

For Parents of Preemies

http://www2.medsch.wisc.edu/childrenshosp/parents_of_preemies/

Answers to commonly asked questions about premature infants.

Parents of Premature Babies: Preemie-L

http://www.preemie-l.org/

Lots of resources. Features links to and information on the popular and active Preemie-L Mailing list and Preemie-L Discussion Forum.

The Preemie Channel

http://www.flash.net/~cyberkid/preemiechannel/index.html

A collection of links especially for parents of premature infants.

Preemie Resource Page

http://members.aol.com/MarAim/preemie.htm

Contains an exhaustive list of links and preemie resources, as well as a short list for those in search of basic information.

Tommy's CyberNursery Preemie Web

http://www.flash.net/~cyberkid/

Site provides a library, picture gallery and personal story of one pre-term infant's birth and growth, as well as a number of premature baby resources that are divided into the following topics: medical, support groups, conditions, articles, chat rooms, off-line resources and more.

Ultrasound, Amniocentesis & Other Prenatal Tests

See also: Medical Imaging/Telemedicine.

3D Ultrasound in Obstetrics

http://myweb.worldnet.net/~henrib/3D_ultra.html

Information about a relatively new ultrasound technique that shows the image in three dimensions instead of just two. This technology is starting to be used in obstetrics to obtain a more precise evaluation of fetal malformations. View 3-D images of a smiling and a yawning fetus. Provides links to other ultrasound sites.

Amniocentesis

http://www.aomc.org/amnio.html

Questions and answers on this prenatal test. Includes benefits and risks.

Medical Ultrasound Imaging WWW Directory

http://home.att.net/~don.christopher/ultrasound.htm

A listing of links and e-mail addresses for people, companies and organizations involved in ultrasound imaging.

Obstetric Ultrasound: A Comprehensive Guide

http://www.ob-ultrasound.net/

Comprehensive and well-written information about what ultrasound is, how it works, and why it is used during pregnancy. This site is authored by Dr. Joe Woo, and is referenced by all of the other ultrasound sites.

Prenatal Tests

http://babyzone.com/prenatal.htm

Describes some of the common and less common prenatal tests, including when and why they are taken, risk factors, method and more.

Ultranet

http://users.quake.net/xdcrlab/Ultrasound.html

Hotlinks to other sites devoted to ultrasound imaging.

Ultrasound and Other Prenatal Diagnostic Tests

http://www.stanford.edu/~holbrook/

Includes information on ultrasound, amniocentesis, percutaneus umbilical blood sampling, chorionic villus sampling, alphagetoprotein screening, cystic fbrosis screening and more.

Ultrasound: What is it?

http://www.bk.psu.edu/faculty/cooper/ultrasnd.html

Basic information from Duke University describing the technology behind ultrasound imaging.

PUBLIC HEALTH

Analysis & Research

International Clearinghouse of Health System Reform Initiatives

http://www.insp.mx/ichsri/

Proposes to study and compare health care reform processes internationally, and to identify the circumstances under which reform succeeds or fails in order to develop methodologies to assess their impact. The site serves to classify, document and dessiminate health policy and reform initiatives and to promote discussion of relevant issues.

Medicine/Public Health Initiative

http://www.sph.uth.tmc.edu/mph/

Seeks to join the fields of public health and medicine in a way that serves both each individual's and the general population's health, and to develop "an agenda of action that cooperatively engages public health and medicine in reshaping health education, research and practice."

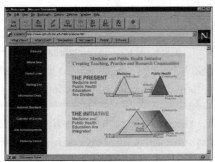

Graphical representation of the mission of the: **Medicine and Public Health Initiative.**
http://www.sph.uth.tmc.edu/mph/

National Public Health Information Coalition

http://nphic.org/

Comprised of senior directors of public health programs, this national organization seeks to promote communication, and to share information and techniques that will advance public health. Site offers information on the Coalition and its activities, presents grant guidelines, a newsletter and information on subscribing to its journal.

Public Health Foundation

http://www.phf.org/

Independent, nonprofit association devoted to initiating and identifying valuable public health research efforts, providing technical assistance and training, and facilitating communication of ideas amongst public health professionals and students from multiple sources. Site offers links to public health databases and related sites, academic links, publications, and a description of programs.

General Resources

BioSites: Public Health Sites

http://www.library.ucsf.edu/biosites/bin/showByTopic.pl?PublicHealth

List of public health resources from BioSites.

HealthWeb: Public Health Page

http://www.lib.umich.edu/hw/public.health.html

Lists resources in biostatistics, environmental health, health administration, health policy, general public health resources, and much more. Links include helpful descriptions of web content.

Links of Interest in Public Health

http://www.il-st-acad-sci.org/health/phlinks.html

Numerous societies and associations, a long list of public health journals, and other links.

The Medical and Public Health Law Site
http://plague.law.umkc.edu/
Public health law cases, articles and course materials.

National Health Information Center
http://nhic-nt.health.org/
Health information referral services. Includes resources database of over 1,100 organizations and government offices, containing contact information, abstracts and other information. Also includes a number of referral documents and a search engine.

Public Health
http://www.hslib.washington.edu/public_health/index.html
Public health databases and other links from the University of Washington.

Public Health Professionals Links
http://hsl.mcmaster.ca/tomflem/pubhlth.html
Collection of links to sites deemed of interest to public health professionals.

Public Health Software, Websites and and Internet Resources in the Public Domain
http://www.jhsph.edu/do/software/
Lots of information and links.

State of New York Department of Health
http://www.health.state.ny.us/
Site contains information for consumers, providers and researchers. Included are a directory of services, how to get New York State vital records information; general health information sheets, health care data for researchers, and a public health forum.

"Virtual" Public Health Center
http://www-sci.lib.uci.edu/~martindale/PHealth.html
Multimedia information resource center.

Global Health Resources & Aid

CARE
http://www.care.org/
International development and relief organization.

Flying Samaritans
http://www.geocities.com/Heartland/Plains/1134/
Volunteer organization that operates free medical clinics in Baja, Mexico. Doctors, dentists, translators, pilots and support personnel travel to the clinics and work as invited teachers. The site provides information about the group, its chapters and the clinics they visit.

Global Health: Key Resources
http://www.pitt.edu/HOME/GHNet/GHKR.html
Collection of resources in areas that relate to public health world-wide.

Interplast
http://www.interplast.org/
Interplast is an affiliation of volunteer surgeons, pediatricians, anesthesiologists, nurses and support personnel who work with developing nations to support and develop a free reconstructive surgery programs for children and adults with birth defects, burns, and other crippling deformities. The organization performs over 1500 free surgeries annually. Information about the organization and its scheduled trips may be found at this site.

MAP International Internet Services
http://map.org/
Website for this nonprofit Christian relief and development organization that helps provide health services to the world's impoverished people.

PanAmerican Health Organization
http://www.paho.org/
This is a public health agency that works to improve health and living standards of the countries of the Americas. There are a number of programs and regional centers. Some of the projects include promoting sanitary engineering, nutrition, perinatology, and the prevention of infectious and foodborne diseases.

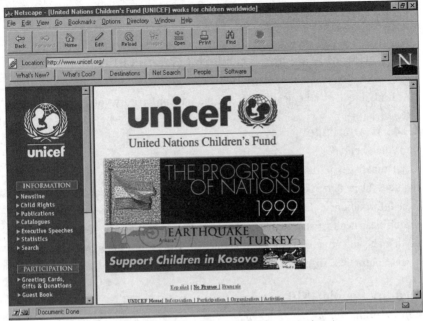

UNICEF: The United Nation's Children's Fund. *http://www.unicef.org/*

Project HOPE
http://www.projhope.org/

"HOPE" stands for Health Opportunities for People Everywhere, and this organization provides health care education and professional assistance to communities in need around the world.

UNICEF
http://www.unicef.org/

Describes the mission and many programs of the United Nations Children's Fund, many of which have health aims.

U.N.'s World Food Programme
http://www.wfp.org/index.html

The mission of this United Nations agency is to provide food to those in need. You can find a description of the WF programs along with hunger statistics.

Government Agencies

Association of State and Territorial Health Officials
http://www.astho.org/about.html

Link directly to the health office of the state or territory you are interested in.

CDC Home Page
http://www.cdc.gov/

Homepage of the Centers for Disease Control and Prevention. The CDC includes 11 centers, institutes and offices, and they can all be accessed from this site. Information includes: help about ill children abroad, diseases, injuries and disabilities, health risks, demographic information, traveler's health, prevention guidelines, and strategies. In addition, this site offers information about vaccines, disease outbreaks, disease data and statistics.

Healthy People 2010
http://www.health.gov/healthypeople/

National initiative to identify and address threats to public health. More eloquently stated: "It is a road map to better health for all that can be used by many different people, states and communities, professional organizations, groups whose concern is a particular threat to health, or a particular population group." Some focus areas include: physical activity and fitness, nutrition, tobacco use, environmental health, food safety, injury/violence prevention and occupational safety.

National Institutes of Health
http://www.nih.gov/

This site offers an overview of the NIH, news and events, and information about the Institutes' health resources including CancerNet, AIDS information and Clinical Alerts. Also provides grant and contract information, scientific resources and links to the various (24) separate institutes, centers and divisions that make up the NIH. It is one of the eight health agencies that comprise the federal government's Public Health Service.

Office of Public Health and Science

http://www.surgeongeneral.gov/ophs/

Information on disease prevention, HIV/AIDS policy, international refugee health watch, minority and women's health issues, the Surgeon General, and physical fitness and health.

United States Public Health Service

http://phs.os.dhhs.gov/phs/phs.html

Use this page to access the U.S. Surgeon General, the public health service agencies (National Institutes of Health, Centers for Disease Control and Prevention, Food and Drug Administration, Administration on Aging, and others), various public health programs, and the Public Health Support Center.

U.S. Department of Health and Human Services

http://www.os.dhhs.gov/

This site describes the Department of Health and Human Services' (DHHS) activities. It supplies links to research, policy and administration divisions, and offers consumers information on a large number of physical and mental health topics, ranging from adolescent to women's health issues.

Home & Occupational Safety

See also: Children's Health/Pediatrics - Child Safety.

Botulism

http://www.seanet.com/~tzhre/botul.htm

Links to sites that discuss botulism and related concerns.

Fire Safety Tips

http://www.fire.ca.gov/cdf_fireprevention.html

Suggestions from the California Department of Forestry and Fire Protection on making your home safe from fire.

Home Safety

http://www.parentzone.com/parents/homesafty/index.htm

Good tips on how to baby-proof the entire house.

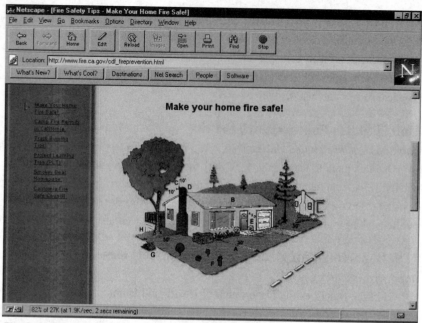

Fire Safety Tips. *http://www.fire.ca.gov/cdf_fireprevention.html*

Medicinal and Poisonous Plants Databases

http://www.wam.umd.edu/~mct/Plants/index.html

Lots of resources.

Occupational Safety & Health

http://www.mic.ki.se/Safety.html

Long list of international sites related to advancing safety and health in the workplace.

Poison Control Answer Book

http://wellness.ucdavis.edu/safety_info/poison_prevention/poison_book/index.html

You can download a PDF file of the Answer Book, look through poison prevention tips, or read about first aid in case of exposure to poisons, allergic reactions and more.

Safety Articles

http://www.kidsource.com/kidsource/pages/k12.safety.poison.html

For parents and others, articles that discuss how they can protect the safety of their K-12 graders.

Safety Related Internet Resources

http://www.christie.ab.ca/safelist/

Includes e-mail addresses, FTP, IRC and gopher sites, electronic publications, mail lists and newsgroups, and a long list of links to websites, alphabetized.

U.S. Department of Labor/Occupational Safety and Health Administration

http://www.osha.gov/safelinks.html

OSHA's list of safety and health Internet sites.

Minority Health Issues

Asthma: A Concern for Minority Populations

http://www.niaid.nih.gov/factsheets/minorasthma.htm

Studies show that inner-city children are experiencing higher rates of asthma than ever before.

Black Health Net

http://www.blackhealthnet.com/

Online health information for African-Americans includes articles and resources on general health, women's health, alternative medicine and fitness; online questions and answers, a discussion forum, a doctor search, history of African-American medicine, and related links.

CancerNet: Cancer Information for Different Ethnic Groups

http://cancernet.nci.nih.gov/ethnic/ethnic_pat.htm

Concentrates on the special health concerns of the following populations: African-American, Alaskan Native, Asian, Hispanic, Native American, Native Hawaiian and Pacific Islander.

Diversity Rx

http://www.DiversityRx.org/HTML/DIVRX.htm

Clearinghouse of information on promoting language and cultural competence to improve the quality of health for minorities, immigrants, refugees and other diverse populations. Lots of resources on cross cultural health care.

Indian Health Service Diabetes Program

http://www.tucson.ihs.gov/

As well as efforts to fight diabetes in the Native American population, the IHS offers ancillary services to tribal health and urban health programs.

The Initiative to Eliminate Racial and Ethnic Disparities in Health

http://www.raceandhealth.omhrc.gov/

The U.S. Federal Government seeks to eliminate disparities experienced by racial and ethnic minority populations by concentrating efforts on the following health status areas: infant mortality, cancer screening and management, cardiovascular disease, diabetes, HIV infection, and child and adult immunizations. Site discusses the disparities, and the initiative's response. Includes charts and statistics.

Just for You: Minority Health

http://www.healthfinder.org/justforyou/minority/

Articles, organizations, timely issues, news, resources and support for consumers and professionals with health questions specific to American Indian, Alaska Native, African-American, Asian-American, Pacific Islander, and Hispanic populations.

Latino Medicine

http://www.latinomed.com/

The purpose of this website is to support and disseminate information to all future Latino physicians interested in serving the Latino community. Includes feature articles and events, site-of-the-day, forum, chat and medical bookstore.

Minority Health Network

http://www.pitt.edu/~ejb4/min/

Minority health resources, including listings by minority group, disease, and demographics. Also provides organizations, grant information and education.

Minority Health Professionals Foundation
http://www.minorityhealth.org/

This organization pools the collaborative resources, scholarship and technology of minority health professional schools. The twelve member institutions of the Foundation include medical, dental, pharmacy, and veterinary medicine schools in historically African-American colleges and universities.

Minority Health Project
http://www.minority.unc.edu/

The Project maintains two databases on minority health issues.

Office of Minority Health Resource Center
http://www.omhrc.gov/welcom.htm

This Office assists the Secretary and the Office of Public Health and Science on public health program activities that affect American Indian and Alaska Native, African-American, Asian-American and Pacific Islander, and Hispanic populations. Its goal is to promote improved health among these racial and ethnic minority populations.

Race, Health Care and the Law
http://www.udayton.edu/~health/

Explores the law's role in improving the health status of minorities in this country. Includes information on health status, access to quality health care, financing, bioethical and other issues.

Organizations

Alpha Center
http://www.ac.org/

Nonpartisan health policy center that serves as a resource for public and private leaders across the country. It offers information, research, analysis, planning and program management in policy-making. At this site, you can view publications written or distributed by the Center, obtain information on state health care policy developments, and find background material on national grant programs which the AC administers.

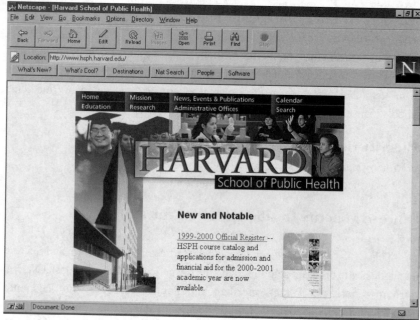

Harvard School of Public Health. http://www.hsph.harvard.edu

American Public Health Association

http://www.apha.org/

This site is a resource for public health professionals and provides information about the Association, as well as a description of legislative affairs and advocacy efforts, news and publications, practice and policy, and public health resources.

Association of Schools of Public Health

http://www.asph.org/

This organization represents the 29 accredited member schools of public health. It seeks to provide a common focus and platform in public health education and accreditation, to assist its member schools to develop and coordinate national health policy, to serve as an information center for those whose interests may overlap those of providing higher education for public health, and, in general, to help meet national goals of health promotion and disease prevention.

Harvard School of Public Health

http://www.hsph.harvard.edu/

Along with a description of the academic program, this site offers news, events, publications and a background on this school.

World Health Organization

http://www.who.int/

Find out about WHO programs, view the *World Health Report*, browse through public information resources and health library.

Publications

American Journal of Public Health

http://www.apha.org/news/publications/journal/AJPH2.html

Peer-reviewed articles in areas of public health; for example, environment, maternal and child health, health promotion, epidemiology, administration, occupational health, education, international health and statistics. Find subscription information, abstracts, editorials and table of contents at this site.

Harvard Public Health Review

http://www.hsph.harvard.edu/review/

Online feature articles, departments, commentary, and archived issues.

Milbank Quarterly

http://www.milbank.org/

A peer-reviewed journal of public health and health care policy published by the Milbank Memorial Fund, which conducts nonpartisan analysis, study, research and communication on significant issues in health policy.

Morbidity and Mortality Weekly Report

http://www2.cdc.gov/mmwr/

This publication of the Centers for Disease Control and Prevention reports on data that is provided by state health departments. You can find back issues, additional publications, related sources, information on diseases and disease trends at this site.

NewsFile

http://www.newsfile.com/

Provides *AIDS Weekly Plus, Antiviral Weekly, Blood Weekly, Cancer Weekly, Disease Weekly,* and other weeklies, many of which cover communicable diseases and public health issues.

Rural Health Care

Agricultural Health and Safety Center
http://agcenter.ucdavis.edu/agcenter/niosh/niosh.html
Links related to agricultural health and safety.

Center for Rural Health and Social Service Development
http://www.siu.edu/~crhssd/
The Center conducts research and training and develops recommendations to improve the health of the rural population. Great section of links.

Federal Office of Rural Health Policy
http://www.nal.usda.gov/orhp/
Promotes better health care service in rural America via research, grants and publications, by promoting federal state and local cooperation, and sponsoring a national clearinghouse for rural health information.

The Issue: Rural Health Care
http://www.fb.com/issues/backgrd/ruralhealth.html
Background and comments from the American Farm Bureau.

National Rural Health Association
http://www.nrharural.org/
Nonprofit association "whose mission is to improve the health and health care of rural Americans and to provide leadership on rural issues through advocacy, communications, education and research."

Research in Action: Improving Health Care for Rural Populations
http://www.ahcpr.gov/research/rural.htm
One-fourth of America's population lives in rural areas which, on the average, have higher poverty rates, and a larger percentage of elderly, yet they have fewer doctors, hospitals, and health resources at their disposal.

Rural Health Network Home Page
http://www.uchsc.edu/sm/sm/rural/index.htm
Site is maintained by a group of medical students striving to create a central information source for students interested in rural health care.

Rural Recruitment and Retention Network
http://www.3RNET.org/

The goal is to find and encourage health professionals to locate practice sites in rural areas.

RuralNet
http://ruralnet.marshall.edu/

Includes an online rural health magazine, rural health resources that include e-mail listings, resources by discipline and disease.

Statistics

America's Lifeline Online
http://www.mindspring.com/~hlthdata/lifeline.html

Images and graphs showing public health risks and statistics.

Center for International Health Information
http://www.cihi.com/

This is a health data reference bureau for the Population, Health and Nutrition Center (PHNC) of USAID's Global Bureau. Health statistics reports, country health profiles, tables, and online data can be accessed here.

Fedstats
http://www.fedstats.gov/

Access to statistics gathered by the various agencies of the Federal government, including the Centers for Disease Control and Prevention, National Institutes of Health, Agency for Health Care Policy and Research, the Health Care Financing Administration, and others.

NAPHSIS
http://www.naphsis.org/

The National Association for Public Health Statistics and Information Systems offers a discussion forum, member training, education and networking.

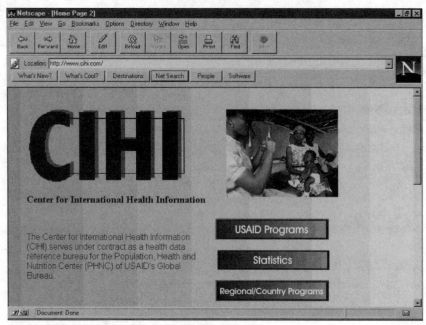

Center for International Health Information. http://www.cihi.com/

National Center for Health Statistics

http://www.cdc.gov/nchswww/default.htm

The NCHS is the primary federal agency responsible for the collection, analysis and dissemination of national health statistics. There are publications, statistical tables, and data files you can download or query, and information on the Center's activities.

Safety and Health Statistics

http://stats.bls.gov/oshhome.htm

From the Bureau of Labor Statistics.

United Nations Population Information Worldwide

http://www.undp.org/popin/

Coordinates population information world-wide. Discusses global population trends, and provides regional data.

Travel Recommendations

See also: Infectious Diseases - Traveler's Health.

Emporiatrics: An Introduction to Travel Medicine

http://indy.radiology.uiowa.edu/Providers/Textbooks/TravelMedicine/TravelMedHP.html

Includes advice to travelers with medical conditions. Note that the most common cause of death to travelers is motor vehicle accidents.

Moon Travel Handbooks

_http://www.moon.com/staying_healthy_

Staying healthy while traveling in Asia, Africa, and Latin America. Includes checklists of health supplies, a directory of traveler's aid organizations, advice on what to eat and drink, signs of illness, and how to get medical assistance.

Outdoor Action Guide to High Altitude Acclimatization and Illnesses

http://www.princeton.edu/~rcurtis/altitude.html

A thorough discussion of the dangers that one can encounter because of high altitude and how to minimize the effect. Preventive medications and aids are described.

QUIZZES, TOOLS & ONLINE CALCULATORS

Alcohol Dependency

Alcohol Use Test
http://www.carebetter.com/
Anonymous, confidential test which determines whether one's level of alcohol use is healthy or abusive.

Quizzes to Help Determine Alcohol Dependency
http://www.recovery.org/aa/aa-related/quizzes.txt
File contains several quizzes, some directed at the individual and others at family members.

Clinical Tools

Clinical Calculators
http://x.medscape.com/Medscape/features/calculators/public/index-calculators.html
Several calculators from Medscape. One helps determine whether hormone replacement therapy would be more of a risk or benefit for individual women, and another helps in determing treatment of patients with community-acquired pneumonia. A third helps with ECG diagnosis of acute myocardial infarction.

Clinical Toolbox
http://dstumpf.net/das/ClinCalc.cfm
How to determine dose, body surface area, mean blood pressure and more.

DoseCalc Services and References

http://www.meds.com/DChome.html

An oncology dosage calculation software program.

Online Clinical Calculator

http://www.intmed.mcw.edu/clincalc.html

This statistical calculator helps researchers determine the Bayesian Analysis of prevalence, sensitivity and specificity of data. It also aids in clinical calculations of estimated blood level, body surface/body mass ratio, weight and measurement conversions.

Online Clinical Calculators from MedStudents

http://www.medstudents.com.br/calculat/index2.htm

These tools help one to determine body surface area, cardiac output, cardiac index, stroke volume, mean arterial pressure, systemic vascular resistance, pulmonary vascular resistance, LV stroke work, oxygen exchange ratio, respiratory quotient, creatinine clearance and many other calculations.

Phys Calculators

http://www.phys.com/c_tools/calculators2/01home/calculators.htm

This site aids in determining body mass index, ideal weight, health risk, caloric and nutrition needs, target heart rate, and calories burned.

Risk Calculator for Hormone Replacement Therapy

http://examroom.medscape.com/Medscape/features/calculators/HRT/HRT1.html

Note: As with all of these online quizzes, this is not meant to replace your personal physician's examination and judgement.

Fitness

The Burn Calculator

http://www.healthyideas.com/walking/burn/

Check to see how many calories you just spent walking.

Calculate Your Body Fat Percentage, Circumference Method

http://www.he.net/~zone/prothd2.html

Enter your measurements to get immediate results.

Caloric Need
http://adam.excite.com/calculator/?calc=calneed&sys=us

Determines your daily caloric needs based on your weight, activity level, and your gender.

Fitness Fundamentals
http://chitrib.webpoint.com/fitness/fundhome.htm

Determine your target heart rate, test your flexibility and strength, and take a general fitness quiz.

LearnWell Fitness Quiz
http://edx.org/h3.htm

This fitness quiz is supposed to be taken after some study; links are provided.

What's Your Fitness I.Q.?
http://www.thriveonline.com/shape/dyngames/gen/shape.fitness.html

Answer a few questions on fitness. You may be surprised at the results.

Health & Longevity

Are You at Risk?
http://www.intelihealth.com/IH/ihtIH?t=8174&p=~br,IHW|~st,8059| ~r,WSIHW000|~b,|*

Cardiac risk assessment test.

Healthy Heart Quiz
http://www.healthyideas.com/healing/quiz/heart/

This quiz is designed to increase your knowledge of heart disease, to help you determine your risk factors, and to stop heart disease before it starts.

Health Risk Assessment
http://greenstone2.sapien.net/

Upon filling out this questionnaire, you will receive a free, personalized health risk assessment.

Johns Hopkins Health Quizzes

http://www.intelihealth.com/IH/ihtIH?t=2415&p=~br,IHW|~st,408
~r,WSIHW000|~b,*|

Test your knowledge of allergies, heart health, weight, pregnancy, blood, hypertension, cholesterol, sleeping, asthma and more at this site.

Longevity Game

http://www.northwesternmutual.com/games/longevity/

Input personal information to receive an estimate on how long you will live, based on research done by the life insurance industry.

Longevity Test

http://www.worldhealth.net/ltest.html

Test helps you determine what lifestyle changes you need to make for increased longevity. You need to have the Shockwave Plugin from Macromedia to take this quiz online.

Lower Your Risk of Colon Cancer

http://www.hsph.harvard.edu/colonrisk/

If you are over 40 years of age and have never had cancer, this test helps to assess your risk for colon cancer. It is one of the most common cancers, and according to this site it is also one of the most preventable.

Self-test for Senility: The Epidemic of the 21st Century?

http://www.frontiersinbiomedicine.com/may7/self-test.htm

Print out this test to take it, and afterwards check your responses.

The Ultimate Cholesterol Quiz

http://www.thriveonline.com/health/dyngames/gen/health.cholesterol.html

Measure what you know about cholesterol.

Mental Health & Personality

Clinical Depression Screening Test

http://sandbox.xerox.com/pair/cw/testing.html

This checklist helps determine if you or someone you know is suffering from clinical depression.

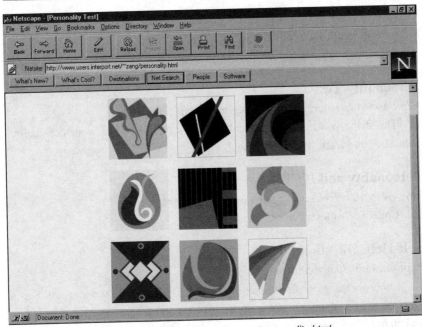

Personality Test. *http://www.users.interport.net/~zang/personality.html*

Emotional Intelligence Quotient

http://www.utne.com/azEQ.tmpl

Do you have that little extra? Or, as the site cautions: "A high IQ may get you into Mensa, but it won't make you a mensch."

The Keirsey Temperament Sorter II

http://www.keirsey.com/cgi-bin/keirsey/newkts.cgi

Identifies you as one of sixteen different personalities.

Online Psychiatry Tests

http://www.med.nyu.edu/Psych/public.html

Determine whether you suffer from depression, anxiety, a sexual disorder, attention deficit disorder or a personality disorder. Information and support links are also provided.

Online Psychology Tests and Quizzes

http://www.helpself.com/quiz.htm

Tests of your emotional IQ, your sexuality, your spirituality, and your intelligence.

Online Stress Test

http://www.health-interactive.com/StressTest.htm

Interactive test determines the amount of stress in your life.

Personality Test

http://www.users.interport.net/~zang/personality.html

The shape you find most appealing says something about your personality. Select one and learn what it "reveals."

Personality and IQ Tests

http://www.davideck.com/online-tests.html

Collection of tests you can take online.

Self-Help Questionnaires

http://mentalhelp.net/guide/quizes.htm

Choose a questionnaire to help determine if you need to see a mental health professional for diagnosis and treatment of attention deficit disorder, depression, and mania (a part of bipolar disorder).

Vulnerability to Stress

http://www.stressfree.com/vlnr_tst.html

Take this test to see your vulnerability to stress.

Miscellaneous

CipherSeek!

http://silcon.com/~nek/cipherseek.html

Hundreds of free online calculators, including health, pregnancy, psychology and diet tools.

Quiz Corner

http://www.naturalland.com/quizzes.htm

Quizzes on garlic, cooking, weight loss, herbs, longevity and more.

Test O'Rama

http://www.spyglasshill.com/References/testorama.htm

Some of these quizzes are just for fun.

Pregnancy

Facts of Life Quiz

http://www.dlcwest.com/~spla/quiz.htm

Interesting quiz tests your knowledge of life in the womb.

OB/Gyn Toolbox

http://www.cpmc.columbia.edu/resources/obgyntools/

Includes tools such as: body surface area calculator, birth weight conversions, creatinine clearance estimation, endometriosis scoring, gestational age calculator, and OB ultrasound analyzer.

The Online Pregnancy Test

http://www.fosml.com/pregnant/index.html

If you're wondering but don't have time to go to the drugstore. Note: works equally well for men and women.

Pregnancy After Age 35

http://www.electra.com/electraquiz/admin/Pregnancy_After_.html

Quiz helps you learn about possible difficulties associated with pregnancy after the woman is age 35.

Pregnancy Calculator

http://www.magma.ca/~rgiffen/PregnancyCalculator.html

Calculate your due date.

Sexuality

Are You a Real Woman/Man?

http://www.helpself.com/real.htm

Test claims to be 98% accurate.

Online Sexual Disorders Screening for Men

http://www.med.nyu.edu/Psych/screens/sdsms.html

Simple 10-question quiz.

Online Sexual Disorders Screening for Women

http://www.med.nyu.edu/Psych/screens/sdsf.html

Answer several questions online.

Online Quiz for Our Sexuality

http://psychology.wadsworth.com/study_center/student/crooksbaur/quiz/

Different aspects of sexuality are explored, from gender issues, to sexual arousal, to love, contraception and atypical activities.

Sexuality Quiz

http://home.netinc.ca/~sexorg/facts/quiz/sexquiz.html

Check your knowledge of sex.

Your Favorite Color is the Key to Your Sexual Life

http://www.gagirl.com/quiz/colours.html

Your favorite color indicates something about your "sexual pattern."

Sleep

Insomnia Quiz

http://www.healthtouch.com/level1/leaflets/sleep/sleep024.htm

Select the symptoms which apply to assess the type and extent of sleep problem you may have.

Sleep Debt Analyzer

http://www.simmonsco.com/sleep.info/quota.html

You cannot train yourself to get by on less sleep. This site discusses "sleep quota," and helps you to determine whether you are getting enough sleep.

Sleep Disorder Help

http://www.sleep-sdca.com/consumer.htm

Self-test for sleep disorders.

Sleep I.Q.

http://www.nhlbi.nih.gov/health/public/sleep/sleep_iq.htm

True-false quiz that tests what you know about sleep.

Sleep Test

http://www.nshsleep.com/test.cfm

Asks questions which will help you detect symptoms that indicate you have a sleep disorder.

Women

Menopause Quiz

http://www.americanwholehealth.com/library/women/whquiz.htm

Test what you know about menopause.

Metabolic Burning Rate

http://www1.ivillage.com/fitness/quiz/0%2C2995%2C7580%2C00.html

This quiz determines your metabolic rate and makes suggestions about your diet habits.

Osteoporosis Evaluation

http://external.aomc.org/osteoporosis/osteoeval.html

Check to see if you may be at risk for this disease.

PMS Inventory Test

http://www.queendom.com/pms1.html

Do you suffer from pre-menstrual syndrome?

RARE, UNKNOWN & GENETIC DISORDERS

Covered in this chapter: General Resources; Genetic Diseases; Rare or Unknown Disorders; Support Groups.

Related chapters: Brain & Brain Disorders; Disabilities; Neurological Disorders; Neuromuscular Disorders; Skin & Connective Tissue/Dermatology.

General Resources

CHID: Combined Health Information Database

http://chid.nih.gov/welcome/welcome.html

Search this database of disease information produced by health-related agencies of the federal government. It offer titles, abstracts, and availability of health information and health education resources.

ChronicIllNet

http://www.chronicillnet.org/

Multimedia information source dedicated to chronic illnesses such as AIDS, cancer, Persian Gulf War syndrome, autoimmune diseases, chronic fatigue syndrome, heart and neurological diseases. Offers general and specific information on diseases and research, facilitates discussion, and serves as a vehicle for data exchange. News, scientific articles, references, personal stories, calendar of events, bulletin board, and other web sources on chronic illness are provided.

Neonatal Diseases and Abnormalities

http://www.mic.ki.se/Diseases/c16.html

This extensive collection of links assembled by the Karolinska Institute includes organizations, indexes and research facilities dealing with genetic, neonatal and developmental disorders such as jaundice, fetal alcohol syndrome, cystic fibrosis and Down syndrome.

Genetic Diseases

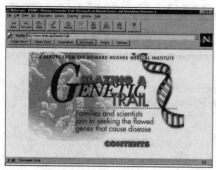

Blazing a Genetic Trail.
http://www.hhmi.org/GeneticTrail/

Blazing a Genetic Trail: Families and Scientists Join in Seeking the Flawed Genes that Cause Disease

http://www.hhmi.org/GeneticTrail/

This report from the Howard Hughes Medical Institute explains genetic disorders and research, including basic genetics. As stated in the foreword, "As a result of this intensive research effort, we should be able in the next century to prevent, cure, or significantly modify the course of many serious genetic illnesses." This report provides insight into the achievement of that goal.

Chromosome Deletion Outreach

http://members.aol.com/cdousa/cdo.htm

The goal of this organization is to provide support for parents of children with rare chromosome disorders, as well as to gather and disseminate information and promote research and a positive community understanding of these disorders. As well as chromosome deletions, information on disorders caused by additions, inversions, translocations and rings is also provided.

GeneClinics: Medical Genetics Knowledge Base

http://www.geneclinics.org/

In its own words, GeneClinics "is an expert-authored, peer-reviewed medical knowledge base consisting of concise descriptions of specific inherited disorders and authoritative, current information on the role of genetic testing in the diagnosis, management, and genetic counseling of patients with these inherited conditions." Search for a disease by name or category. Provides the following information: summary, diagnosis, clinical description, differential diagnosis, management, genetic counseling, molecular genetics, resources, references, and profile history.

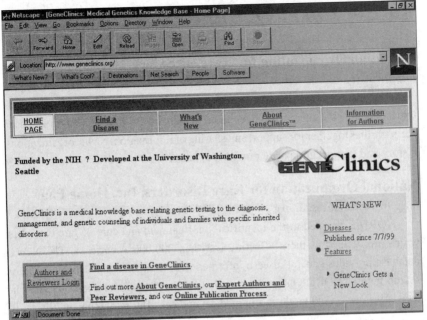

GeneClinics: Medical Genetics Knowledge Base. http://www.geneclinics.org/

Genetic Disorders & Birth Defects Sri Lanka Collection

http://infolanka.com/org/genetics/

Site is for the general public along with patients, students, doctors and researchers.

Genetic Information and Patient Services, Inc.

http://www.icomm.ca/geneinfo/index.html

Descriptions of disorders, links to information or support group websites, resources and encouragement. Section entitled "All About Genetics" covers genes, genetic testing, and genetic counseling. This humble-looking sight contains a lot of information.

Glossary

http://www.icomm.ca/geneinfo/glossary.htm

Definitions of words describing genetic disorders and birth defects.

Yahoo! Genetic Disorders

http://dir.yahoo.com/Health/Diseases_and_Conditions/Genetic_Disorders/

Alphabetical listing of dozens of different genetic disorders.

Rare or Unknown Disorders

Canadian Organization for Rare Disorders
http://www.bulli.com/~cord/

Rare disorders are difficult to diagnose and often untreatable. CORD provides understandable information on over 5,000 rare disorders, and links individuals and their families together for support and sharing of information. News, organizations, history and support groups are provided at this site.

National Organization for Rare Disorders, Inc. Home Page
http://www.rarediseases.org/

NORD is devoted to the identification, treatment and cure of rare disorders, which are defined as those affecting less than 200,000 Americans. The NORD database provides general disease information and organizational links based on search items. "NORD Online," a newsletter, describes government activity and legislative news. Action-alerts and medical updates offer research news.

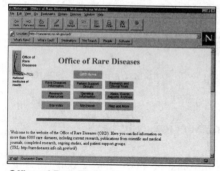

Office of Rare Diseases.
http://cancernet.nci.nih.gov/ord/

Office of Rare Diseases
http://cancernet.nci.nih.gov/ord/

Information on over 6,000 rare diseases. Includes current research, publications from scientific and medical journals, completed research, ongoing studies, and patient support groups.

Rare Genetic Diseases in Children
http://mcrc22.med.nyu.edu/murphp01/homenew.htm

This is a support-resources directory for parents whose child suffers from rare genetic disorders. Links to hospice groups, death and dying support sites, parent-to-parent groups, respite care information, mailing lists, numerous newsgroups and bulletin boards. Both disease-specific and more general support links may be found.

Unknown and Rare Conditions
http://www.kumc.edu/gec/support/unknown.html

Links to websites of interest to those researching unknown and rare conditions.

Unknown and Rare Disorders/Diseases

http://www.dubuque.net/~manemann/

This site was created to serve those who suffer from an unknown disorder. Individuals describe their own or their family-member's unusual case history, with the hope that another reader will recognize the symptoms and respond with advice and answers about the unknown affliction.

Support Groups

Abiding Hearts

http://cu.imt.net/~hearts/

This site provides support and encouragement for parents and others related to those who are continuing their pregnancy even after receiving an adverse prenatal diagnosis. Offers literature, networking, and videos to help in preparing for the birth.

Alliance of Genetic Support Groups

http://www.geneticalliance.org/

Contact information, newsletter, and resources. The Alliance is a national coalition of consumers, professionals and genetic support groups to voice the common concerns of children, adults and families living with, and at risk for, genetic conditions.

Genetic/Rare Conditions Support Groups and Information

http://www.kumc.edu/gec/support/

Information on genetic conditions or birth defects for professionals, educators, and individuals. Site provides lists, national and international organizations, condition categories, genetic counselors/clinical geneticists, children and teen sites, and more.

A Heartbreaking Choice

http://www.erichad.com/ahc/

This site is for parents who chose to interrupt a wanted pregnancy after a poor prenatal diagnosis. Includes suggested readings, support groups, poetry, articles and personal stories. Chat room provided.

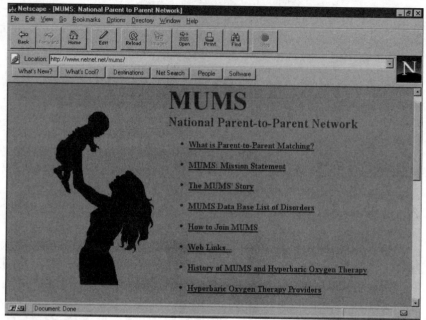

MUMS: National Parent-to-Parent Network. http://www.netnet.net/mums/

MUMS: National Parent-to-Parent Network

http://www.netnet.net/mums/

This network matches up parents and families of children with any disorder, medical condition, mental or emotional disorder, or rare diagnosis. Site provides a listing of disorders, newsletter and information.

Online Genetic Syndrome Support Groups

http://members.aol.com/DNAcutter/sgroup.htm

This directory of support groups is arranged alphabetically, by disease or condition.

Organizations and Support Groups

http://www.kumc.edu/gec/support/grouporg.html

Sites for those interested in or affected by genetic and rare conditions.

SEXUAL & REPRODUCTIVE HEALTH

Covered in this chapter: Abortion; Adolescents; Adoption; Condoms; Contraception; Fertility; General Resources; Herpes; Safe Sex; Sexual Disorders; Sexually Transmitted Diseases; Transgender Issues.

Related chapters: HIV/AIDS; Men's Health; Pregnancy & Childbirth; Women's Health.

Abortion

Abortion
http://www-polisci.mit.edu/BostonReview/BR20.3/thomson.html

This essay originally appeared in the *Boston Review* and discusses abortion from a standpoint of bioethics.

Abortion Clinics Online
http://www.gynpages.com/

Abortion providers are listed by state and category. Links to sites, some of which argue the ethics of abortion.

Abortion Law
http://hometown.aol.com/abtrbng/index.htm

This page seeks to help people get a background and understanding of abortion law in America, no matter what their views on the issue. It presents key court rulings, state laws, a glossary of terms and other resources.

Center for Bioethics: Abortion Resources
http://www.med.upenn.edu/~bioethic/library/resources/abortion.html

Abortion and reproductive rights, abortion issues links, newsgroups, risks and complications, and description of *Roe vs. Wade*.

International Society of Abortion Doctors

http://alpha.nedernet.nl/~ngva/isadindex.htm

Society statutes, practical guide, agenda and related links.

Partial Birth Abortion: All Sides

http://www.religioustolerance.org/abo_pba.htm

Appears to be a fair-minded discussion of this controversial issue.

Pro-Choice Views

http://prochoice.about.com/

Links and articles.

Pro-Life Views

http://prolife.about.com/

Links and articles.

Adolescents

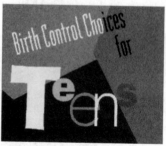

http://www.plannedparenthood.org/
TEENISSUES/BCCHOICES/
BCCHOICES.HTML

Birth Control Choices

http://www.plannedparenthood.org/TEEN ISSUES/BCCHOICES/BCCHOICES.HTML

Birth control methods are assessed in terms of comfort, effectiveness, safety and affordability.

Coalition for Positive Sexuality

http://www.webcom.com/~cps/

Information for teens.

Sex, Etc.

http://www.sxetc.org/

Online magazine written for teens, by teens.

Teenwire

http://www.teenwire.com/

Sexuality and relationship information for teenagers. Helpful guides, news, articles, quizzes and charts; ask the expert section; world views on sex and dating.

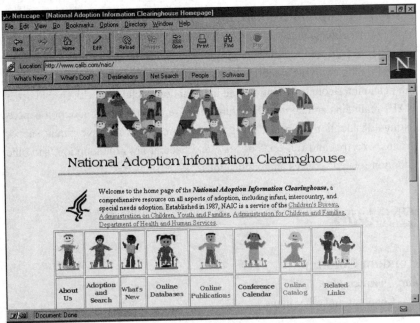

National Adoption Information Clearinghouse. *http://www.calib.com/naic*

Adoption

Adoption Policy Resource Center
http://www.fpsol.com/adoption/advocates.html

Legislative news and analysis, adoption and subsidy information, legal resources, and links to related websites.

AdoptioNetwork
http://207.226.25.92/

Information for the adoption community. Includes chat groups, frequently asked questions, and news. Sections for birthparents, for adoptees and for parents.

Faces of Adoption: America's Waiting Children
http://www.adopt.org/adopt/

The National Adoption Center (NAC) and Children Awaiting Parents (CAP) bring children waiting to be adopted "online" by posting their photographs and descriptions. Site offers a wealth of information about adoption. Chat, mail list and links.

National Adoption Information Clearinghouse
http://www.calib.com/naic

Site was created by the federal government to give professionals and the general public easily-accessible information on all aspects of adoption, including infant and inter-country adoption, and the adoption of children with special needs. NAIC maintains an adoption literature database, a database of adoption experts, listings of adoption agencies, crisis pregnancy centers, adoptive parent support groups, excerpts and full texts of State and Federal laws on adoption, and other adoption-related services and publications.

Condoms

Condom Country
http://www.condom.com/

Condoms and other items.

Condom Shop
http://geewiz.com/std.html

Frequently asked questions (FAQs) and information from the Department of Health and Human Services.

Condomania Online
http://www.condomania.com/

News, safe sex information and products.

Condoms Express
http://www.webcom.com/~condom/express/express.html

Frequently asked questions (FAQs), products, tips and ordering information.

Female Condom
http://wso.williams.edu/orgs/peerh//sex/safesex/femcon.html

Illustration shows how to use the female condom.

The Female Condom
http://www.nau.edu/~fronske/fcondom.html

Describes this form of birth control and how to use it.

Female Health Foundation

http://www.femalehealth.com/

Information on Reality, the female condom, from the company that manufactures it.

Official Condom Directory

http://users.deltanet.com/users/agkid/

Place to go for links to condom sites on the Internet.

Contraception

Ann Rose's Ultimate Birth Control Links Page

http://gynpages.com/ultimate/

Extensive links to information for individuals of all ages to make informed decisions about sexual activity and potential childbearing.

Contraception

http://www.powerup.com.au/~fpq/contraception.html

Describes different forms of contraception and their success rates.

Contraceptive Guide

http://www.mjbovo.com/Contracept/index.htm

Covers various methods of birth control.

Emergency Contraception Website

http://opr.princeton.edu/ec/ec.html

Information on emergency contraception and how to find locations where you can get it. Answers some important questions about emergency contraceptives and how they work. Reference to news and publications.

The Hall of Contraception

http://desires.com/1.6/Sex/Museum/museum1.html

The museum shows over 600 different IUD's, sponges, condoms and other contraceptive devices.

The History of Contraception
http://rtt.colorado.edu/~mcck/Home.html
> Interesting information on birth control throughout history.

Myths about Birth Control
http://www.pixi.com/~521teen/117.htm
> Geared to adolescents.

Nature's Method
http://www.familyplanning.net/
> Known as the "ovulation method." Claims to be 98 to 99 percent effective.

Successful Contraception
http://www.arhp.org/success/
> Guide to choosing the form of contraception that will work best for you.

A Woman's Guide to Contraception and Responsible Sex
http://www.epigee.org/guide/
> Advantages and disadvantages of different methods of birth control, educational materials, pregnancy resources and more.

Fertility

4Fertility
http://www.4fertility.com/
> Links to fertility sites on the Internet. Includes resources and discussions, clinics and related topics.

Atlanta Reproductive Health Centre WWW
http://www.ivf.com//index.html
> Information on infertility, polycystic ovaries, in vitro fertilization, endometriosis and pelvic pain treatment options. Includes frequently asked questions, off-site links and a chat room.

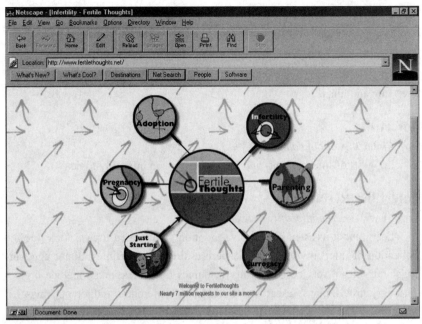

Fertile Thoughts. http://www.fertilethoughts.net/

Family Helper
http://www.helping.com/family/helper.html

Information on infertility and adoption. Also provides resources on post-adoption issues which may arise.

Fertile Thoughts
http://www.fertilethoughts.net/

A web community for infertile couples and couples seeking to build a family through medical treatment of infertility. Major discussion topics include pregnancy, adoption, infertility, parenting and surrogacy. The site includes chat rooms, bulletin boards, advocacy and insurance information, as well as professional directories showing adoption agencies, day care, surrogacy agencies, doctors, lawyers and therapists by state.

Fertilitext
http://www.fertilitext.org/

Information about infertility and reproductive issues to those pursuing fertility treatment.

Ferti.Net

http://www.ferti.net/

Information for health care professionals, researchers and patients interested in assisted fertilization and human reproduction. Infertility and infertility treatment literature and links.

Infertility

http://infertility.about.com/

Long list of Internet links and feature articles on infertility topics.

Infertility Resources

http://www.ihr.com/infertility/index.html

Learn about assisted pregnancy, adoption, and related topics; look through collection of infertility articles, and peruse directory of clinics, donor egg, surrogacy and legal services. Infertility resources for professionals include organizations, journals, news, research and treatment, conferences and job openings.

Spermatology WWW Home Page

http://numbat.murdoch.edu.au:80/spermatology/spermhp.html

Information on the science of sperms. Links to research facilities and utilities, spermatological images, journals, cloning information, conferences and more.

Surrogacy.com

http://www.surrogacy.com/online_support/

E-mail discussion lists and support groups on surrogacy topics, for donors, surrogate mothers, parents through assisted reproductive technology, and others.

General Resources

ALT.SEX FAQ

http://www.halcyon.com/elf/altsex/longdex.html

Straightforward answers to many sex questions.

HealthGate Healthy Sexuality

http://www.healthgate.com/healthy/sexuality/fs.index.html

All sorts of information about sexuality, from sensation, to contraception, to sexually transmitted diseases.

Planned Parenthood Federation of America

http://www.plannedparenthood.org/

Resources on sexual and reproductive health and education, including contraception, birth control, family planning, pregnancy, sexually transmitted diseases and reproductive rights.

Planned Parenthood Local Affiliate

http://www.plannedparenthood.org/zip.htm

Enter your zip code to get information about local clinics and services.

Rainbow Query

http://www.glweb.com/rainbowquery/

Features approximately 200 categories of information relating to gay, lesbian, bisexual and trangender human sexuality.

Sex Laws

http://www.geocities.com/CapitolHill/2269/

Legislation and religious rules that deal with sexual practices.

Sexuality

http://sexuality.about.com/

Internet links and spotlighted features.

Herpes

Café Herpe

http://www.cafeherpe.com/

A genital herpes resource. Find information, products and online support groups.

Genital Herpes and Pregnancy Information

http://noah.cuny.edu/pregnancy/march_of_dimes/stds/herpesis.html

Public health information on genital herpes and the impact it can have on pregnancy.

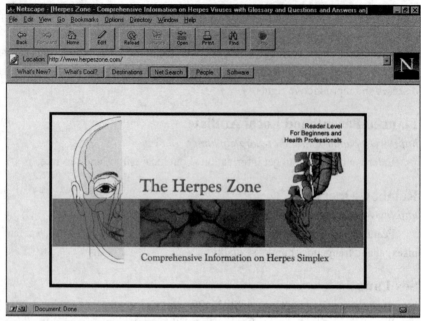

The Herpes Zone. *http://www.herpeszone.com/*

Herpes Alternative Approaches

http://www.AltHerpes.com/

Lots of social and support groups, the basics of herpes, and links to sites presenting alternative therapy options.

Herpes Zone

http://www.herpeszone.com/

All about herpes and how to manage it once you have it. Includes questions and answers, and resources.

Safe Sex

Safe(r) Sex: Information and Education

http://www.med.jhu.edu/jhustd/safesex.htm

Links to safe sex resources. Most of these sites provide information for lay people on condom use and other safe sex practices.

Safer Sex Options

http://www.montrose-clinic.org/education/safersex.htm

Suggestions and alternatives to unprotected intercourse.

Safer Sex Page

http://safersex.org/

Discusses what "safer sex" is and encourages condom use.

Sexual Disorders

See also: Addiction; Men's Health; Mental Health.

Gender as Illness: Issues of Psychiatric Classification

http://www.transgender.org:80/tg/gic/ictltext.html

This paper examines issues of gender identity and expression in light of current definitions of mental illness.

Sexual Compulsives Anonymous

http://www.sca-recovery.org/

Includes an explanation of the group's purpose, which is to help people who wish to recover from a sexual compulsion, along with support information, tools and online meetings.

Sexual Disorders

http://mhsource.com/disorders/sexual.html

List of consumer questions on various sexual issues with answers from an expert, articles and resources.

Sexual Dysfunction

http://eee.oac.uci.edu/96s/class/p121da/dysfunc.html

Female and male sexual dysfunctions, causes, and case examples.

Sexual Masochism and Sadism

http://mentalhelp.net/disorders/sx90.htm

Brief description of symptoms.

Sexually Transmitted Diseases

See also: HIV/AIDS chapter.

Allabout Center: Sexual Diseases

http://www.icemall.com/allabout/sexdis.html

Links to sites about sexually transmitted diseases.

American Social Health Association

http://www.ashastd.org/

The mission of this group is to stop sexually transmitted diseases (STDs) and their harmful consequences to individuals, families and communities. Site offers STD information, answers to frequently asked questions, support groups, and hotline information.

Ask NOAH About: Sexually Transmitted Diseases

http://Noah.cuny.edu/stds/stds.html

Information resources cover the basics of STDs, including prevention, statistics, testing, treatment and types of diseases.

Johns Hopkins University STD Research Group

http://www.clark.net/pub/jhustd/

General information on sexually transmitted diseases and on research being undertaken by the Johns Hopkins group. Site also offers patient education, HIV/AIDS related sites, and covers special topics which include gonorrhea, chlamydia, syphilis, trichomonas, herpes, and genital warts. Additional topics cover more general health topics.

SHAPE: Sexual Health Advocate Peer Education Website

http://www.hsc.missouri.edu/~shc/helthed4.htm

Offers information on sexually transmitted diseases, safer sex principles and practices, and how to improve communication skills.

STD Glossary

http://www.ashastd.org/abc/

Medical and scientific technology relating to sexually transmitted diseases.

Transgender Issues

Ingersoll Gender Center
http://www.ingersollcenter.org/

This is a nonprofit agency supporting the transsexual, transvestive and transgender community. It offers therapy and peer counseling pertaining to issues of daily living, changes in lifestyle, preparation for surgery, and post-operative care. The site offers a variety of resources, as well as human interest material.

Notes on Gender Transition
http://www.avitale.com/

Discusses issues regarding gender dysphoria, transsexualism, transgenderism, Gender Identity Disorder and gender role transition. Essays, articles, and links.

Sexual Identity and Gender Identity Forum
http://php.indiana.edu/~mberz/ttt/faqs/glossary

This pamphlet is designed to provide and define some basic common terms used in the gender and sexual identity communities.

Transgender Community Forum
http://members.aol.com/onqgwen/

Contains chat and conference rooms, resource library, frequently asked questions, message boards, community resources, web links and news.

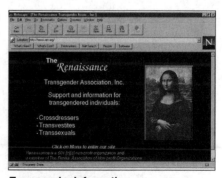

Transgender Information
http://www.ren.org/

Support and information for cross-dressers, transvestites and transsexuals, from the Renaissance Education Association, Inc.

Transgender Information.
http://www.ren.org/

SKIN & CONNECTIVE TISSUE / DERMATOLOGY

Acne

AcneCures
http://www.acnecures.com/

Information about acne treatments, alternative acne therapies, pimple prevention, acne in teens, newsgroups and chat rooms.

In Your Face!
http://kidshealth.org/kid/normal/acne.html

What acne is and what to do about it, for teenagers.

Eczema

Ask NOAH about Eczema
http://www.noah.cuny.edu/dermatology/derm.html#eczema

Lots of links to information on eczema, arranged in an easy-to-negotiate outline.

Eczema Informant
http://ei.addr.com/

Information for those who suffer from eczema. Includes medications, news and research, along with the use of nutritional and herbal supplements.

Ehlers-Danlos Syndrome

Ehlers-Danlos National Foundation
http://www.ednf.org/
   Emotional support and information for those who suffer from Ehlers-Danlos and their families. Includes a newsletter. Ehlers-Danlos syndromes are a heritable connective tissue disorders, characterized by articular (joint) hypermobility, skin extensibility and tissue fragility.

Ehlers-Danlos Syndrome
http://www.familyvillage.wisc.edu/lib_e-ds.htm
   Links to web resources and chat site.

Genetic/Metabolic Disorders: Ehlers-Danlos Syndrome
http://www.mc.Vanderbilt.Edu/peds/pidl/genetic/ehlers.htm
   Fact sheet on this group of disorders.

General Resources

Ask NOAH About: Dermatology
http://www.noah.cuny.edu/dermatology/
   Choose from the list of dermatological conditions, which range from the serious to the cosmetic.

Black Skin
http://www.aad.org/_vti_bin/shtml.exe/aadpamphrework/black.html/map
   This online pamphlet discusses certain skin conditions that are more common in black people than in white people.

Department of Dermatology
http://tray.dermatology.uiowa.edu/home.html
   The University of Iowa's Department of Dermatology has created a point of access to an impressive number of dermatology-related websites, image banks, organizations, etc. Also offers an introduction to basic dermatology, a tutorial in diagnosis, and the *Dermatology Online Journal*.

Dermatology

http://dermatology.about.com/

Skin disorders from the serious to the every-day, questions and answers, support groups, feature articles and more.

Dermatology and Allergology Journals

http://www.sciencekomm.at/journals/medicine/dermat.html

Link to 57 journals on the web.

Dermatology Image Database

http://tray.dermatology.uiowa.edu/
DermImag.htm

Images of various skin conditions.

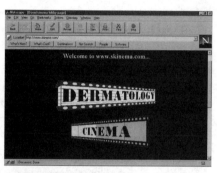

Dermatology in the Cinema

http://www.skinema.com/

Dermatologist and film buff Dr. Reese has assembled examples of skin lesions and conditions found in movies to unite his two interests. Entertaining.

Dermatology in the Cinema. *http://www. skinema.com/*

Dermguide.com

http://www.dermguide.com/derm/

Dermatology Internet search.

HealthWeb Dermatology Page

http://www.medlib.iupui.edu/cicnet/derma/derma.html

Includes a list of dermatologic disease resources, including educational resources, electronic publications, online discussion groups, organizations, and miscellaneous dermatological resources. The Dermatological Disease Resources section contains selected chapters and articles from books and journals, related websites, clinical trial information and contacts, and National Institutes of Health reports.

InfoDerm

http://www.galderma.com/

Learn about skin and skin disorders, connect to support groups, find a dermatologist, and link to other resources.

Interactive Dermatology
http://interactive.dermato.com.br/

Mailing lists, image index, books, chat groups and medical topics of interest to dermatologists.

An Introduction to Basic Dermatology
http://www.vh.org/Providers/Lectures/PietteDermatology/
BasicDermatology.html

Images for dermatologists.

Matrix Dermatology Resources
http://matrix.ucdavis.edu/

Access the archives of RxDerm, an online discussion group for dermatologists. There are also texts and tutorials created for dermatology students on diseases of the skin, common viral and common bacterial infections, skin tumors and more.

Mayo Clinic Skin Conditions
http://www.mayohealth.org/mayo/library/htm/tocskinc.htm

Articles on skin conditions directed at the consumer audience, on everything from warts, to wrinkles, to understanding the health clues provided by your fingernails.

Patient Information Pamphlet Index
http://tray.dermatology.uiowa.edu/PIPs/PIP-Index.htm

Covers a number of skin conditions, from acne to warts.

Project Dermatology Online Atlas
http://www.medic.mie-u.ac.jp/derma/bilddb/db.htm

The goal of this project is to create a hypermedia textbook of dermatology.

Skin and Connective Tissue Diseases
http://www.mic.ki.se/Diseases/c17.html

The Karolinska Institute has provided visitors to this site with a very long list of basic dermatology organizations and resources, as well as links to sites discussing specific skin and connective tissue conditions.

Skin Deep

http://grossbart.com/sd/index.htm

Contains text from Dr. Ted Grossbart's book of the same name which considers emotions a major factor in skin problems. Chapters include, "Our Skin: Listening and Responding to the World Around You," "Why Me? The Skin Has Its Reasons," "Breaking the Itch/Scratch Cycle," and "The New Psychopsoriasis."

Hair Loss (Alopecia)

See also: Men's Health - Hair Loss.

Alopecia Areata

http://angelfire.com/wa/Victor2/alopecia.html

General information and frequently asked questions about alopecia areata, a disease characterized by hair loss that is suspected to be the result of an autoimmune system disorder. Information about diagnosis, prevalence, research and treatment, along with related websites.

Alopecia Research and Resources

http://npntserver.mcg.edu/default.htm#npindex-2.1000

This website is devoted to helping people with abnormal hair loss, also known as alopecia. It offers information and an opportunity to share personal stories, as well as guidelines for managing the disorder. There is a special focus on helping children with alopecia.

Living with Hair Loss

http://www.arcnewmedia.com/hairloss/

Web author Sheila Jacobs lost her hair due to alopecia areata, and has written a book and conducted seminars to help others cope and treat their baldness. This website lists organizations, articles, books, videos, newsgroups and bulletin boards to which people suffering from alopecia may turn for support and information.

Leprosy

What Is Leprosy
http://www.leprosymission.org/what.htm

The cause, cure and prevalence of this disease, also known as Hansen's.

A World without Leprosy
http://www.who.int/lep/

Information on leprosy from the World Health Organization. Describes the global leprosy situation, the most endemic countries, disease and treatment. Links to the Leprosy Discussion list, and other relevant research and publications.

Lupus

Circle of Friends: Autoimmune Disease and Lupus Support Group
http://members.aol.com//mycircle/index.htm

E-mail group that offers emotional support to people who suffer from lupus and other autoimmune disorders.

Living with Lupus
http://internet-plaza.net/lupus/

The homepage of the Lupus Foundation of America includes frequently asked questions, a research and resource library, and general information about the causes, symptoms, testing and treatment of lupus. Site features a calendar of events, chapter activities and contacts, and also has a helpful and friendly health forum where you can post questions, help others with answers to their questions, and share experiences, expertise, and/or support.

Lupus
http://lupus.miningco.com/

Loads of links to resources on lupus, including treatment, support, organizations, research, clinical trials, and related sites.

Lupus Around the World

http://www.mtio.com/lupus/

Includes a main forum and chat group on lupus, a discussion of lupus procedures, advocacy efforts, lupus in the media, and "ask a doctor." Also offers many links to organizations, support groups, medical and educational sites, and regional lupus groups.

Lupus Home Page

http://www.hamline.edu/~lupus/

The Lupus Foundation of America provides general and clinical information, news briefs, lists of organizations, conferences, and meetings. Two mailing lists are also maintained, LUPUS-L (primarily for patients) and LUPUS-R (primarily for researchers). To subscribe, send e-mail to: *listproc@piper.hamline.edu* with the message "SUBSCRIBE LUPUS-L *Yourfullname*" or "SUBSCRIBE LUPUS-R *Yourfullname*," depending on which list you wish to join.

Lupus Letter

http://www.balch-lupus.com/

Online version of this newsletter that contains lupus questions and answers, interviews, feature articles, advice on diet, books and more.

Lupus Living

http://www.medcheck.org/lupus.html

Basic information on lupus and lots of links.

Nikki's Lupus Home Page

http://members.aol.com/NikkisCats/Lupus.html

Commonly asked questions about lupus, information, links and one patient's personal story.

Non-English Links to Lupus

http://www.mtio.com/lupus/l5index.htm

Lupus sites in many different languages.

Select Resources for Compassionate Care of Lupus (SLE)

http://cerebel.com/lupus/overview.htm

Includes a clinical overview of lupus, lupus nephritis treatment issues, lupus books, survey and more.

Organizations

American Academy of Dermatology
http://www.aad.org/

Provides member information, continuing medical education, and Melanoma-Net, an educational program for patients and dermatologists.

American Society of Dermatology
http://www.asd.org/

This site offers legislative updates, advocacy, meeting and membership information.

Dermatology Foundation
http://www.dermfnd.org/

The Foundation raises funds to promote research in skin cancer and other diseases of the skin, hair, and nails.

Internet Dermatology Society
http://www.telemedicine.org/ids.htm

This site is geared to dermatologists world-wide. Its goal is to facilitate communication and share research results by creating an information clearing-house. Besides Society information, this site offers an electronic textbook of dermatology, global dermatological grand rounds, Internet teledermatology triage, dermatology lectures and mailing lists. It also has links to the Women's Dermatologic Society and other groups.

National Skin Centre, Singapore
http://www.nsc.gov.sg/commskin/nsc.html

Patient information as well as Centre activities and treatment programs for skin diseases. List of academic activities, research and scientific publications; meeting and conference news and announcements.

Society for Investigative Dermatology
http://www.sidnet.org/index.htm

Nonprofit organization for the advancement of research of skin, hair, nails and mucous membrane conditions.

Pigmentation

International Albinism Center

http://lenti.med.umn.edu:80/iac/

This site of the International Albinism Center at the University of Minnesota provides a link to an electronic copy of *Facts about Albinism*, as well as links to related websites.

National Incontentia Pigmenti Foundation

http://medhlp.netusa.net/www/nipf.htm

The NIPF is organized to encourage research and education about incontentia pigmenti, a rare genetic disease for which there is no cure. The disease initially manifests itself in the skin of newborn infants. This website describes both the disease and Foundation activities.

Porphyria

American Porphyria Foundation Page

http://www.enterprise.net/apf/

The porphyrias are a group of rare metabolic diseases with many symptoms appearing in the skin, as well as in the neurologic system. This site offers in-depth information for patients and the public on porphyria, including information on suggested diet and drug treatment.

Porphyria Web Links

http://darwin.clas.virginia.edu/~rjh9u/aip.html

This site offers about a dozen links to web pages related to this skin and neurologic disease, including an entry about King George III, who is believed to have suffered from this affliction.

Shelly's Porphyria Page

http://members.xoom.com/shelhill/index.html

Personal story and porphyria information, remarks about porphyria and diet, chronic pain, the patient's bill of rights, and tips on how to find a good doctor.

Porphyria: A Patient's Guide

http://www.uq.edu.au/porphyria/

Description of the different types of porphyria, diagnosis, treatment and management options. Both safe and unsafe drugs are identified, and specific therapies are described.

Psoriasis

National Psoriasis Foundation

http://www.psoriasis.org/

Offers general information and frequently asked questions on psoriasis, with statistics, photos and description. Includes psoriasis therapies and case histories, research efforts, Foundation activities, meetings, publications, and links to other psoriasis sites on the web.

Psoriasis and Self Help

http://www.pinch.com/skin/

Psoriasis information and forum, with short-cuts to searching skin-disease newsgroups and databases.

Psoriasis Research

http://www.tecc.co.uk/psoriasis/

Questions and answers about psoriasis and psoriasis cures, personal accounts, celebrities who suffer from psoriasis, newsgroups about the skin condition, and related sites.

Scleroderma

Coping with Crest

http://hometown.aol.com/REDAPRIL4/index.html

CREST syndrome is another term for scleroderma, which is a disease that results in hardening of the skin and multiple organs due to over-deposit of collagen. CREST includes a complex of symptoms, generally: Calcinosis (calcium deposits on the skin), Raynaud's (decreased circulation), Esophageal dysfunction, Sclerodactyly (fingers become hard and shiny), and Telangiectasia (tiny blood vessels show through the skin). Site was created by a scleroderma patient and includes information on living with the disease, as well as clinical material.

I Have Scleroderma

http://www.ihavescleroderma.com/

Personal stories of those who have scleroderma. Art page displays poetry, short stories, and provides information on visual artists who suffered from the disease.

Scleroderma from A to Z

http://www.sclero.org//

There are over 400 pages and 1,500 links to scleroderma medical and world-wide support group information, available in eight different languages.

Scleroderma Federation

http://www.scleroderma.org/

Scleroderma is a chronic, autoimmune disease of the connective tissue that is generally classified as a rheumatic disease. Site offers facts, support groups, literature, chat and scleroderma links.

Sjogren's Syndrome

See also: Eyes/Optometry & Ophthalmology - Dry Eye Syndrome.

Sjogren's Syndrome

http://www.silcom.com/~sblc/sjogrens.html

Alphabetized list of links to sites with information on Sjogren's syndrome and dry eye.

Sjogren's Syndrome Foundation
http://www.sjogrens.com/

This site acts as an information clearinghouse for Sjogren's syndrome, an incurable autoimmune disorder where the body attacks its own moisture-producing glands causing dry eyes, dry mouth, and potentially worse effects.

Skin Cancer
See also: Cancer/Oncology.

Melanoma Patients' Information Page
http://www.mpip.org/

Includes selected patient information geared toward specific stages of the cancer, news, bulletin board and chat room, research library, glossary, and many links to related sites.

Skin Cancer: The Facts
http://www.jas.tj/skincancer/

Basics on skin cancer and how to protect yourself. Includes frequently asked questions, links to other sites and discussion groups.

Sweating (Hyperhidrosis)

Hyperhidrosis
http://www.parsec.it/summit/hyper1e.htm

Hyperhydrosis is excessive sweating in one or more localized portions of the body. This rare affliction has several manifestations and its cause is unknown. The website offers an overview and description of the disease, its symptoms and treatment options. The page is also available in Italian and German.

Patient Information: Hyperhidrosis
http://www.dermnet.org.nz/dna.hyperhidrosis/hyper.html

Description of this disorder, and tips on management and treatment.

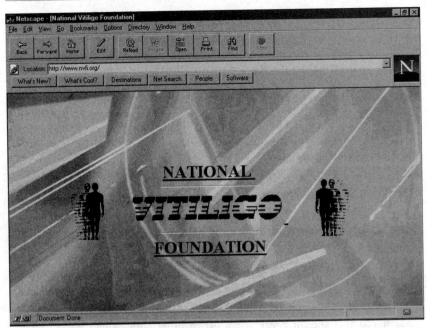

National Vitiligo Foundation. http://www.nvfi.org/

Vitiligo

A Handbook for Patients with Vitiligo

http://www.nvfi.org/handbook.htm

Addresses some of the most common questions about vitiligo.

National Vitiligo Foundation

http://www.nvfi.org/

Vitiligo is a spontaneous irregular depigmentation of skin which, while it does not have serious health consequences, does cause much suffering because of social consequences. The National Vitiligo Foundation site describes efforts to promote education and research, and offers support and information for patients and their families. In addition, there are links to other websites and information on mail lists related to vitiligo.

Vitiligo

http://www.skinsite.com/info_vitiligo.htm

Brief description of the definition, causes, course and treatment of this skin disorder.

Xeroderma Pigmentosum

NORD Information on Xeroderma Pigmentosum
_http://www.stepstn.com/nord/rdb_sum/339.htm_

General information about this group of rare inherited skin disorders characterized by a heightened reaction to sunlight (photosensitivity).

Xeroderma Pigmentosum
http://www.icondata.com/health/pedbase/files/XERODERM.HTM

Clinical information from the Multimedia Medical Reference Library.

Xeroderma Pigmentosum Society, Inc.
http://xps.org/

Xeroderma pigmentosum sufferers are unable to tolerate ultraviolet radiation (especially sunlight). The Society seeks to promote awareness of and research into XP, and to support patients and their families. You may obtain a copy of the Society newsletter at this site, or check out a list of other publications, organizations, newsgroups and individuals that may be contacted for further information.

SLEEP & SLEEP DISORDERS

Dreams

The Association for the Study of Dreams
http://www.asdreams.org/

Nonprofit organization dedicated to the study of dreams and dreaming. Site provides membership and conference information, a journal called Dreaming, an online magazine and forum called *Dream Time*, news and discussion, books, educational resources and more.

Dr. Dream's Resources for People Who Dream
http://www.dr-dream.com/

How to remember your dreams, how to understand them, and many other dream materials.

Dreams and Nightmares
http://www.freezone.co.uk/zeb1/index.html

Site assists you with understanding your dreams and provides resources on dream-related topics such as dream analysis, sleep remedies, hot links and organization contact information.

Dreams FAQ
http://www.faqs.org/faqs/dreams-faq/

Several collections of frequently asked questions about dreams, covering general comments, a discussion of lucid dreaming, dream interpretation, the paranormal and other topics.

The Dream Tree
http://dreamtree.com/

A resource center for dreamers that includes global dreaming news, different views on dreams, dreams in art and literature, and a dream discussion forum.

DreamWeaver's Web
http://www.webcom.com/dreamwvr/

Jungian dream analysis. Includes a searchable dream index resources, information on dream symbols, and an interactive dream workbook.

Electric Dreams
http://www.dreamgate.com/electric-dreams/

Dream sharing community and information network includes articles on dreams and interpretation, links and more.

Gothic Skywalker's Dream Analysis
http://www.geocities.com/TimesSquare/Dungeon/3913/dream.html

Step-by-step guide to help you understand your dreams.

Iris Publishing
http://www.Iris-Publishing.com/

Dream discovery and sleep/insomnia help.

Working (and Playing) with Dreams
http://www.rider.edu/users/suler/dreams.html

Includes syllabus of a clinical psychology course on dreams, as well as essays and a number of exercises.

General Resources

Normal Sleep Cycle
http://www4.umdnj.edu/med/slepsymp.html

Discusses the different stages in the sleep cycle. Suggestions on how to prepare for a good night's sleep, and brief description of different sleep disorders and their symptoms.

Simmons Company Sleep Information

http://www.simmonsco.com/sleep.info/

Describes the stages of sleep, especially the third level, or REM sleep, during which dreaming occurs. Also offers a sleep test and a sleep quota calculator, and resources on various sleep studies and dreams.

Sleep

http://www.asda.org/journal.html

This professional publication of the American Sleep Disorder Association contains articles ranging from clinical investigations of sleep/wake disorders and medical problems during sleep, to investigations of the basic physiological and biochemical events and anatomical structures involved in normal and abnormal sleep.

Sleep Disorder Centers of America

http://www.sleep-sdca.com/

Resources for physicians and hospitals, as well as information for consumers on sleep disorders and sleep medicine.

Sleep Home Pages

http://bisleep.medsch.ucla.edu/

Resources for the general public, patients and professionals about sleep, sleep disorders, sleep research and more. Includes a number of forums on clinical and research aspects of sleep. Lots of links.

Sleep Medicine Home Page

http://www.cloud9.net/%7Ethorpy/

Many links to sites, including sleep-related newsgroups and discussion groups. An alphabetical listing of sleep disorders is available, along with information broken down into the following topics: clinical practice, professional associations, journals, sleep research sites, government information, medications, meetings, centers around the world, book reviews and organizations.

The Sleep Well

http://www.stanford.edu/~dement/

This large index of sleep resources includes research, journals, information on snoring, sleep disorders, dreams, organizations, sleep aids and more.

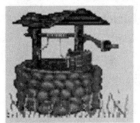

The Sleep Well. *http://www.stanford.edu/~dement/*

SleepDocs Online
http://www.cloud9.net/%7Ethorpy/sleepdoc.html

For a fee, you can send in a question about sleep and sleep disorders to a sleep specialist certified by the American Board of Sleep Medicine. Topics include snoring, sleep apnea, insomnia, sleeping pills, melatonin, jet lag, sleepwalking, nightmares and more.

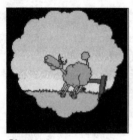

Sleepnet.
http://www.sleepnet.com/

Sleepnet
http://www.sleepnet.com/

"Everything you wanted to know about sleep disorders but were too tired to ask." Lots of links, sleep forums, support groups, dream discussion, professional organizations and news.

Sleep/Wake Disorders Canada
http://www.geocities.com/HotSprings/1837/

Information about sleep and an introduction to sleeping disorders, including frequently asked questions, diagnosis, books, online and off-line resources.

Humor

Lighter Side of Sleep
http://www.stanford.edu/~dement/sleephumor.html

Humorous anecdotes and sleep jokes.

Insomnia

Insomnia
http://www.saonet.ucla.edu/health/healthed/HANDOUTS/insomnia.htm

This handout offers a brief description of insomnia, its causes, symptoms and treatments.

Insomnia
http://www.4women.org/faq/Insomnia.htm

Questions and answers about insomnia.

Insomnia? Just Go to Sleep and Forget About It

http://www.well.com/user/mick/insomnia/

Suggestions for insomniacs.

Insomnia Quiz

http://www.healthtouch.com/level1/leaflets/sleep/sleep024.htm

Simple quiz helps you identify if you have a sleeping problem that merits professional help.

Redbook: How to Feel Rested on Too Little Sleep

http://redbook.women.com/rb/health/features/66slee11.htm

Tips on napping and other ways to energize.

SleepMedic

http://sleepmedic.com/

Secrets for better sleep, including relief of insomnia and stress.

Melatonin

Melatonin Central

http://www.melatonin.com/

Frequently asked questions about melatonin and what it may do for you, melatonin and medical conditions, and purchasing information.

Melatonin Mania

http://www.sciam.com/explorations/040196explorations.html

Article from *Scientific American* discusses the popular claims about melatonin and "separates the facts from the hype."

Narcolepsy

Center for Narcolepsy Research

http://www.uic.edu/depts/cnr/index.htm

General facts about narcolepsy including research, information and support.

Cure Narcolepsy Now!

http://www.cloud9.net/~thorpy/NARCO.HTML

Narcolepsy affects approximately 1 person out of 2000. This site seeks to encourage the communication and funding of research to cure narcolepsy.

Stanford University Center for Narcolepsy

http://www-med.Stanford.EDU/school/Psychiatry/narcolepsy/

Presents symptoms, medications, publications and research findings for this sleeping disorder. Explains the basic mechanisms of the disease, and offers links and information about the Center's research activities.

YAWN: Young Adults with Narcolepsy

http://www.yawn.org/

Offers news, education, support and advocacy group information on narcolepsy, especially for young people with this disorder.

Organizations

American Sleep Disorder Association

http://www.asda.org/

A professional medical association representing practitioners of sleep medicine and sleep research. Site provides information on membership, educational opportunities and accreditation, as well as patient information on sleep disorders and their treatments.

National Sleep Foundation

http://www.sleepfoundation.org/

Includes information on sleep disorders, sleep links, publications, activities and projects of the Foundation.

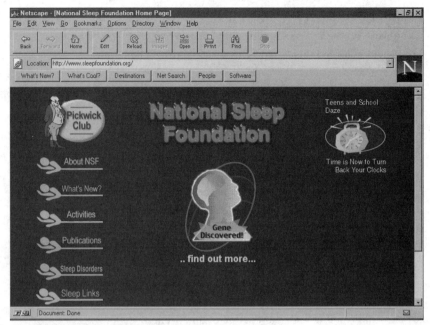

National Sleep Foundation. http://www.sleepfoundation.org/

Restless Leg Syndrome

Restless Leg Syndrome Support Site
http://www.rls.org/

Patient information, medical facts, support groups and research on restless leg syndrome (RLS), which can lead to severe insomnia and escessive daytime sleepiness.

Restless Legs Syndrome Foundation, Inc.
http://www.stepstn.com/nord/org_sum/77.htm

Basic information from the National Organization of Rare Disorders, with contact information.

Restless Legs Syndrome Information
http://www.ninds.nih.gov/patients/disorder/restless/restless.htm#description

Briefly describes RLS, its treatment and prognosis.

Vitamin Dispenser: Restless Leg Syndrome

http://www.prevention.com/healing/vitamin/ail/restlesslegs/?lec

Provides information on nutrients which may help this disorder.

Sleep Apnea & Snoring

Airway Examples

http://www.sleep-breathing.bc.ca/airway.htm

Illustrates the air passage as it appears during primary snoring, as well as snoring with accompanying mild, moderately severe, and severe obstructive sleep apnea.

A.W.A.K.E. New York

http://www.bway.net/~marlene/awake.html

Includes articles as well as information on local meetings. Sleep apnea is the cessation of breathing for a short period of time while sleeping.

Causes of Snoring

http://www.sleep-breathing.bc.ca/osa1.htm

The causes of snoring are divided into intrinsic factors, which are unique to the individual, and into extrinsic factors, which are related to the individual's environment and life style.

Central Sleep Apnea Informational Page

http://members.aol.com/blackcover/csa.html

Site answers frequently asked questions, describes symptoms and treatments, and offers a list of links as well as a glossary of sleep-related terms. Includes the personal account of one patient's experience with the diagnosis and treatment of sleep apnea.

Mark's Sleep Apnea Page

http://www.winternet.com/~mbiegert/apnea.htm

Long list of questions about sleep apnea and what can be done about it. Lots of helpful information gathered by someone who has suffered from the disorder.

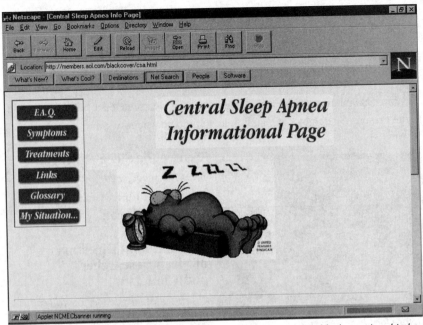

Central Sleep Apnea Informational Page. http://members.aol.com/blackcover/csa.html

Phantom Sleep Page
http://www.newtechpub.com/phantom/

Discusses sleep apnea, snoring, and other sleep problems.

Sleep Apnea Information Clearinghouse
http://www.pilgrimvoices.com/apnea/

Includes apnea questions and answers, articles, stories, links, tips, support and chat, as well as the the Epworth Sleepiness Scale, a survey and the opportunity to submit your questions to a sleep specialist.

Snoring & Sleep Apnea
http://www.sleep-breathing.bc.ca/prod01.htm

People who snore may be at risk for sleep apnea. This site educates the public on the implications of snoring, and describes treatments that are available.

Snoring: Measures to Silence the Sawing
http://www.healthyideas.com/children/remedies/virtped.snoring.html

Suggestions on what you can do if your child snores, and when it may be advisable to see a physician.

Research

BiblioSleep
http://www.websciences.org/bibliosleep/

Presents citations and abstracts on published sleep-related articles from 1992 to the present. Search by date, author, keyword and category.

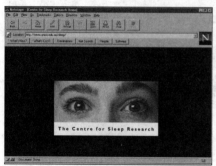

Centre for Sleep Research.
http://www.unisa.edu.au/sleep/

Centre for Sleep Research
http://www.unisa.edu.au/sleep/

Poetry, art, research, publications and more. A beautifully-designed site.

International Directory of Sleep Researchers and Clinicians
http://www.websciences.org/directory/

Select a geographical area or enter an individual's last name to search this global directory.

Sleep and Health
http://www.websciences.org/sleepandhealth/

Research and clinical perspectives.

SURGERY

Anesthesiology

American Society of Anesthesiologists
http://www.asahq.org/
Information for the general public and the anesthesiology profession, Society news, continuing education and links.

Anesthesiology
http://anesthesiology.about.com/
Links to associations, commercial sites, companies, critical care sites, discussion groups, frequently asked questions, patient education sites and much more. "Spotlight" features selected resources and articles.

Anesthesiology Clinical Manuals and Resources
http://www.anes.ccf.org:8080/lab2.htm
Educational pamphlets on: *Anesthetic Management of the Latex-Allergic Patient, ENT Anesthesia, Neuroanesthesia,* and *Anesthesia for Orthopedic Surgery.*

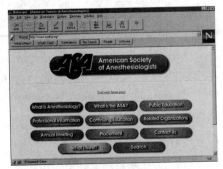

Anesthesiology Journals
http://www.sciencekomm.at/journals /medicine/ana.html
Links to information about forty different anesthesiology journals.

American Society of Anesthesiologists.
http://www.asahq.org/

GASNet

http://gasnet.med.yale.edu/

The Global Anesthesiology Server Network (GASNet) is for the anesthesiology community world-wide. Abstracts, journals, newsletters, meetings, book reviews, discussion groups, software and video library, further links to anesthesiology organizations and information sites are all provided at this site. The reference area includes the *Global Textbook of Anesthesiology*.

The Journal *Anesthesiology*

http://www.anesthesiology.org/

This is the journal of the American Society of Anesthesiologists.

Virtual Anaesthesia Textbook

http://gasnet.med.yale.edu/vat/VAT.html

The goal of the Virtual Anaesthesia Textbook (VAT) is to create and maintain a comprehensive set of links to all known anaesthesia-related Internet information, for health care professionals.

Virtual Museum of Anesthesiology

http://umdas.med.miami.edu/aha/vma

Historical images, written works, information and resources regarding the history of anesthesiology. Includes a portrait gallery and images of early anesthetic equipment and devices, as well as written archives.

Wright's Anesthesia and Critical Care Resources on the Internet (ACCRI)

http://www.eur.nl/FGG/ANEST/wright/

Site provides a link to the ACCRI discussion group on anesthesiology and critical care topics. This thorough and precise site includes news and a featured Internet site of the month, a discussion list, FTP sites, peer-reviewed journals, other gopher resources, and an exhaustive list of hundreds of anesthesiology websites around the world. A bibliography and non-net educational resources (mostly software and CD-ROM) are offered as well.

Cardiac Surgery

See also: Heart & Veins/Cardiovascular.

Cardiac Surgery

http://www.cardio-info.com/lnksusrg.htm

Many links to cardiology and cardiac surgery sites.

Cardiac Surgery

http://www.doctorpage.com/Diseases_and_Conditions/html/cardiac_surgery.h tm

Links to information on cardiac surgery, including how to find a surgeon.

Cardiac Surgery Glossary

http://www.musc.edu/chp-clin/ect/glossary.htm

Defines important terms and acronyms encountered in perfusion technology, open heart surgery, and cardiology.

Cardiac Surgery in the Adult

http://www.ctsnet.org/doc/3174

Online textbook. Requires advanced browser capability.

Heart Disease Online

http://www.dencats.org/heart/disease.htm

Congenital heart disease, heart valve disease, coronary artery disease, heart failure and related heart surgical topics are discussed.

Heart Surgery Forum

http://www.hsforum.com/

Journal for cardiac surgery professionals. Contains subscription information, e-mail forums, literature searches, a learning center, links and much more.

Surgery for Coronary Artery Disease

http://www.geocities.com/HotSprings/1652/surgery.html

Explains coronary bypass surgery, as well as vein and arterial grafts.

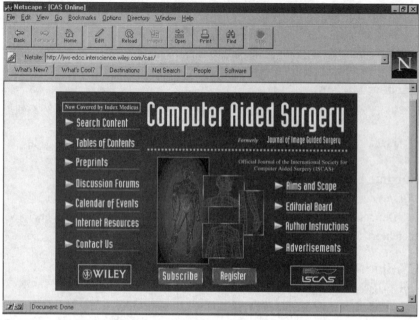

Computer Aided Surgery. *http://journals.wiley.com/cas/*

Cataract Surgery

See also: Eyes/Optometry & Opthalmology - Cataracts.

Cataract Surgery

http://www.steen-hall.com/cataract.html

Overview of the eye and cataracts, and explanation of cataract surgery and patient follow-up. Prepared for patients.

Cataract Surgery: Frequently Asked Questions

http://www.ascrs.org/patient/catafaq.html

Common questions are answered by the American Society of Cataract and Refractive Surgery, for patients.

Cataract Surgery Techniques

http://www.eyenet.org/public/faqs/cataract/cat_techniques.html

Describes different types of cataract surgical procedures. Includes Quicktime movie clips.

History of Cataract Surgery

http://www.eyenet.org/public/museum/history.html

Details on the history of this procedure. The earliest written reference to cataract surgery is found in Sanskrit manuscripts dating from the 5th century BC, but the past 50 years have shown remarkable refinements.

Computers and Surgery

Computer Aided Surgery

http://journals.wiley.com/cas/

Search text, view table of contents, join discussion forums and learn how to subscribe to this journal.

International Society for Computer Aided Surgery

http://www.iscas.org/

Site provides the missions, aims, goals, activities and membership requirements for this nonprofit organization that seeks to encourage the scientific and clinical advancement of computer-aided surgery and related medical interventions throughout the world.

Internet Resources of Computer Aided Surgery

http://www.aist.go.jp/NIBH/~b0673/english/cas.html

Offers web resources regarding future technology in surgery, such as computerized surgical planning, surgical navigation, image-guided sugery, surgical robotics and virtual reality in medicine.

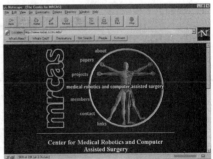

Medical Robotics and Computer-Assisted Surgery

http://www.mrcas.ri.cmu.edu/

Site provides online versions of published papers, describes projects under development, links and member information.

Medical Robotics and Computer-Assisted Surgery. *http://www.mrcas.ri.cmu.edu/*

Video Surgery

http://www.mindspring.com/~videosur/

Video surgery may be used for treatment of heartburn, hiatal hernias, gastro-esophogeal reflux disease and inguinal hernias. Information on common health problems, their causes and treatment, and answers frequently asked questions.

Virtual Environments and Real-Time Deformations for Surgery Simulation

http://www.cc.gatech.edu/gvu/visualization/surgsim/

The goal of this project is to explore deformations of organs in a surgery scene while emphasizing real-time interaction.

What is Computer Aided Surgery?

http://www.aist.go.jp/NIBH/~b0673/english/cas_about.html

Basic questions and answers.

Dental and Oral Surgery

See also: Dentistry.

American Academy of Otolaryngology Head and Neck Surgery

http://www.ent.net.org/

Website for the world's largest organization of physicians dedicated to the care of ear, nose and throat disorders. It offers patient information, clinical indicators, research, a journal, meeting and education information, organization links and even a virtual museum.

Columbia-Presbyterian Medical Center School of Dental and Oral Surgery

http://cpmcnet.columbia.edu/dept/dental/

Information about the Columbia program, courses and tutorials in dental ethics, dental informatics, dental trauma, oral pathology and more.

Department of Oral and Maxillofacial Surgery

http://itsa.ucsf.edu/~ucomfs/omfs.html

Describes the University of California at San Francisco residency training and predoctoral programs, OMFS curriculum, research and faculty. Links to Internet sites on related topics.

Maxillofacial Surgery Resources on the Web

http://bpass.dentistry.dal.ca/mfsurg.html

Maxillofacial resources on the Internet, with a description of the sites.

Oral and Maxillofacial Surgery Online

http://www.omfs.org/

This journal is free to professionals. The site provides access to news, feature articles, patient health information, discussion forums, meeting information, and related links.

Oral Surgery Center

http://cust.iamerica.net/molar/

Links to maxillofacial surgery departments at academic institutes and to related dentistry and medical sites. There is also a maxillofacial graphic-of-the-month.

General Surgery

American College of Surgeons

http://www.facs.org/

Information for members and for the general public. Link to the *Journal of the American College of Surgery*, and other publications.

AskPhysicians.com

http://www.askphysicians.com/

Post your question about any surgical procedure to the bulletin board.

Association of Women Surgeons

http://www.womensurgeons.org/

The mission of this organization is "to inspire, encourage, and enable women surgeons to realize their professional and personal goals."

General Surgery

http://www.vh.org/Providers/ClinRef/FPHandbook/09.html

From the Family Practice Handbook of the University of Iowa, this site discusses wound management, pre-op and post-op care. Some sections include the general surgical treatment of abdominal pain, appendicitis, gall bladder disorders, burns and more. Written in outline form.

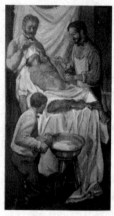

International Museum of Surgical Science
http://www.imss.org/

View displays on over 4,000 years of surgical history. One exhibit allows viewers to play "interactive antique illness" to see how they would fare having an illness in 19th century America.

Medscape Surgery Home Page
http://surgery.medscape.com/Home/Topics/surgery/surgery.html

Surgery articles, news, discussions and links.

International Museum of Surgical Science. http://imss.org/

Questions to Ask Your Doctor Before You Have Surgery
http://www.ahcpr.gov/consumer/surgery.htm

Checklist of questions that should be answered and understood before you undergo a surgical operation, and the reasons for asking them. Assembled by the Agency for Health Care Policy and Research. Additional resources are also listed.

Surgery
http://surgery.about.com/

Select from a long list of surgical specialtes, or link to journals, organizations, and collections of frequently asked questions.

Your Surgery.com
http://www.yoursurgery.com/

This is a multimedia database of the most common surgical procedures, for patient education. Select the surgery you are interested in, and you can view images and animations, receive information on symptoms, anatomy of the area, description of the surgical procedure, potential complications and recovery.

Neurosurgery

See also: Brain & Brain Disorders.

Angel Neurosurgical Information

http://www.usc.edu/hsc/neurosurgery/angel.html

This site from the University of Southern California Department of Neuro-surgery offers information for consumers, residents, students, and neuropracti-tioners.

Brain Surgery Information Center

http://www.brain-surgery.com/

"Everything you wanted to know about brain surgery. . . almost." The goal of this site is to provide usable, non-technical information about the conditions which require brain surgery. It offers a primer on brain tumors, information on aneurysms, hemorrhages, and other sources of "brain attack." The site also describes the brain surgery patient's experience.

The Center for Spine Surgery at NYU

_http://mcns10.med.nyu.edu/spine/spine_main.html_

Includes information about some spinal disorders and their treatment.

Department of Neurosurgery at NYU

http://mcns10.med.nyu.edu/index.html

This site serves as a resource center for patients suffering from neurological disorders, their families and health care professionals. Electronic consultations are invited, and the site also provides access to support groups for individuals who have undergone neurosurgery. The Neurosurgery Internet Grand Rounds includes actual case studies.

MedMark Neurosurgery

http://www.medmark.org/ns/

Many links to neurosurgery sites. Includes a long list of associations/societies, as well as links to academic department/divisions, consumer information, general neurosurgery information, journals, and material on different neurosurgical specialties.

NeuroNews

http://www.neurosurgery-neff.com/

This site is a resource for physicians and interested lay people and provides information on neurosurgical patient care, education, treatments of diseases of the nervous system, and research.

Neurosurgery://On-Call

http://www.neurosurgery.org/splash.html

This website for the American Association of Neurological Surgeons and Congress of Neurological Surgeons is divided into professional and public pages. The former contains education, news, journals, library, and meeting information, while the latter contain patient resources which explain neurosurgery and neurosurgical news topics, assistance in locating a neurosurgeon, and issues of particular concern to patients.

NeuroWorld

http://neuroworld.com/

"Global portal" to neurology, neurosurgery, neuroradiology and related areas. For neuromedical professionals, provides links to clinical topics, library of resources and journals, news, chapters and online textbooks.

Topics in Neurosurgery

http://neurosurgeon.com/

Specific links to sites in the field of neurosurgery, and a global directory of neurosurgeons.

Orthopedic Surgery

American Academy of Orthopaedic Surgeons

http://www.aaos.org/

Member information, as well as information for the public and media.

American Association of Hip and Knee Surgeons

http://www.aahks.org/

Contains mostly member and conference information, along with links to related orthopedic sites on the Internet.

Online Clinic for Sports Medicine and Orthopedic Surgery

http://www.sports-medicine.com/

Dr. Zeman will answer your medical questions for a small fee, and he offers free general advice and tips on heel pain, carpal tunnel syndrome, knee pain, tennis elbow, spine and hip pain, shin splints and sprained ankles. Special section on golf injuries, accidents and legal medicine.

Orthopaedic Surgery Residency Ring

http://www.webring.org/cgi-bin/webring?ring=orthosurg;list

Jump to any of thirty-six different sites of interest to orthopedic surgery residents.

Orthopedic Surgery Mailing List

http://www.sechrest.com/ortho/index.html

Site provides information on the orthopedic mailing list, but also membership directory, newsgroups, orthopedic surgery grand rounds, FTP site, and numerous related links. To subscribe, send e-mail to: *orthopedic-request@weston.com* with the following message: "SUBSCRIBE *Yourfirstname Yourlastname.*"

OrthoSearch

http://www.orthosearch.com/servlet/BackBone/0/4/1

Search the web for orthopedic surgery and related information.

Pain Management

See also: Pain & Pain Management chapter.

Chronic Pain Q and A

http://www.neurosurgery.org/pubpages/patres/faq_chronicpain.html

Frequently asked questions about chronic pain and the neurosurgeon's role in treating it.

Pain Control after Surgery

http://text.nlm.nih.gov/ftrs/pick?ftrsK=0&collect=ahcpr&dbName=apmp&t=845876946

Patient brochure from the Agency for Health Care Policy Research explains the goal of pain control after surgery, and the types of treatment you may receive.

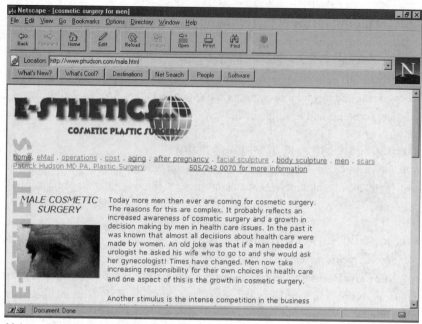

Male cosmetic surgery at: **E-STHETICS**. http://www.phudson.com/

Plastic and Reconstructive Surgery

American Society for Aesthetic Plastic Surgery

http://surgery.org/

Describes the most common cosmetic surgery procedures and offers advice on selecting a qualified surgeon. Site is geared to anybody considering a cosmetic surgical procedure, from eye-lid surgery to "body contouring."

Cosmetic Surgery Online Information

http://www.mayo.edu/staff/plastic/Cosmetic/CSOLMain.html

Site discusses who may be a candidate for cosmetic surgery, what the surgery will entail, and a description of various cosmetic surgical procedures.

Cosmetic.org

http://www.cosmetic.org/

For consumers and professionals. Learn about cosmetic procedures, including what is safe, what to expect, and what to ask for when consulting with your doctor. Chat online, or send a question to an expert.

E-STHETICS

http://www.phudson.com/

Information on aging, plastic surgery after pregnancy, male cosmetic surgery, facial and body sculpturing and scar revision. Details about major operations such as facelifting, liposuction, breast enlargement and abdominoplasty (tummy tuck). Choose a problem or an operation to review. Chat room and message board are also provided.

Interplast

http://www.interplast.org/

Interplast is an affiliation of volunteer surgeons, pediatricians, anesthesiologists, nurses and support personnel who work with third world nations to support and develop a free reconstructive surgery programs for children and adults with birth defects, burns, and

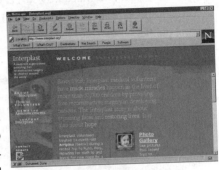

Interplast. *http://www.interplast.org/*

other crippling deformities. The organization performs over 1500 free surgeries annually. Information about the organization and the trips it has scheduled may be found at this site.

Plastic Surgery Information Service

http://www.plasticsurgery.org/

Site is maintained by the American Society of Plastic and Reconstructive Surgeons and the Plastic Surgery Educational Foundation. It provides news, the latest advances and techniques, professional information, statistics, and a referral service.

Plastic Surgery Network

http://www.plastic-surgery.net/

Offers information on procedures and doctor referrals.

P-Link, the Plastic Surgery Link

http://www.nvpc.nl/plink/

Provides numerous links to societies, journals, academic and medical organizations, newsgroups, research programs, and more related to plastic surgery. Subjects include aesthetics, hand surgery, traumatology, reconstructive surgery, micro-surgery, craniomaxillofacial surgery, and others.

Procedures at a Glance

http://www.plasticsurgery.org/surgery/cosmetic.htm

Online brochure describes basic cosmetic surgical procedures. Includes the length of time, side effects, risks, recovery, and duration of results.

University of Iowa Plastic Surgery

http://www.surgery.uiowa.edu:80/surgery/plastic/

Reconstructive and cosmetic surgical procedures for potential patients and the general public.

World Plastic Surgery

http://www.ipras.org/

The International Plastic, Reconstructive and Aesthetic Surgery website. Contains a long list of links and details on the organization's activities.

TRANSPLANTATION

Bone Marrow

See also: Cancer/Oncology - Bone Marrow Transplantation.

Bone Marrow Donors Worldwide

http://WWW.BMDW.ORG/

Collects information on bone marrow donors from 43 donor and cord blood registries in 30 countries, and seeks to match them up with BMT recipients.

The Bone Marrow Foundation

http://www.bonemarrow.org/

Patient aid, resources, frequently asked questions, literature, and "ask the expert."

Bone Marrow Transplantation Branch

http://www.hrsa.dhhs.gov/osp/dot/bone.htm

This group oversees the National Marrow Donor Program, and helps patients suffering from leukemia or other blood diseases to find matching unrelated volunteer marrow donors for transplants. The NMDP also performs research.

National Bone Marrow Transplant Links

http://comnet.org/nbmtlink/

Information for those considering undergoing a bone marrow transplant. This site offers a resource guide, survivor's guide, frequently asked questions, and information on stem cell transplant for breast cancer patients.

National Marrow Donor Program Online
http://www.marrow-donor.org/index.html
> Donor information, patient information, and facts for the media.

Ethics

Bioethics: Xenotransplantation
http://www.ccf.org/ed/bioethic/biocon10.htm
> Xenotransplantation involves the use of live, non-human animal cells, tissues and organs in human patients.

Campaign for Responsible Transplantation
http://www.crt-online.org/
> This organization believes that xenotransplantation poses a grave danger to humans because of the risk of transferring deadly viruses. Because they believe there are alternatives, they seek a complete ban on xenotransplantation. Site offers press releases, legal petitions, news, publications and resources, links, and information on how to join.

Can We Transplant Organs from Animals?
http://whyfiles.news.wisc.edu/007transplant/index.html
> Information and discussion of cross-species transplantation.

Transplant Ethics
gopher://info.med.yale.edu:70/11/Disciplines/Disease/Transplant/Ethics
> Documents discussing the ethics of presumed consent, financial incentives for organ donors, and the preferred status for organ donors.

Financial Help

Current Patient Campaigns
http://transplants.org/patient/tblpatie.html
> Information about individuals who need financial help to pay for transplantation costs. Posted by the National Foundation for Transplants.

Financial Assistance

http://www.transplantawareness.org/resguide/chap20.htm

Hints on where to get help to pay for transplantation costs, post-transplant care and medications.

Financing Your Transplant

http://207.239.150.10/patients/101%5Ffinance.htm

Discusses medical and non-medical costs for transplantation procedures; common funding sources, and programs which help pay for the cost of care after transplantation.

Indigent Drug Programs

http://www.insulin-free.org/articles/drugprogs.htm

Some information on programs that help people who can't afford medications.

Let COTA Help You

http://www.cota.org/helpyou/helpyou.html

Information on how to apply for assistance from the Children's Organ Transplant Association.

National Transplant Assistance Fund

http://www.transplantfund.org/

Offers educational information, expertise for patients raising money for transplants, and financial support via medical assistance grants.

General Resources

CenterSpan

http://www.centerspan.org/

Transplant news, Internet resources, online abstracts, publications, and a tutorial for health care professionals. Full articles from the journal, *Transplantation*, are available for all members of the American Society of Transplantation or the American Society of Transplant Surgeons.

Division of Transplantation
http://www.hrsa.dhhs.gov/osp/dot/

The Division of Transplantation (DOT) of the Health Resources and Services Administration, Department of Health and Human Services, manages the Organ Procurement and Transplantation Network and other organ transplant registries. DOT also provides assistance to organ procurement organizations and acts in the area of public education. This site provides facts and statistics about solid organ and bone marrow transplantation, including technical data, health guidelines, a description of the donation and transplantation processes, and links to further organizations and publications.

Division of Allergy, Immunology and Transplantation
http://www.niaid.nih.gov/research/dait.htm

DAIT supports research in genetics and transplantation for several reasons: 1) to clarify the organization and the mechanisms of expression of the genes on which immune function depends; 2) to characterize the protein products of the genes; 3) to determine the manner in which these gene products condition the responses to foreign antigens; and 4) to develop and facilitate engraftment of transplanted organs and tissue.

Emory Transplant Center
http://Picasso.eushc.org/transplant/homepage.cgi

Donation information and links for patients and their families.

Experimental Organ Preservation
http://sapphire.surgery.wisc.edu/preservation/

The primary interests of this lab located at the University of Wisconsin Clinical Sciences Center are in organ preservation and transplantation, and associated fields. Specific organs they are interested in preserving include the kidney, liver, heart, lung, intestine and pancreas.

Giving Life
http://www.ama-assn.org/sci-pubs/journals/archive/jama/vol_280/no_13/pp1007.htm

This web page from the *Journal of the American Medical Association* (*JAMA*) provides information on donating your organs and tissues, and why it is so valuable.

Glossary of Terms
http://www.niaid.nih.gov/publications/transplant/glossary.htm
Terms used in transplantation science, from "allogeneic" to "xenogeneic."

NIT Patient Education Program
http://www.transplantation.com/patient.htm
Provides ten online brochures, in both English and Spanish, which were created to fully inform the potential transplant patient about the transplant process, to influence the patient to take an active role in caring for his or her pre- and post-transplant health, and to improve the transplant outcome.

Organ Donation/Transplantation
http://www.midland-memorial.com/organweb.htm
Website links, with brief descriptions.

Surviving Transplantation
http://www.stjosephs.london.on.ca/SJHC/programs/mental/survive/
An online book that is a guide to coping for people who are undergoing a major organ transplant.

Transplant Centers with Web Sites
http://transweb.org/reference/sites/centers.htm
Although the majority of the centers listed are located in North America, there are also links to websites of transplant centers found in Asia, Europe and the Philippines.

The Transplant Journey
http://www.transweb.org/journey/index.html
A multimedia guide to the transplantation process.

Transplant Resources
http://www.uchsc.edu/ctrsinst/organtx/resource.htm
Links to transplant-related sites and to transplant centers with a web presence.

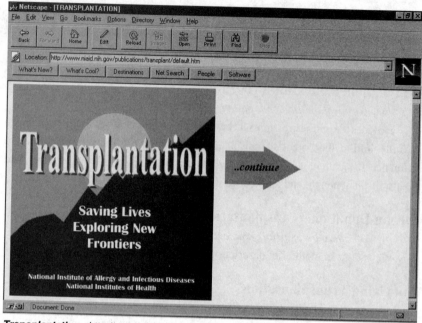

Transplantation. http://www.niaid.nih.gov/publications/transplant/default.htm

Transplantation

http://www.niaid.nih.gov/publications/transplant/default.htm

Online brochure that provides an overview of the ways scientists are resolving the problems facing transplantation today, the accomplishments of NIAID-supported investigators, and the prospects for the future when transplantation will involve not just organs and tissues, but cells and genes.

Transplantation on the Web

http://hageman.trnovo.kclj.si/transplant/transweb_e.html

Web resources related to organ and tissue transplantation. Includes not only general resources, but also links to transplantation centers, donor organizations and organ banks, brain death resources, information on histocompatability and bone marrow transplantation.

TransWeb

http://www.transweb.org/

All about organ transplantation and donation. This site includes news, research and patient information, personal stories of transplants, as well as frequently asked questions and answers. Additional resources, organizations and a library search are also available.

Heart/Heart & Lung

Heart and Heart-Lung Transplant
http://thedailyapple.com/Level3/ds3/cardiov/trhmdv3.htm

Approximately 2,300 heart transplants are performed each year in the United States, and about 500 people receive heart-lung transplants. This site provides public and patient information on what happens during a transplant, who can have it, risks, cost and more.

Heart Transplantation
http://heartdisease.about.com/msubtx.htm?pid=2750&cob=home

Collection of Internet links with brief description.

Heart Transplantation at UCLA
http://www.nursing.ucla.edu/Userpages/mwoo/special/htx.htm

Evaluation and management, pre- and post-transplant protocols, patient selection criteria, policies and procedures.

Heart Transplants and Statistics
http://www.americanheart.org/Heart_and_Stroke_A_Z_Guide/htrans.html

Basic information from the American Heart Association.

The International Society for Heart & Lung Transplantation
http://www.ishlt.org/

Society and program information, transplant registry, heart-failure registry and access to statistics.

Jon's Heart Transplant Page
http://www.geocities.com/Heartland/Hills/2571/CHFtransplant.htm

Site addresses basic questions regarding heart transplantation.

My Heart Transplant
http://jensoft-cs.com/heart.htm

One heart transplant recipient's experience, thoughts and support group information.

Questions about Heart and Lung Transplantation

http://www.transweb.org/qa/qa_txp/faq_heartlung.html

Answers common questions and provides statistics.

Kidney and Pancreas

Insulin-Free.org

http://www.insulin-free.org/

This site seeks to be a comprehensive and current source of information about immunology and transplantation as they relate to diabetes. The organization's goal is to ensure access to pancreas transplantation, and to make islet transplantation a clinical reality for all diabetics.

Kidney Transplant/Dialysis Association

http://www.ultranet.com/~ktda/index.shtml

This organization is dedicated to providing financial aid, information, and emotional support to chronic renal disease patients and their families. Site contains patient information, pen pals, information on how to join and on how to help out.

Kidney Transplant

http://www.niddk.nih.gov/health/kidney/summary/transpla/transpla.htm

Provides contact information for kidney transplantation resources, from the National Institute of Diabetes and Digestive and Kidney Diseases.

My Kidney/Pancreas Transplant

http://members.aol.com/OhLarry922/home.html

Personal story, list of hospitals and centers that perform kidney/pancreas transplants, chat group information and links to related sites.

Pancreas Transplantation

http://www.diabetesmonitor.com/transplt.htm

Article from the *Diabetes Monitor*, with links.

A Small Part of Me

http://home.ici.net/~kenneth/aspomka.htm

Information on a book authored by a man who donated his kidney to his brother.

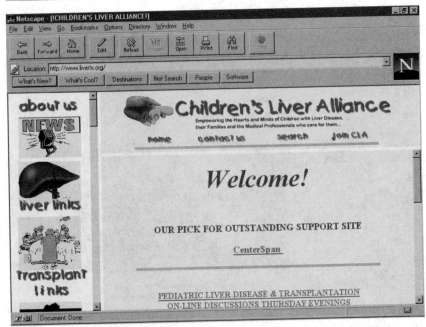

Children's Liver Alliance. http://www.livertx.org/

Tissot Family Kidney Transplant Stories

http://www.tissotfamily.com/kidney.html

A personal page created to promote living-donor kidney transplantation.

Transplant Patient Partnering Program

http://www.ktppp.com/

Support for transplant patients, their families and caregivers. The history of kidney transplants is presented, along with finding a kidney, the finances involved, rejection, and much more information on the pre- and post-transplant experience.

Liver

Children's Liver Alliance

http://www.livertx.org/

This is the largest pediatric liver organization world-wide. It is dedicated to empowering children with liver disease, their families and the medical professionals who care for them. Liver links, transplant links, news, newsletter and chat room.

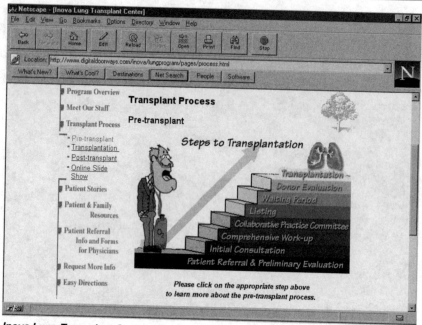

Inova Lung Transplant Center. http://www.digitaldoorways.com/inova/lungprogram/

Facts and FAQs on Liver Transplantation

http://sadieo.ucsf.edu/alf/alffinal/infoltxfaqs.html

This online pamphlet addresses some common questions about liver transplantation.

Hepatitis Haven

http://www.tiac.net/users/birdlady/hep.html

Set up for those who have chronic hepatitis, this site contains personal stories and pictures of individuals suffering from hepatitis, a directory of doctors and support groups, tips for receiving Social Security, and liver transplant information.

Liver Transplant Links

http://www.livertx.org/txlinks.html

Long list of alphabetized links to transplantation sites.

Lung

Inova Lung Transplant Center
http://www.digitaldoorways.com/inova/lungprogram/

An overview of this center's lung transplant program, as well as facts on various aspects of transplantation. Site has patient and family resources, describes the transplant process, offers patient stories and links. For patients who may need a lung transplant, people who are recipients, family members, friends, physicians, and allied health professionals.

Physical Therapy in Lung Transplantion
_http://www.apta.org/pt_journal/abstracts/down.html_

Abstract of an article that appeared in _Physical Therapy._

Second Wind Lung Transplant Association, Inc.
http://www.2ndwind.org/

Member information, transplantation self-help programs, patient stories and links to personal web pages, frequently asked questions, and mailing list archives (for members).

Medications

Post-Transplant Medications
http://www.geocities.com/Athens/Oracle/5231/posttx.html

Information on financial assistance available to individuals who may need aid in obtaining prescription medications.

Transplant Medications
_http://www.transweb.org/reference/articles/drugs/drug_index.html_

Information on several drugs used in transplant cases.

What Types of Medications Will I Be Taking?
http://www.transplantation.com/instruct.htm

Descriptions of the immunosuppressive drugs commonly used following transplants, along with instructions and potential side effects.

Organizations

American Society of Transplantation
http://www.a-s-t.org/

New name for the American Society of Transplant Physicians.

Children's Organ Transplant Association
http://www.cota.org/

COTA's primary mission is to ensure that no U.S. citizen is ever denied a life-saving transplant or access to a transplant waiting list due to the lack of funds.
National Foundation for Transplantation
http://transplants.org/

Information, financial support and patient advocacy.

National Institute of Transplantation
http://www.transplantation.com/

Information on the Institute and its many programs, which cover all scientific areas of organ transplantation, including laboratory and clinical research as well as professional and public education.

Transplant Awareness
http://www.transplantawareness.org/

This nonprofit organization promotes organ donation by marketing products that will promote organ donation and increasing awareness among the general population. All of the profit from the sale of their merchandise goes toward increasing organ and tissue transplantation awareness.

Transplantation: Organizations
http://www.rotrf.org/35es.htm

Links to a number of transplant organizations.

The Transplantation Society
http://www.transplantation-soc.org/

Forum for physicians and scientists to discuss transplantation issues. Site provides a journal, abstracts, meeting and membership information.

United Network for Organ Sharing

http://www.unos.org/

This site provides facts and statistics about organ transplantation. "Transplant 101" offers answers to common patient concerns. Information on specific organs, data on survival, prevalence, and a brief history of transplantation are available. Also find UNOS resources and policy proposals, events, legislation, publications and related websites.

VIRTUAL MEDICINE & MULTIMEDIA

> *Covered in this chapter*: Anatomy; Brain; Heart; Interactive Medicine; Links; Mental Health; Multimedia & References; Projects & Software; Surgery; Visible Human.
>
> *Related chapters*: Biomedicine; Medical Imaging/Telemedicine; Surgery.

Anatomy

Anatomy of the Human Body
http://rpisun1.mda.uth.tmc.edu/mmlearn/anatomy.html
Online book of anatomy.

Digital Anatomist Program Interactive Atlases
http://www9.biostr.washington.edu/da.html
Interactive atlases of the brain, neuro system, thoracic organs, and knee. With colorful graphics, radiological images and three-dimensional (3-D) animations.

The Interactive Ankle
http://rpiwww.mdacc.tmc.edu/cgi-bin/ankle_engine
Learn to identify bone, muscle, nerve and vein parts in the human ankle.

Normal Radiologic Anatomy
http://www.vh.org/Providers/TeachingFiles/NormalRadAnatomy/Text/RRadM1 title.html
X-ray, computed tomography (CT), magnetic resonance (MR) and ultrasound images of the head and neck, thorax, abdomen, pelvis, upper and lower extremities.

Skull Module
http://www.csuchico.edu/anth/Module/skull.html
Characteristic features of skull bones are identified, and animations are available to learn some of the trickier three-dimensional views.

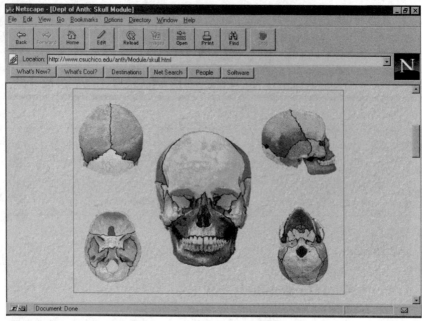

Skull Module. http://www.csuchico.edu/anth/Module/skull.html

Three Dimensional Medical Reconstruction

http://www.crd.ge.com/esl/cgsp/projects/medical/

A collection of movie clips showing various medical reconstructions, such as colon, lung, brain, torso and skull "fly-throughs." Images were gathered from slice data from medical imaging modalities, such as magnetic resonance or computed tomography. The two-dimensional slice data from these scanners was used as input for the three-dimensional reconstructions.

Virtual Anatomy Project

http://www.vis.colostate.edu/library/gva/gva.html

Site describes this Colorado State University program to generate a 3-D geometric database of the human body.

The Virtual Body

http://www.medtropolis.com/vbody/

Using Macromedia's Shockwave technology (information on how to use this plugin supplied), view downloadable presentations of the brain, heart, digestive system and skeleton.

Virtual Tour of the Ear

http://ctl.augie.edu/perry/ear/ear.htm

Learn about hearing, ear anatomy function and ear disorders. A number of images and diagrams, with text.

Brain

Dissections of the Real Brain

http://www.vh.org/Providers/Textbooks/BrainAnatomy/BrainAnatomy.html

Images and diagrams, with minimal text. Main chapters include the spinal cord, meninges, blood vessels, cerebellum, brain stem, and cerebral hemispheres.

Human Brain Project

http://WWW-HBP.scripps.edu/Home.html

The Human Brain Project is a long-term research initiative to create a database containing a full range of information about the brain, behavior, and related technological services. Its goal is to help scientists learn how various aspects of the brain function together. This site at Scripps Research Institute is the "master server," and connects to 21 other research institutions which have contributed to the Brain Project Database. Some of the projects currently being undertaken include language/brain mapping, a neural simulation project, a study of the action of drugs on the nervous system, and a 3-D reconstruction of the cerebral cortex.

The Human Brain: A Mystery to Itself

http://library.advanced.org/26463/

Fun, interactive site to learn about the brain. Includes games and articles of human interest. Available in English or Spanish.

A Short Tour of the Brain

http://werple.mira.net.au/~dhs/brain.htm

From the Alzheimer's Web, a short tour of the brain with animated graphics.

The UW Human Brain Project

http://www1.biostr.washington.edu/BrainProject.html

This project's goal is to develop a system for organizing, visualizing, integrating and sharing information about human language function.

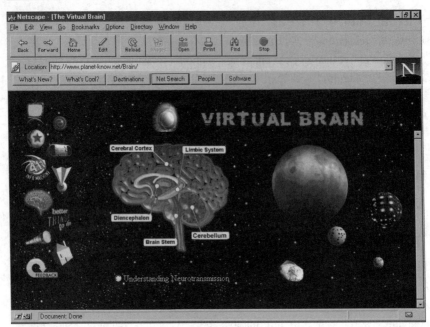

The Virtual Brain. http://www.planet-know.net/Brain/

The Virtual Brain

http://www.planet-know.net/Brain/

Identifies the parts of the brain, and discusses the affects various mind-altering drugs have on them.

Whole Brain Atlas

http://sig.biostr.washington.edu/projects/brain/

Computed tomography (CT), magnetic resonance (MR) and other radiographic images of a normal brain and of brains from patients with cerebrovascular disease, neoplastic disease, degenerative disease, and inflammatory or infectious diseases. The images may be accessed in sequence, and specific views and anatomic parts of the brain may be selected. The accompanying neuroimaging primer is geared towards those without a technical background. "Tours" and time-lapse "movies" are also provided.

Heart

The Heart: An Online Exploration
http://sln.fi.edu/biosci/heart.html

This is a great site for the general public and especially children to learn everything about the heart: anatomy, development, function and health tips. Find images and movies depicting open heart surgery and blood flow, along with recordings of actual heartbeats. Less scientific topics such as the heart in literature and poetry, healthy recipes and exercises are also included.

Interactive Medicine

Interactive Patient
http://medicus.marshall.edu/medicus.htm

This site is a teaching tool for physicians, residents and medical students. Simulating an actual patient encounter, the patient's chief complaint is provided, and it is up to the user to ask the proper questions to obtain additional history, physical exam information, tests, and x-rays, then to come up with a diagnosis and treatment plan. The diagnosis and treatment plan are submitted over the web, and feedback is provided.

Net Medicine
http://www.netmedicine.com/

Features the Cyberpatient Simulator ("see if you can save the patient"), as well as Medfinder search, EKG of the Month, Radiology Rounds and Pediatric Topics.

Outline of the Virtual Hospital
http://www.vh.org/Misc/Outline.html

This site is self-described as a continuously updated digital health sciences library that provides patient care support and distance learning to practicing physicians and other professionals. The Virtual Hospital's search engine allows you to search the entire library database to learn about disorders, symptoms, treatments, and support organizations. Information for patients provides instructional and educational materials by title, organ system, and department. Information for health care providers also includes continuing medical education courses, conferences, a physician consultation and referral center.

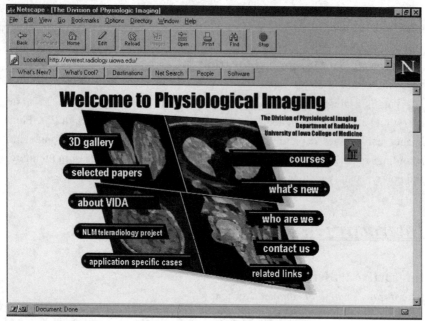

Physiological Imaging. http://everest.radiology.uiowa.edu/

Physiological Imaging
http://everest.radiology.uiowa.edu/

Three-dimensional gallery of movies, images, research papers, tutorials and case studies.

The Virtual Autopsy
http://www.le.ac.uk/pathology/teach/VA/

Try your hand at determining the cause of death for a number of cases. Designed for medical students.

Links

4 Sources and Resources in Medical VR
http://www.informatik.umu.se/~jwworth/4Resources

Huge list of medical virtual reality research and institution sites, products, datasets, conferences, journals and organizations.

Bioport
http://bioport.com/

"Your transporter to the world of virtual medicine."

iMedical: Interactive Medical Center
http://www.imedical.com/

Striving to be a the most complete website about medicine around.

Medicine and Virtual Reality: A Guide to the Literature
http://www.hitl.washington.edu/kb/medvr/

Provides keywords, selected citations, journals, conferences, patents, research centers, commercial organizations, and more.

MedWebPlus: Virtual Reality in Medicine
http://www.medwebplus.com/subject/Virtual_reality_in_medicine.html

Links to a number of sites of topical interest.

Virtual Reality in Medicine
http://www.eng.iastate.edu/~stefanch/575_presentation.html

Collection of links to projects using virtual reality principles to aid in surgical training, augmented reality, preoperative planning, and telemedicine.

Mental Health

Virtual Environments in Clinical Psychology and Neuroscience
http://www.psicologia.net/pages/book2.htm

Information on this published book and how to buy it. Site provides preface, introduction, table of contents and abstracts of papers included in the book.

Virtual Reality Exposure Therapy
http://www.cc.gatech.edu/gvu/virtual/Phobia/

This site describes research into the use of virtual reality devices in therapy which involves exposing a patient to anxiety-producing stimuli while letting the anxiety fade away in an effort to free the patient from his or her phobia. In this case, the patient is exposed to a virtual environment, which can be controlled more easily. An animation designed to help patients who have a fear of elevators is provided.

The Virtual Body Project
http://www.ehto.be/ht_projects/vrepar/vrbody.htm

European site on body image disturbances uses virtual reality techniques in treatment.

Virtual Reality Therapy
http://www.virtuallybetter.com/links.htm

Includes links to several sites that use virtual reality in treating psychological disorders, as well as links to mental health sites. From Virtually Better, Inc.

Multimedia & References

Glossary of Terms
http://www.informatik.umu.se/~jwworth/7.Glossary.html

Defines terms used in virtual reality and medicine.

Multimedia Catalog of the Spencer S. Eccles Health Sciences Library
http://www-medlib.med.utah.edu/webpac-bin/wgbroker?new+-access+top.kw

Contains images, illustrations, animations, videos and sounds related to the health sciences. The multimedia items are designed to be re-purposed for educational and nonprofit use.

Multimedia Medical Reference Library
http://www.med-library.com/medlibrary/

Connect and search this library for software, images, audio files, medical school links, journals and hospitals.

Multimedia Teaching Files
http://www.vh.org/Providers/TeachingFiles/MultimediaTeachingFiles.html

Teaching files for health care providers.

Multimedia Textbooks
http://www.vh.org/Providers/Textbooks/MultimediaTextbooks.html

Links to dozens of multimedia textbooks on line, covering anatomy and genetics, pediatric medicine and cancer topics.

Virtual Hospital

http://www.vh.org/

A digital health sciences library that contains hundreds of books and brochures for health care providers and patients.

Virtual Reality in Medicine: A Survey of the State of the Art

http://www.informatik.umu.se/~jwworth/medpage.html

Online paper.

Projects & Software

3D Virtual Colonoscopy

http://www.cs.sunysb.edu/~vislab/projects/colonoscopy/colonoscopy.html

A trip through the colon, courtesy of data gathered by the Visible Human Project.

Make Your Own Visible Woman

http://www.crd.ge.com/esl/cgsp/projects/makevw/

Site tells you how to use the Visualization Toolkit to create surface models of the bone and skin from the Visible Woman's CT data and publically available software.

Medicine Meets Virtual Reality

http://amainc.com/MMVR/MMVR.html

Information on this annual conference. MMVR2000 will have a special focus on computer-based tools that magnify the subtle aspects of the healing process.

Project Hippocrates

http://www.cs.cmu.edu/afs/cs/project/mrcas/www/hippocrates.html

This site describes a project whose goal is to develop less invasive, computer-assisted surgical robots, in this case for hip replacement surgery. A biomechanics-based surgical simulator will help surgeons determine the results of a proposed surgical plan which, when combined with the precision of surgical robots, will allow for the ideal surgery.

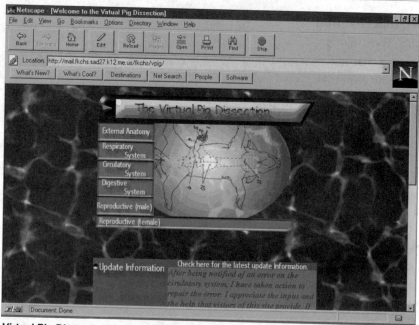

Virtual Pig Dissection. http://mail.fkchs.sad27.k12.me.us/fkchs/vpig/

VIDA: Volumetric Imaging Display and Analysis
http://everest.radiology.uiowa.edu/vida/vidahome.html

Software package for the manipulation, display, and analysis of multi-dimensional image data sets. Lots of links to other medical imaging sites on the Internet.

Virtual Pig Dissection
http://mail.fkchs.sad27.k12.me.us/fkchs/vpig/

Good learning tool for anatomy. Diagrams identify external anatomy, and the respiratory, circulatory, digestive and reproductive systems of pigs.

Virtual Reality in Medicine and Biology Group
http://www.shef.ac.uk/~vrmbg/

This group's projects, past and present, focus on knee topics.

Visible Embryo Project
http://www.ucalgary.ca/UofC/eduweb/virtualembryo/

The Human Developmental Anatomy Center's Visible Embryo Project provides computer-generated models and a prototype database containing embryo images for research and teaching.

Visualization Toolkit
'http://www.kitware.com/vtk.html
Computer software for 3-D visualization. Used for medical images.

VREPAR Project
http://www.psicologia.net/
Virtual reality in medicine, European site.

"Whole Frog" Project
http://george.lbl.gov/ITG.hm.pg.docs/Whole.Frog/Whole.Frog.html
This is a project that uses computer-based 3-D visualization to explore the anatomy of a frog.

Surgery

See also: Surgery - Computers and Surgery.

Vesalius
http://www.vesalius.com/
Internet-based resource for surgical education. Vesalius relies primarily on graphical communications to explore and explain concepts in surgical anatomy, pathology and intervention. Content is divided into clinical folios ("short, educational narratives") and image archives ("a hierarchically-structured repository of anatomical and surgical illustrations, photographs, and radiological images").

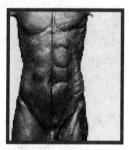

Vesalius.
http://www.vesalius.com/

Virtual Environments and Real-Time Deformations for Surgery Simulation
http://www.cc.gatech.edu/gvu/visualization/surgsim/
This project explores deformations of organs in a surgery scene while emphasizing real-time interaction.

Visible Human

Center for Human Simulation
http://www.uchsc.edu/sm/chs/

View images, animations and 3-D models which show what the Visible Human Database can be used for. Browse through the Visible Human Male or the Visible Human Female. The Center for Human Simulation seeks to facilitate the collaboration of anatomists, radiologists, computer scientists, engineers, physicians and educators to promote the application of this and other anatomical data to basic and clinical research, clinical practice and teaching.

A Guided Tour of the Visible Human
http://www.madsci.org/~lynn/VH/

Describes the project and how it may be used as a learning tool.

Human Anatomy On Line
http://www.ucar.edu/staffnotes/12.94/vizman.html

Access to the Visible Man.

Marching Through the Visible Man
http://www.crd.ge.com/esl/cgsp/projects/vm/

This hypertext paper describes the methodology for using the Visible Male's computed tomography (CT) data to create models of the skin, bone, muscle and bowels.

Marching through the Visible Woman
http://www.crd.ge.com/cgi-bin/vw.pl

This is a companion paper to Marching Through the Visible Man, and it describes the on-going efforts to process the computed tomography data obtained from the National Library of Medicine's Visible Woman Project, which used the cadaver data of a 59-year-old woman. In contrast with the Visible Man whose cross-section images are 1 mm apart, the Visible Woman's CT slices are .3 mm apart.

Visible Human Knee Images

http://www.rad.upenn.edu/rundle/InteractiveKnee.html

This site provides sagittal and axial radiological views of the human knee. Selecting and clicking on a part of the image pulls up a closer view with descriptive text that describes definitions, location, and activity.

Visible Human Female/Visible Human Male Browsers

http://www.uchsc.edu/sm/chs/

Select "Browsers" in the menu, then select either the Visible Male or Visible Female to get to a coronal image that was reconstructed from the Visible Human Database of transverse images. These transverse images can be viewed separately.

Visible Human Male Products

http://www.uchsc.edu/sm/chs/vhm.html

This site offers sample images, reconstructions and animations of the Visible Human Male, as well as VHM products and specs, and access to the Visible Human Male Browser.

Visible Human Project

http://www.nlm.nih.gov/research/visible/visible_human.html

The U.S. National Library of Medicine project to create complete, anatomically detailed, 3-D representations of the male and female bodies online. Currently, the project includes collecting traverse computed tomography, magnetic resonance and cryosection images of representative male and female fresh and frozen cadavers. Some collections of images are available at this site, and samples may be found at NLM's FTP site: *ftp://nlmpubs.nlm.nih.gov*. Scaled-down versions are available as *.gif images on the NLM gopher, on the Research Projects Page, and in the Visible Human Project Section as *.jpg files. These use CT, MRI, x-rays and photographs of cross slices. The plan is that eventually any anatomical part can be viewed separately from the body. The relationship of organs and other structures can be observed as well. According to one NLM representative, it takes two weeks to download all of the information from the Internet and it might take up 15 gigabytes of computer space. However, access to data is free on the Internet.

WOMEN'S HEALTH

Advocacy & Reproductive Rights

Center for Reproductive Law and Policy

http://www.crlp.org/searchworld.html

The Center for Reproductive Law and Policy believes that reproductive rights are human rights with which every woman is endowed. This site provides information on the Center's global efforts.

Findings: The Women's Healthcare Advocacy Service

http://www.findings.net/index.html

"Encouraging women to make thoughtful choices about their health by providing them with information and support."

National Organization for Women

http://www.now.org/

NOW has information on women's abortion rights (including position statements, actions women can do, actions NOW has done, and news and issue information), on violence against women, and on general, non-medical political and social issues.

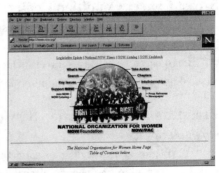

National Organization for Women.
http://www.now.org

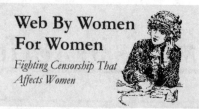

Web by Women for Women.
http://www.io.com/~wwwomen/

Web by Women for Women
http://www.io.com/~wwwomen/

Information on pregnancy, contraception, abortion, censorship, sexuality and menstruation. Search engine and links. Site is very concerned that censorship of tabooed topics may suppress discussion on issues of great importance.

WHAM!
http://www.echonyc.com/~wham/

Women's Health Action and Mobilization, a women's rights advocacy group.

Breast Cancer

Avon Breast Cancer Awareness Crusade
http://www.avoncrusade.com/

Information about breast cancer (see "Resource Center") and about Avon's crusade. Includes library, news, support groups, glossary and common questions.

Breast Cancer Answers
http://www.medsch.wisc.edu/bca/

Frequently asked questions (FAQs) and resources, clinical trials and hot topics. Also allows viewers to submit a cancer question via e-mail.

Breast Cancer Condition Center
http://www.mediconsult.com/mc/mcsite.nsf/conditionnav/breast~section introduction

Breast cancer-specific resources include educational material, support groups, medical news, clinical trials, drug information, articles, a glossary and web links.

Breast Cancer Information Service
http://trfn.clpgh.org/bcis/

Information about the diagnosis, treatment and prevention of breast cancer, as well as information on insurance issues and support groups. Includes an online tutorial and a chat room.

Breast Cancer Lighthouse

http://www.visualman.com/gsm/breast.htm

Describes a CD-ROM resource on the diagnosis and treatment of breast cancer.

Breast Cancer NCI Statements

http://www.oncolink.upenn.edu/disease/breast/cancernet/

Statements, citations and abstracts on breast cancer from the National Library of Medicine's CANCERLIT database.

Breast Cancer Network

http://www2.cancer.org/bcn/index.html

Resources and information from the American Cancer Society on breast cancer and breast reconstruction. Includes a glossary, research updates, patient support organizations and summaries of advocacy efforts and awareness campaigns.

Breast Cancer Research Foundation

http://www.bcrfcure.org/

This organization funds clinical and genetic research into the causes and treatment of breast cancer.

Breast Cancer: Women's Health

http://womenshealth.about.com/msubbreastcancer.htm

Great list of links to a variety of breast cancer topics, with descriptions.

Breast Self Exam

http://trfn.clpgh.org/bcis/GeneralInfo/bse.html

It is recommended that women examine their breasts for signs of a suspicious lump once a month. This site explains why, when and how to examine your breasts.

BreastCancer.Net

http://www.breastcancer.net/

Subscribe to receive a free e-mail news summaries, or check out recent headlines and stories on breast cancer. Also provides links and information on support groups and treatment centers by state.

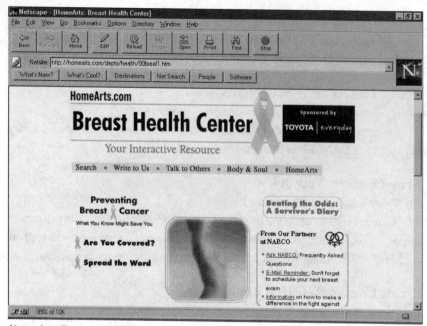

HomeArts Breast Health Center. http://homearts.com/depts/health/00breaf1.htm

BSE

http://www.intranet.ca/~stancar/bse2.htm#bse2

Easy instructions on how to perform a monthly self-exam. Includes illustrations.

Common Questions about Breast Cancer

http://www.y-me.org/faq.html

Answers to 25 frequently asked questions.

Community Breast Health Project

http://www-med.stanford.edu/CBHP/

Patients' stories, medical information, and advice on coping.

Educare Inc., Breast Health and Breast Cancer Network

http://www.CancerHelp.com/ed/

Patient and clinical resources.

HomeArts Breast Health Center

http://homearts.com/depts/health/00breaf1.htm

Feature articles, find a doctor by state, learn more about breast cancer, menopause and related topics. Also contains a breast cancer patient's diary, frequently asked questions, and a service that reminds you via e-mail when you are due for your next breast exam.

Lifetime Chats: Breast Cancer Forum

http://www.lifetimetv.com/chat/frameset.shtml/unmoderated_chats.html

Choose "Breast Cancer," and join in this chat room.

National Action Plan on Breast Cancer

http://www.napbc.org/

Site provides information on this group, which is a partnership of governmental and non-governmental sectors devoted to creating a comprehensive plan for eradicating breast cancer. It also serves as a gateway to breast cancer resources, including clinical trials, frequently asked questions, and other information.

NCI/PDQ Physician Statement: Breast Cancer

http://www.oncolink.upenn.edu/pdq_html/1/engl/100013.html

Information on breast cancer for physicians and other health care professionals.

OncoLink: Breast Cancer

http://www.oncolink.upenn.edu/disease/breast/

Provides general information on cancer in general, and breast cancer specifically. Discusses causes, risk factors, screening, diagnosis, prevention and treatments available. Additional information on genetic and hormonal connections.

An Ounce of Prevention. . . How to Do a Self-Exam

http://www.columbia.edu/cu/sister/SelfExams.html

A thorough description of how to do a breast self-examination.

Yahoo! Breast Cancer Links

http://dir.yahoo.com/Health/Diseases_and_Conditions/Breast_Cancer/

Provides hundreds of links to breast cancer sites on the Internet.

Y-Me National Breast Cancer Organization

http://www.y-me.org/

Facts and support for individuals with breast cancer, frequently asked questions, and breast self-examination instructions.

Cervical Cancer

Annual Pap Smear E-mail

http://www.papsmear.org/

The College of American Pathologists will send you an e-mail reminder when you are due for an annual cervical exam. Information on Pap smears, and other health care issues.

Cervical Cancer

http://oncolink.upenn.edu/specialty/gyn_onc/cervical/

Frequently asked questions, screening information, cervical cancer news, treatment information and psychosocial support.

National Cervical Cancer Coalition

http://www.nccc-online.org/

Coalition that campaigns to educate the public about the many benefits, limitations and reimbursement difficulties related to the cervical cancer screening test, the Pap smear, new cervical/gyn technologies, treatments, and research.

Pap Test

http://www.erinet.com/fnadoc/pap.htm

Hypertext information about the Pap test which is used to identify cancer signs in cervical cell smears. Claims that the Pap is "the only cancer screening test which has decreased the incidence and mortality. . . of a cancer."

Understanding Cancer of the Cervix

http://www.cancerbacup.org.uk/info/cervix.htm

Booklet written for patients to help them better understand cervical cancer. It describes the cervix, disease etiology, symptoms, diagnosis, types of cancer, and treatments. In addition, it helps patients understand what to expect and provides a list of recommended reading and organizations.

Diet & Nutrition

Fitness and Nutrition Information for Women Fifty Plus
http://www2.utep.edu/~joannel/

A few links that women over 50 years old may want to browse.

Healthy and Natural Cooking for Women
http://www.health4her.com/recipes/recipe4.html

Recipes, articles, questions and answers, glossary and more. Site is maintained by a company that sells natural products for women.

Information for Women on Food Safety, Nutrition and Cosmetics
http://vm.cfsan.fda.gov/~dms/wh-toc.html

Good collection of sites targeting specific age groups, conditions, life situations, and other concerns. From the U.S. Food and Drug Administration, Center for Food Safety and Applied Nutrition.

Nutrition and Health Campaign for Women
http://www.eatright.org/womenshealth/

From the American Dietetic Association. The Campaign seeks to educate women about how making informed food choices can help them to decrease their risk of heart disease, breast cancer, osteoporosis, diabetes, and obesity; and it advocates for nutrition research on women's health issues.

Soy and Human Health
http://www.ag.uiuc.edu/~stratsoy/expert/askhealth.html

Provides facts about soybean nutrition. Includes information about soy and women's health issues, such as breast cancer, menopause, and osteoporosis.

WISHES: Women's Issues: Self-Help, Education, Support
http://www.perigee.net/~mgross/

Diet and nutrition issues of concern to women. Includes eating disorders, ten reasons not to diet, cellulite, premenstrual syndrome and diet, cravings, and more.

Women and Nutrition: A Menu of Special Needs
http://www.parenthoodweb.com/parent_cfmfiles/comments.cfm/649

Bulletin board on women's nutrition.

Endometriosis

Atlanta Reproductive Health Centre WWW/ Endometriosis Association

http://www.ivf.com/endoassn.html

Site provides good explanation and description of this puzzling disease, support for patients, research in finding a cure, as well as information about this international organization.

Clinical Articles on Endometriosis

http://www.nezhat.com/end_arts.htm

Abstracts with full citations.

Endometriosis Association

http://www.EndometriosisAssn.org/

Homepage for a self-help organization that provides information and support to women and girls with endometriosis, educates the public as well as the medical community about the disease, and conducts and promotes research related to endometriosis.

Endometriosis Information and Links

http://www.frii.com/~geomanda/endo/

Contains a thoughtful selection of links for learning about endometriosis. Includes frequently asked questions, information on communicating with your doctor, and "other interesting reading."

Endometriosis Multimedia Gallery

http://www.ivf.com/galendo.html

Images and a downloadable video.

Endometriosis Online Support Friends

http://www.geocities.com/HotSprings/Spa/4318/endo1.html

Seeks to be a haven for women coping with endometriosis. Includes support forum, chat room, e-mail list, survivor stories, facts and links.

WITSENDO: Endometriosis Mailing List Information

http://www.ivf.com//witsend.html

To subscribe, send e-mail to: *LISTSERV@listserv.dartmouth.edu* and in the first line of the message, write: "subscribe Witsendo *Lastname, firstname.*"

General Resources

Atlanta Reproductive Health Care WWW: Women's Health

http://www.ivf.com/womhtml.html

Great resource. Offers an enormous amount of information on women's health issues, including breast disease, endometriosis, gynecologic cancer, pregnancy, contraception, menopause, infertility, and other health conditions.

HealthGate Healthy Women

http://www.healthgate.com/healthy/woman/index.shtml

Articles on women's health issues.

National Women's Health Information Center

http://www.4woman.org/

NWHIC is a free information and resource service on women's health issues designed for consumers, health care professionals, researchers, educators, and students. It answers frequently asked questions, and offers dictionaries and journals, special groups, and news.

National Women's Health Resource Center

http://www.healthywomen.org/

A national clearinghouse for information and resources on women's health. Its intent is to educate health care consumers with easy-to-understand and comprehensive information, so that they make wise decisions. Includes a bulletin board, women's resources, questions and answers, e-mail list and links. Members will receive the *National Women's Health Report* and several other perks, but the health information at this site is available to all.

Natracare Guide to Women's Health Resources on the Internet

http://www.indra.com/natracare/guide.html

Sites are divided into general women's health, breast-related links, reproduction-related links, and others.

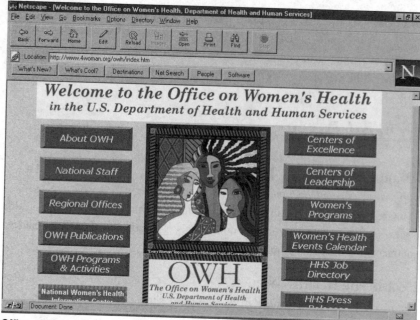

Office of Women's Health. *http://www.4woman.org/owh/index.htm*

Office of Women's Health

http://www.4woman.org/owh/index.htm

Part of the U.S. Department of Health and Human Services, the OWH works to redress the inequities in research, health care services, and education that have placed the health of women at risk. It also coordinates women's health research, health care services, policy, and public and health care professional education across the agencies of the HHS, collaborating with other government organizations, consumer and health care professional groups.

Reproduction and Women's Health

http://www.med.upenn.edu/~crrwh/ScientificSites.html

Links are divided into the following topics: upcoming meetings, scientific societies, journals, research centers, governmental agencies, medical sites, e-mail discussion groups, databases, special interest sites, Internet and grant information, and population centers.

Women and Health Resources

http://www.igc.apc.org/women/activist/health.html

Lists and describes several organizations with websites that provide health information and advocacy efforts.

WomenCare

http://www.womencare.com/

Site is maintained by an OB/GYN Nurse Practitioner who provides patient information on women's health issues.

WomenIcon

http://www.newsfile.com/protect/cwh/scripts/paysite/icon_wom.cgi

Newsfile search of over 40,000 full text articles. Search world news, journal news or research news. Enter search criteria, or select from a long list of women's issues.

Women's Health Center

http://wellweb.com/WOMEN/WOMEN.HTM

Includes recommended medical tests for women, information on menopause and hormone replacement therapy, and much more.

Women's Health Hot Links

http://www.libov.com/

Online newsletter that provides the media with information on women's health.

Women's Health Issues

http://feminist.com/health.htm

"Reading room" provides links organized into general women's health issues, breast cancer, reproductive health, women and AIDS. In addition, describes how to do a breast self-examination.

Yahoo! Women's Health Links

http://www.yahoo.com/Health/Women_s_Health/

Women's health issues, by topic.

Gynecological Cancers

The Gynecologic Oncology Group
http://www.gog.org/

Links to information on various gynecological cancers, and the activities of GOG. This is a national organization dedicated to clinical research in the field of gynecologic cancer. The purpose is to improve the treatment of gynecologic cancer through research into surgery, radiation therapy, chemotherapy, pathology, immunology and/or gynecologic nursing.

OncoLink: Gynecologic Cancers
http://oncolink.upenn.edu/disease/gynecologic1/

Links and information on cervical cancer, endometrial and uterine cancers, fallopian tube cancer, gestational trophoblastic disease, ovarian cancer, vaginal cancer, and vulvar cancer.

What You Need to Know about Cancer of the Uterus
http://rex.nci.nih.gov/WTNK_PUBS/uterus/index.htm

This is a National Cancer Institute booklet for women that describes the symptoms, diagnosis, and treatment of cancer of the uterus. It also has information about resources and sources of support to help women cope with this cancer.

Hysterectomy & Myomectomy

Alternatives to Hysterectomy
http://www.netreach.net/~hysterectomyedu/

Designed for women who have been told they need a hysterectomy but who are looking for alternative treatments. It suggests alternative medical and surgical treatments to consider, depending on which disease the patient has.

Fibroid Uterine Treatment Center
http://www.fibroid.com/index.html

Alternatives other than hysterectomy. Patient information, physician center, technical and licensing information.

Hysterectomy: Know Your Options

http://www.healthywomen.org/qa/hysterectomy.html

Important basic concerns about hysterectomy, including medical reasons, risks and recovery.

Hysterectomy Support Group of the HERS Foundation

http://www.ccon.com/hers/

Provides full, accurate information about hysterectomy, its adverse effects and alternative treatments. HERS is an independent, nonprofit international women's health organization. It offers free information, telephone counseling, physician and legal referral, a reading list and a lending library, as well as networking for women.

The Hysterectomy Hoax

http://repmed.com/html/introduction.html

Ninety percent of these procedures are unnecessary. Site helps you to recognize and understand the reasons for this.

INTRADESIGN: Hysterectomy Discussion Group

http://www.intradesign.com/forums/hyst/

Hysterectomy support forum. Links to related sites.

Outpatient Uterine Myomectomy

http://www.inciid.org/myomectomy.html

Describes uterine fibroids and myomectomy, the operation whereby they are removed.

Radical Hysterectomy: A Guide to Patient Care

http://gynoncology.obgyn.washington.edu/Documentation/Rad%20Hyst.html

Booklet for patients describes the surgery, hospital stay and recommended follow-up care for hysterectomy.

Interstitial Cystitis

Intercyst.Org

http://www.intercyst.org/

Support for all who suffer from interstitial cystitis, including patients, family members, doctors and friends.

Interstitial Cystitis Association
http://www.ichelp.com/

Interstitial cystitis is chronic inflammation of the bladder, and it most commonly affects women. This site provides and introduction to IC, and includes self-help and diet information, resources and other related issues. Connect to the IC treatment and medications guide, and to the IC terminology guide.

Interstitial Cystitis Network
http://www.ic-network.com/

A huge amount of information for patients, researchers and health care professionals. Answers basic and specific questions on interstitial cystitis, offers a number of live chats and message boards, provides a thorough patient handbook, as well as to support links and a research library.

Menopause

Better Health Profiles: Menopause
http://fbhc.org/Patients/BetterHealth/Menopause/home.html

Introduction to menopause, understanding estrogen and progesterone, health changes after menopause, symptoms and frequently asked questions.

Birthing the Crone: Menopause and Aging Through an Artist's Eyes
http://www.birthingthecrone.com/

Artistic rendering of menopause. The Crone is redefined as "fully actualized woman . . . the fulfillment of female life experience and wisdom." Includes links, workshops, and other resources.

FAQ about Menopause/NAMS
http://www.menopause.org/faq.htm

Discusses "natural" products, hormone replacement therapy, nondrug approaches to treating the symptoms of menopause and related topics. Part of the site of the North American Menopause Society.

Female Menopause
http://www.midlife-passages.com/menopaus.htm

Read online articles about menopause, estrogen and related topics.

A Friend Indeed

http://www.pangea.ca/~afi/

Information on this "support group through the mail"; i.e., a newsletter that provides understandable and reliable information about the menopause transition. Published eight times a year.

Meno Times

http://web.aimnet.com/~hyperion/meno/menotimes.index.html

A quarterly journal dedicated to alternative approaches to treating osteoporosis and other effects of menopause.

Menopausal Exercises

http://www.naturalland.com/nv/wom/menex.htm

The right kind of physical activity can ease the symptoms of menopause.

Menopause Matters

http://world.std.com/~susan207/

Information on the treatment of problems arising at menopause.

ThirdAge

http://www.thirdage.com/cgi-bin/rd/goto/health/women/whi/sex_assess.html

Discusses a women's sexuality in the context of menopause. Includes a quiz that will assessy sexual difficulties.

Yoga and Menopause

http://www.hotflashyoga.com/

Downloadable video files demonstrating Katonah Yoga and its poses which, when mastered, provide relief for certain symptomatic discomforts associated with menopause.

Menstruation

The Cycles Page

http://www.io.com/~brenda/cycles/

Free, anonymous web-based application that keeps a record of women's past cycles and predicts their menstruation and ovulation dates for the next six months.

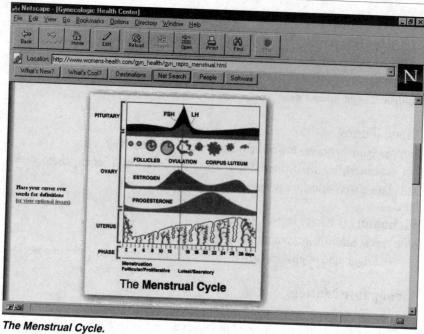

The Menstrual Cycle.
http://www.womens-health.com/gyn_health/gyn_repro_menstrual.html

Menstrual Cramps
http://womenshealth.about.com/msubcramps.htm
Links to articles on menstrual cramps and what can be done to provide relief.

The Menstrual Cycle
http://www.womens-health.com/gyn_health/gyn_repro_menstrual.html
Discusses each phase of the menstrual cycle.

Menstruation Disorders
http://www.ohsu.edu/cliniweb/C13/C13.371.491.html
Search for research articles on amenorrhea, dysmenorrhea, menorrhagia, oligomenorrhea, and premenstrual syndrome.

Menstruation: A Parents' Guide for Preparing Daughters
http://www.mayohealth.org/mayo/9805/htm/mens.htm
Suggestions on ways to discuss menstruation that will help your daughter handle menarche with confidence.

Museum of Menstruation and Women's Health

http://www.mum.org/

Presents menstrual physiology, customs and products. Also find art related to menstruation. Definitely out of the ordinary.

Premenstrual Syndrome

http://www.mayohealth.org/mayo/9609/htm/pms.htm

Good article on the causes of premenstrual syndrome (PMS), nutritional and other remedies.

The Red Spot

http://onewoman.com/redspot/

Although not a medical or clinical site, it includes menstruation biology information, as well as a discussion of cultural and historical aspects of periods, personal stories, frequently asked questions, and links.

S.P.O.T.: The Tampon Health Website

http://critpath.org/~tracy/spot.html

Healthier tampons and tampon alternatives.

Tampax Community

http://www.tampax.com/

Resources ("Body Matters"), chat room and web zine for teens.

Obstetrics/Gynecology

See also: Pregnancy & Childbirth.

Gynaecology, Obstetrics and Paediatrics

http://www.sciencekomm.at/journals/medicine/gyna.html

Links to nearly 200 journals.

Links of Interest to Obstetrics and Gynecology

http://www.museum.state.Il.us/isas/oblink.html

Academic departments, e-mail lists, societies, journals, and links to sites which focus on maternal-fetal issuess, general gynecology, reproductive endocrinology, oncology and related topics.

MedMark: Obstetrics and Gynecology
http://members.iWorld.net/medmark/obgy/
> Links to sites of interest to health professionals, patients and researchers.

MedWebplus: Gynecology
http://www.medwebplus.com/subject/Gynecology.html
> Hundreds of links, organized by by topic.

Yale Library: Obstetrics and Gynecology
http://info.med.yale.edu/library/sir/select.php3?prof_subject=Medicine~ Obstetrics+and+Gynecology
> Selected Internet resources, for patients and health care professionals.

Osteoporosis
See also: Bones/Orthopedics - Osteoporosis.

Calcium: Reference Guide
http://www.cybervitamins.com/calcium.htm
> Recommended daily allowances, symptoms of calcium deficiencies, sources, and signs of toxicity.

Osteoporosis
http://dpalm2.med.uth.tmc.edu/ptnt/00000767.htm
> Bone basics, risk factors, prevention, and good food sources of calcium.

Osteoporosis
http://text.nlm.nih.gov/nih/cdc/www/43.html
> National Institutes of Health Consensus Development Statement on Osteoporosis.

Osteoporosis Awareness Center
http://www.bergenimaging.com/osteo/index.html
> Find out about this disease which effects one in four women, and one in eight men. A recent survey suggests that few women have more than a passing knowledge of this disease or its consequences.

Postmenopausal Osteoporosis: Prevention
http://www.silcom.com/~dwsmith/boned394.html
Alternatives to estrogen replacement therapy.

Ovarian Cancer

Cancer of the Ovary
http://www.vic.com/~smokyweb/hall&martin/
ovarycan.htm
Basics about ovarian cancer, for patients.

National Ovarian Cancer Coalition
http://www.ovarian.org/
Lots of information and support, including real-time chat, discussion groups, and mail lists. Resources and personal stories.

OncoLink: Ovarian Cancer
http://www.oncolink.upenn.edu/specialty/gyn_onc/
ovarian/
Support groups and information on ovarian cancer screening, treatment options, causes and ovarian cancer news. Also contains general information on cancer and the link between hormones and cancer.

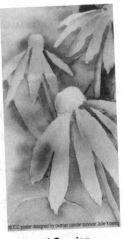

NOCC poster designed by ovarian cancer survivor Julie Koenig

National Ovarian Cancer Coalition.
http://www.ovarian.org/

Ovarian Cysts

Ovarian Cysts
http://www.vic.com/~smokyweb/hall&martin/ovarian.htm
Information for patients about ovary cysts, which are extremely common and may be very painful.

Ovarian Cysts and Tumors
http://www.mayohealth.org/mayo/9612/htm/ovarian.htm
Patient information from the Mayo Clinic.

Ovarian Cysts - Images

http://www.pta.net.au/sgeg/ovcyst.htm

Shows some images of benign cysts.

Professional Groups

American Medical Women's Association

http://www.amwa-doc.org/

Organization of women physicians and medical students dedicated to caring for women patients.

Association of Women Surgeons

http://www.womensurgeons.org/

This organization supports the professional and personal needs of female surgeons at various stages in their career, from residency through retirement.

Journal of American Medical Women's Association

http://www.jamwa.org/

Site displays the current table of contents and full-text article from present issue, subscription information, past and upcoming journals, and more.

INDEX